Nutrition and Dietary Patterns: Effects on Brain Function

Nutrition and Dietary Patterns: Effects on Brain Function

Guest Editors

Roser Granero
Gemma Guillazo-Blanch

MDPI

Basel • Beijing • Wuhan • Barcelona • Belgrade • Novi Sad • Cluj • Manchester

Guest Editors

Roser Granero
Departament de Psicobiologia i Metodologia de les Ciències de la Salut
Universitat Autònoma de Barcelona
Bellaterra (Cerdanyola del Valles)
Barcelona
Spain

Gemma Guillazo-Blanch
Departament de Psicobiologia i Metodologia de les Ciències de la Salut
Institut de Neurociències
Universitat Autònoma de Barcelona
Bellaterra (Cerdanyola del Valles)
Barcelona
Spain

Editorial Office
MDPI AG
Grosspeteranlage 5
4052 Basel, Switzerland

This is a reprint of the Special Issue, published open access by the journal *Nutrients* (ISSN 2072-6643), freely accessible at: https://www.mdpi.com/journal/nutrients/special_issues/QUNNH0K00E.

For citation purposes, cite each article independently as indicated on the article page online and as indicated below:

Lastname, A.A.; Lastname, B.B. Article Title. *Journal Name* **Year**, *Volume Number*, Page Range.

ISBN 978-3-7258-3937-7 (Hbk)
ISBN 978-3-7258-3938-4 (PDF)
https://doi.org/10.3390/books978-3-7258-3938-4

Contents

About the Editors

Roser Granero

Roser Granero is a Full Professor at the Autonomous University of Barcelona (UAB), Department of Psychobiology and Methodology of Health Sciences. She leads the Neurosciences Program "Psychoneurobiology of Eating Disorders and Addictive Behaviors" at the Bellvitge Biomedical Research Institute (IDIBELL) in Spain. She is also a researcher in the CIBERobn Group (Center for Biomedical Research in Network on the Physiopathology of Obesity and Nutrition, Instituto de Salud Carlos III).

Gemma Guillazo-Blanch

Gemma Guillazo-Blanch is a Full Professor at the Autonomous University of Barcelona (UAB) where she works in the Department of Psychobiology and Methodology of Health Sciences. She is the Principal Investigator of the CogniDiet research group at the Institute of Neuroscience of the UAB (INc-UAB) in Spain.

nutrients

MDPI

Editorial

Nutrition and Dietary Patterns: Effects on Brain Function

Roser Granero *,† and Gemma Guillazo-Blanch †

Departament de Psicobiologia i Metodologia de les Ciències de la Salut, Institut de Neurociències, Universitat Autònoma de Barcelona, 08193 Barcelona, Spain; gemma.guillazo@uab.cat

* Correspondence: roser.granero@uab.cat

† These authors contributed equally to this work (co-first authorship).

1. Introduction

Dietary habits are strongly associated with neuropsychological functioning. Etiological studies suggest that healthy cardiometabolic status is a protective factor against vascular dementia [1] and neurological disease [2], and balanced nutrition may slow the rate of cognitive decline with age [3]. These associations are observed throughout life. First, poor dietary quality during the fetal and early postnatal period negatively impacts neurodevelopment in early life (especially in cases of deficiencies in essential nutrients and protein-energy malnutrition) [4]. Second, dietary patterns in early childhood have been associated with differences in brain morphology, neurodevelopment, and cognitive performance [5]. Long-term longitudinal studies have also linked dietary patterns in childhood to posterior cognitive performance during pre-adolescence [6]. Third, studies on the elderly (in the general population, hospital settings, or long-stay units) have observed that nutritional status has a significant influence on vital and functional prognosis and that a balanced diet is associated with better performance in tests assessing memory, attention, reasoning skills and other executive functions [7]. Studies of the impact of diet and nutrition on age-related cognitive decline are a growing field.

In recent years, nutrition research has increasingly emphasized the major impact of sociocultural factors on dietary practices, including preferences for specific foods, selective eating, and different cooking styles. For example, the Western diet is characterized by large amounts of saturated fats, refined sugars, and processed foods and has been linked to impaired learning and memory [8]. Conversely, dietary patterns like those typical of the Mediterranean [9–11] and Nordic countries [12] may be important protective factors for cognitive health. Etiological research suggests that the potential of these diets for brain function may be mediated by their particular anti-inflammatory, lipid-lowering, antioxidant, gut–brain-axis modulating, and ligand activities in cell signaling pathways.

However, while most studies have observed a strong relationship between nutritional habits, eating behaviors, and biopsychosocial dysfunction, this has not always been the case. The theoretical models used in these studies may explain some of these discrepancies. For instance, the classical model of homeostatic feeding posits that individuals ingest food when they perceive that their energy resources are depleted and stop eating (or abstain from) when those energy levels are restored. This traditional theory does not account for the implications of psychosocial functioning. Current models of eating behavior are substantially more complex, encompassing a broader range of constructs, including homeostatic balance, eating habits, food choices/motives, nutrition practices, and dieting. According to these newer models, eating behavior and dietary decision-making are driven by complex interactions between various motivational, affective, and social factors, including the availability of certain foodstuffs, sociocultural contexts, cognitive influences, and internal

Received: 26 February 2025
Accepted: 3 March 2025
Published: 28 March 2025

Citation: Granero, R.; Guillazo-Blanch, G. Nutrition and Dietary Patterns: Effects on Brain Function. *Nutrients* **2025**, *17*, 1169. https://doi.org/10.3390/nu17071169

emotional states such as boredom and stress. Plassmann and colleagues present an interdisciplinary framework for dietary decision-making in which three broad systems interact [13]: (a) the physiology of homeostatic drivers, which regulate eating based on energy needs and the availability of specific foods; (b) the neuroeconomics of dietary decision-making, which is regulated by the connections between the central nervous system and emotions and environmental variables; and (c) the emerging research on the role of the gut microbiome in reward-based dietary decision-making, which has attracted so much interest in the fields of nutrition and neurology. It is known that the combination of bacteria and other microorganisms residing in the gut makes a major contribution to host health through the mediation of homeostatic and reward processes [14,15]. Scientific advances in sequencing and bioinformatics have enabled a more accurate study of communication mechanisms between the microbiome, brain, and behavior [16].

This Special Issue provides evidence for the complex relationships between nutrition and multiple biopsychosocial dysfunctions and the neurobiological basis of these interactions. The study by Arata and colleagues specifically focuses on the underlying mechanisms of the effects of androgens on body weight and appetite in females, considering the role of endogenous oxytocin (OT) (contribution 1). This peptide hormone and neuropeptide is produced in the hypothalamus, is released by the posterior pituitary, and is involved in several processes (including lactation, parturition, mother-infant interaction, psychosocial function, and regulation of eating behaviors) [17]. Arata et al.'s study consisted of a controlled assay on rats and showed that the effects of androgens on OT may be affected by the estrogen milieu and that elevated OT levels may blunt the appetite and help to prevent obesity under estrogen-deficient conditions.

Other areas of particular interest explored in this Special Issue include the relationship between nutrition and neurocognition in eating disorders (EDs) and other physical and psychiatric conditions. Special attention is given to the underlying processes of dietary habits that support the maintenance and progression of cognitive function.

2. Nutrition, Neurocognition and ED

It is well known that persistent disturbances in eating behavior can lead to the onset and progression of several mental illnesses, which can increase the likelihood of comorbid cardiometabolic disorders. Several common biological pathways have been identified that explain these comorbidities between poor-quality diets and mental disorders, including oxidative stress, hypothalamic–pituitary–adrenal axis dysregulation, and regulation of monoamine and overall neuronal function [18,19]. EDs are mental conditions strongly associated with alterations in nutrition and eating habits. Epidemiological and clinical research show that anorexia nervosa, bulimia nervosa, and binge eating have a significant impact on personal well-being, including physical disturbances (gastrointestinal, renal, and cardiovascular problems), psychological distress (mood and anxiety disorders) and social issues (loss of relationships and isolation). Compared to healthy control groups, eating disorder samples exhibit specific brain markers, including impaired neurocognitive processes, altered functional connectivity, and even different brain structures. Moreover, specific impairments in executive functions, sensitivity to reward and punishment, and neurobiological mechanisms (disturbances in neurotransmitter functions such as dopamine, serotonin, and endogenous opiates) have also been related to the onset and persistence of eating behavior-related problems.

This Special Issue includes studies providing new evidence for the complex relationship between nutrition patterns, EDs, and brain function. First, Krug et al. (contribution 2) present a critical narrative review of multiple neurocognitive findings from experimental work on the most prevalent ED subtypes. The neuropsychological processes covered by their study include cognitive flexibility, central coherence, attentional bias, reward processing, inhibitory control, emotion regulation, and impulsivity. The ED subtypes examined in their study include anorexia nervosa, bulimia nervosa, and binge eating, among others. Cognitive functioning among overweight individuals was also reviewed and analyzed. The authors conclude that some neuropsychological processes seem to be transdiagnostic across multiple EDs and weight issues, such as impulsivity, lack of cognitive flexibility, emotion management difficulties, and impaired reward processing. In contrast, other such processes seem more specific to certain ED subtypes, such as an enhanced focus on detail in anorexia nervosa and heightened attention bias toward food-related stimuli in bulimia nervosa and binge eating. This review covers the latest scientific evidence on neurocognitive factors across the most prevalent ED subtypes, thus contributing to developing more nuanced therapeutic approaches that address both the unique (specific) and shared (transdiagnostic) neurocognitive patterns driving disordered eating behaviors.

The second study included in this Special Issue, published by Seelarbokus and colleagues (contribution 3), explores the prevalence of food addiction in stroke patients, as well as its association with the main risk factors of vascular stroke (dyslipidemia, hypertension, diabetes, and obesity). Food addiction is commonly characterized by the persistent and uncontrollable over-consumption of (hyper)palatable foods despite the adverse consequences (such as obesity and increased cardiovascular risk). The term "addiction" is based on neurobiological evidence suggesting that certain components of (hyper)-palatable foods (salt, sugars, and fats) may induce addictive behaviors by activating dopamine reward systems in the brain [20]. Food addiction is not included as an eating disorder in the principal diagnostic taxonomies, but it has been strongly associated with disordered eating. Seelarbokus et al. analyzed data gathered from N = 101 patients who were consecutively hospitalized for a first stroke event in a neurovascular unit (mean age of 62.8, 61 men and 40 women). Based on a self-report questionnaire, the prevalence of participants who were screened positive for food addiction was 5%, while 38.6% reported at least one symptom. The most strongly related vascular risk factor with food addiction was dyslipidemia, followed by diabetes. The authors note the importance of administering standardized measurement tools to identify the presence of food addiction (not only as a specific diagnosis but also as the key symptom criteria) during the routine evaluation of stroke patients. They suggest that treatment units should include multidisciplinary teams of neurologists, dietitians, and psychiatrists/psychologists specialized in disordered eating in order to develop precise treatment strategies, particularly considering that stroke is ranked as the second leading cause of death in the Global Burden of Disease.

The third study in this Special Issue was conducted by Ciancarelli and colleagues (contribution 4) and focused on stroke patients. Their systematic review provides cumulative evidence of the benefits of neuro-nutrition as an adjuvant strategy in personalized nutritional interventions aimed at improving post-stroke neuroplasticity and neurorehabilitation. The review identifies nutrients and dietary patterns supporting recovery by mitigating oxidative stress, inflammation, and gut–brain axis disturbance. Special attention is paid to the role of minerals in oxidative/nitrosative stress, the effects of antioxidant and anti-inflammatory diets (such as Mediterranean and Ketogenic), the description of stroke-induced modifications of the gut-bran axis and dysbiosis, and gut microbiota as a potential target for post-stroke functional recovery.

Reivan-Ortiz et al. (contribution 5) explore the underlying mechanisms and mediating links contributing to body mass index (BMI) and eating disorder (ED) severity based on a large set of variables, including emotion regulation capacity, impulsiveness, anxiety and stress levels, and decision-making performance. Their study examines a broad spectrum of ED subtypes, including bulimia nervosa, binge eating, night eating syndrome, and other specified feeding and ED. Path analysis revealed that BMI was directly associated with ED severity and that ED symptomatology mediated the relationship between BMI and emotion regulation strategies, impulsivity, reasoning skills, and stress levels. The authors conclude that the structural coefficients were invariant across sexes, but differences were identified based on ED subtypes. These findings highlight the important role of nutrition education in managing food-related anxiety and fears and in preventing the onset and progression of ED.

Estévez et al. (contribution 6) carried out a study among a large population-based sample (N = 1076 men and women aged between 18 and 61) to test the mediating role of coping strategies (including emotion regulation capacity) in the relationship between metacognition, impulsivity, and EDs. The authors confirm that coping partially mediates the associations between executive functioning and ED severity. One strength of this study is its focus on metacognition. This concept refers to beliefs, awareness, understanding, and interpretation regarding one's thought processes, which have been defined as central targets in metacognitive therapy, having been strongly associated with a greater likelihood of multiple psychopathologies and negative emotions (including anxiety, depression, and ED). The findings of this research support the use of metacognitive therapy (a third-wave cognitive therapeutic approach aimed at improving ED outcomes by modifying metacognitive beliefs that perpetuate states of selective attention fixation, rumination, and worry). Previous studies have also proposed an integrated cognitive behavioral therapy complemented with metacognitive therapy for treating different ED subtypes [21,22].

This Special Issue also includes two systematic reviews of the effect of Transcranial Direct Current Stimulation (tDCS) on two ED types, namely anorexia nervosa (contribution 7) and binge eating (contribution 8). tDCS is a non-invasive technology that is currently used in many areas of medicine for the treatment of various neurological and psychiatric disorders (including EDs). The procedure is based on stimulation of the cerebral cortex using low-intensity electrical currents by means of sponge electrodes with opposite polarities (anode and cathode) soaked in saline and applied to the scalp. Sessions typically last between 15 and 30 min. The capacity of tDCS for modulating cortical activity in humans has been extensively studied, as has its impact on perceptual, cognitive, and behavioral functions. However, the number of studies in the field of EDs is limited. The two reviews included here summarize the evidence on how tDCS can influence neurofunctional reorganization and behavioral changes by altering cortical excitability in anorexia nervosa and binge eating. They conclude that tDCS is well-suited for neuromodulatory treatment of EDs as it helps to reduce cognitive biases related to eating (such as body dissatisfaction and drive for thinness), and also to improve eating practices, modify food intake and enhance body composition (especially weight recovery in anorexia nervosa). Interestingly, tDCS has also been proven to be effective in reducing depression and anxiety levels and for increasing self-esteem and global psychological adjustment.

3. Diet, Cognition and Bio-Psychological Illness

Other studies in this Special Issue focus on how eating patterns contribute to physical and neuropsychological functioning among diverse populations. Maury and colleagues (contribution 9) assessed serum homocysteine and inflammatory cytokines (IFN-γ, IL-6, IL-1β, TNF-α) as potential biomarkers for alleviating depression among veterans with Gulf War Illness (also called Gulf War Syndrome). This illness, of debated etiology and pathophysiology, is a complex neuropsychological condition characterized by chronic pain and fatigue, hypertension, insomnia, cognitive impairment (such as reduced coordination and memory problems), and negative mood symptoms. Post-traumatic stress disorder and depression are two highly probable comorbid disorders in relation to Gulf War Illness [23].

Maury et al. analyzed data recruited from N = 33 veterans who met clinical criteria for the syndrome (11 women and 22 men, mean age ~ 54 yrs). The findings from a clinical trial showed that after a one-month dietary plan aimed at reducing excitotoxicity and increasing micronutrients, more than half of the participants reported a significant reduction in depression symptom levels. The authors thus conclude that serum homocysteine and cytokine IFN-γ may serve as possible biomarkers for alleviating depression using a low-glutamate diet that could complement effective pharmacological and psychological therapies [24].

Tsuji and colleagues (contribution 10) assessed the role of L-carnosine in CD157 knockout (KO) mice, a murine model for autism spectrum disorder (ASD). Carnosine is a dipeptide molecule composed of the amino acid beta-alanine and histidine, which is highly concentrated in the muscles, the gastrointestinal tract, and the brain. It is commercially available as a nutritional supplement for recovery from fatigue, given its potential antioxidant, anti-inflammatory, and neuroprotective properties, improving brain functioning and protecting the central nervous system. Animal (rodent) models have indicated that L-carnosine may be involved in stress-induced corticosterone responses and anxiety behaviors. Tsuji et al.'s findings are consistent with this hypothesis and have interesting implications for psychiatry, as this molecule may relieve anxiety by suppressing stress-induced hyperresponsivity in a subgroup of individuals with ASD. Previous research has also observed that L-carnosine may be deficient among children with ASD [25,26], but results demonstrating its effectiveness in this regard are inconsistent [27].

Talik and colleagues employed a double-blind placebo-controlled methodology to study the effects of guarana on cognitive performance, motivation, mental energy, mental fatigue, mood parameters, and the effect of this component and the role of sympathetic activation (contribution 11). Guarana is a climbing plant in the Sapindaceae family native to the Amazon basin. It is typically used as a dietary supplement or herb due to the stimulant properties of its seeds [28]. Previous studies have found that guarana seeds may enhance cognitive performance (alertness, vigilance, reaction time, and attention) [29] among the general population ([30] and within clinical samples of patients with fatigue and pain symptoms [31]. Guarana also has anti-inflammatory, antioxidant, and anti-aging effects [32] and may promote wound healing [33]. Studies on the benefits of guarana for psychological well-being, anxiety, and mood have also yielded promising results [34].

Lacasa et al. analyzed the benefits of beta-glucan on fatigue, unrefreshing sleep, anxiety and depression symptoms, and health-related quality of life in patients diagnosed with myalgic encephalomyelitis (also called chronic fatigue syndrome) by means of a randomized double blind placebo-controlled trial (contribution 12). This syndrome is a serious, long-lasting illness causing widespread pain, physical and mental exhaustion, and severe fatigue that prevents individuals from performing typical everyday activities [35]. It has been defined as a complex neurological disease with widely varying recovery rates [36,37]. In a sample of N = 67 patients consecutively recruited from a single outpatient tertiary referral center, Lacasa and colleagues observed that beta-glucan helped to reduce cognitive fatigue symptoms, with major beneficial effects all along the gut microbiota–immune–brain axis. Interestingly, the authors suggest that this positive effect could be extended to a disease model of cognitive decline.

This Special Issue also includes a review by Daida and colleagues (contribution 13) on the role of diet and energy perturbations in the emergence of neurodevelopmental and neurodegenerative disorders mediated by isoforms of glucose transporters, concretely GLUT3 (a protein that in humans is encoded by the SLC2A3 gene). GLUT3 is mainly found in the brain and is responsible for transporting glucose across the plasma membranes of mammalian cells (it was originally designated as the neural glucose transporter [GLUT]). In the first part of the study, Daida et al. detail the expression and function of GLUT3 in human and animal models, after which they describe how maternal diet and genetic modifications of GLUT3 influence the propensity to develop neurodevelopmental disorders. This study contributes to current systematic reviews exploring the role of GLUT3 as a biomarker to aid diagnosis and prognostication of diverse severe physical conditions, such as carcinoma [38–41] and cardiomyopathies [42], as well as other reviews on the role of GLUT3 in psychopathological conditions such as depression [43] and Alzheimer's disease [44].

A final area of special scientific interest is the role of nutrition in the neurological functioning of professional athletes. Since peak sports performance relies on adequate cognitive functions [45], nutritional habits are crucial. The high demands of professional sports have led to research on reducing cognitive decline before, during, and after exercise. Recent reviews have concluded that sport plays a relevant role in neuropsychological performance (attention, information processing speed, inhibitory control, cognitive flexibility, working memory and decision-making) and that specific nutrients and diets contribute to cognitive and motor abilities. For example, vitamins (B, E, D, and C), minerals (iodine, zinc, iron, and magnesium), carbohydrates (glucose), lipids (omega-3 fatty acids), and alkaline and protein-based supplements have shown improvements, while low energy availability is associated with poor physical and cognitive performance [46]. Two studies in this Special Issue area contribute to this research area. First, Finnegan and colleagues (contribution 14) explore the knowledge of performance dietitians and nutritionists on implementing nutritional plans to support athletes with recovery from concussion (also called mild traumatic brain injuries). Second, Morton et al. (contribution 15) explore the neuroprotective effect of supplementation with a functional blend of phytonutrients containing blackcurrant, L-theanine, and pine bark extract, as well as how high-intensity interval exercise performed during ozone exposure can boost cognitive processes. Specifically, the authors analyze inflammation, Brain-Derived Neurotrophic Factor (BDNF), and neurocognition in healthy male cyclists following polyphenol supplementation and exercise in an ozone-polluted environment.

4. Conclusions

In summary, nutrition is a complex, crucial part of health and development that influences brain function via several networks. Adequate dietary practices help reduce neuroinflammation and oxidative stress and increase brain insulin sensitivity and the derived neurotrophic factor. Contrarily, poor-quality diets have been linked to a range of negative health outcomes, including neurological alterations that significantly contribute to long-term global disability and a lower quality of life. Multiple lifestyle factors, especially dietary patterns, have been associated with alterations in various brain systems and functions. This Special Issue provides new evidence on the impact of nutrition on various aspects of neurological function and the potential cognitive impairment associated with ED. The studies published in this issue analyze how dietary patterns and their biochemical compounds impact neuropsychological functioning. The findings provide a solid foundation for designing accurate measurement tools to detect early cognitive decline related to ED and to develop effective evidence-based interventions tailored to the specific needs of these patients.

Author Contributions: Conceptualization, writing—original draft preparation, writing—review and editing: R.G. and G.G.-B. All authors have read and agreed to the published version of the manuscript.

Funding: R.G. is supported by the Catalan Institution for Research and Advanced Studies (ICREA-Academia, 2021-Programme).

Conflicts of Interest: The authors declare no conflicts of interest with respect to the content, authorship, and/or publication of this Editorial.

List of Contributions

1. Arata, M.; Tamura, K.; Aoki, H.; Noguchi, H.; Takeda, A.; Minato, S.; Yamamoto, S.; Kinouchi, R.; Yoshida, K.; Yamamoto, Y.; Et Al. The Effects of Testosterone on Hypothalamic and Serum Oxytocin Levels Are Affected by the Estrogen Milieu in Female Rats. *Nutrients* **2024**, *16*, 2533. https://doi.org/10.3390/nu16152533.
2. Krug, I.; Dang, A.B.; Lu, E.; Ooi, W.L.; Portingale, J.; Miles, S. A Narrative Review on the Neurocognitive Profiles in Eating Disorders and Higher Weight Individuals: Insights for Targeted Interventions. *Nutrients* **2024**, *16*, 4418. https://doi.org/10.3390/nu16244418.
3. Seelarbokus, B.A.; Rabat, Y.; Lalanne, C.; Sibon, I.; Berthoz, S. Food Addiction: Prevalence, Severity, and Impact on Vascular Stroke Risk Factors in a French Hospital-Based Sample. *Nutrients* **2024**, *16*, 4327. https://doi.org/10.3390/nu16244327.
4. Ciancarelli, I.; Morone, G.; Iosa, M.; Cerasa, A.; Calabrò, R.S.; Tozzi Ciancarelli, M.G. Neuronutrition and Its Impact on Post-Stroke Neurorehabilitation: Modulating Plasticity Through Diet. *Nutrients* **2024**, *16*, 3705. https://doi.org/10.3390/nu16213705.
5. Reivan Ortiz, G.G.; Elizalde, B.; Tapia, C.; Granero, R. Psychoneurological Links Contributing to Body Mass Index and Eating Disorder Severity. *Nutrients* **2025**, *17*, 296. https://doi.org/10.3390/nu17020296.
6. Estévez, A.; Momeñe, J.; Macía, L.; Iruarrizaga, I.; Olave, L.; Aonso-Diego, G. The Mediating Effect of Coping Strategies and Emotion Regulation in the Relationship between Impulsivity, Metacognition, and Eating Disorders. *Nutrients* **2024**, *16*, 1884. https://doi.org/10.3390/nu16121884.
7. Chmiel, J.; Gladka, A.; Leszek, J. The Effect of Transcranial Direct Current Stimulation (tDCS) on Anorexia Nervosa: A Narrative Review. *Nutrients* **2023**, *15*, 4455. https://doi.org/10.3390/nu15204455.
8. Chmiel, J.; Kurpas, D.; Rybakowski, F.; Leszek, J. The Effectiveness of Transcranial Direct Current Stimulation (tDCS) in Binge Eating Disorder (BED): Review and Insight into the Mechanisms of Action. *Nutrients* **2024**, *16*, 1521. https://doi.org/10.3390/nu16101521.
9. Maury, A.A.; Holton, K.F. Biomarkers Associated with Depression Improvement in Veterans with Gulf War Illness Using the Low-Glutamate Diet. *Nutrients* **2024**, *16*, 2255. https://doi.org/10.3390/nu16142255.
10. Tsuji, T.; Furuhara, K.; Guo, E.; Wu, Y.; Zhong, J.; Higashida, H.; Yamamoto, Y.; Tsuji, C. Oral Supplementation of L-Carnosine Attenuates Acute-Stress-Induced Corticosterone Release and Mitigates Anxiety in CD157 Knockout Mice. *Nutrients* **2024**, *16*, 2821. https://doi.org/10.3390/nu16172821.
11. Talik, T.N.; Penna, E.M.; Hack, B.P.; Harp, A.; Millard-Stafford, M. Effects of Acute Guarana (Paullinia cupana) Ingestion on Mental Performance and Vagal Modulation Compared to a Low Dose of Caffeine. *Nutrients* **2024**, *16*, 1892. https://doi.org/10.3390/nu16121892.
12. Lacasa, M.; Alegre-Martin, J.; Sentañes, R.S.; Varela-Sende, L.; Jurek, J.; Castro-Marrero, J. Yeast Beta-Glucan Supplementation with Multivitamins Attenuates Cognitive Impairments in Individuals with Myalgic Encephalomyelitis/Chronic Fatigue Syndrome: A Randomized, Double-Blind, Placebo-Controlled Trial. *Nutrients* **2023**, *15*, 4504. https://doi.org/10.3390/nu15214504.
13. Daida, T.; Shin, B.-C.; Cepeda, C.; Devaskar, S.U. Neurodevelopment Is Depend.ent on Maternal Diet: Placenta and Brain Glucose Transporters GLUT1 and GLUT3. *Nutrients* **2024**, *16*, 2363. https://doi.org/10.3390/nu16142363.
14. Finnegan, E.; Daly, E.; Ryan, L. Nutritional Considerations of Irish Performance Dietitians and Nutritionists in Concussion Injury Management. *Nutrients* **2024**, *16*, 497. https://doi.org/10.3390/nu16040497.
15. Morton, L.; Paton, C.; Braakhuis, A. The Effects of Polyphenol Supplementation on BDNF, Cytokines and Cognition in Trained Male Cyclists following Acute Ozone Exposure during High-Intensity Cycling. *Nutrients* **2024**, *16*, 233. https://doi.org/10.3390/nu16020233.

References

1. Axelsson, E.; Wallin, A.; Svensson, J. Patients with the Subcortical Small Vessel Type of Dementia Have Disturbed Cardiometabolic Risk Profile. *J. Alzheimers Dis.* **2020**, *73*, 1373–1383. [CrossRef]
2. Hu, J.R.; Abdullah, A.; Nanna, M.G.; Soufer, R. The Brain-Heart Axis: Neuroinflammatory Interactions in Cardiovascular Disease. *Curr. Cardiol. Rep.* **2023**, *25*, 1745–1758. [CrossRef]
3. Gorelick, P.B.; Scuteri, A.; Black, S.E.; DeCarli, C.; Greenberg, S.M.; Iadecola, C.; Launer, L.J.; Laurent, S.; Lopez, O.L.; Nyenhuis, D.; et al. Vascular contributions to cognitive impairment and dementia: A statement for healthcare professionals from the American Heart Association/American Stroke Association. *Stroke* **2011**, *42*, 2672–2713. [CrossRef]
4. Borge, T.C.; Aase, H.; Brantsæter, A.L.; Biele, G. The importance of maternal diet quality during pregnancy on cognitive and behavioural outcomes in children: A systematic review and meta-analysis. *BMJ Open* **2017**, *7*, 1016777. [CrossRef] [PubMed]
5. Mou, Y.; Blok, E.; Barroso, M.; Jansen, P.W.; White, T.; Voortman, T. Dietary patterns, brain morphology and cognitive performance in children: Results from a prospective population-based study. *Eur. J. Epidemiol.* **2023**, *38*, 669–687. [CrossRef] [PubMed]
6. Ramírez-Salazar, S.A.; Herren, C.; McCartney, J.; Ortiz García, J.G. Dietary Insights in Neurological Diseases. *Curr. Neurol. Neurosci. Rep.* **2021**, *21*, 55. [CrossRef] [PubMed]
7. Smyth, A.; Dehghan, M.; O'Donnell, M.; Anderson, C.; Teo, K.; Gao, P.; Sleight, P.; Dagenais, G.; Probstfield, J.L.; Mente, A.; et al. Healthy eating and reduced risk of cognitive decline: A cohort from 40 countries. *Neurology* **2015**, *84*, 2258–2265. [CrossRef]
8. Bhave, V.M.; Oladele, C.R.; Ament, Z.; Kijpaisalratana, N.; Jones, A.C.; Couch, C.A.; Patki, A.; Garcia Guarniz, A.L.; Bennett, A.; Crowe, M.; et al. Associations Between Ultra-Processed Food Consumption and Adverse Brain Health Outcomes. *Neurology* **2024**, *102*, e209432. [CrossRef]
9. Siervo, M.; Shannon, O.M.; Llewellyn, D.J.; Stephan, B.C.M.; Fontana, L. Mediterranean diet and cognitive function: From methodology to mechanisms of action. *Free Radic. Biol. Med.* **2021**, *176*, 105–117. [CrossRef]
10. Dominguez, L.J.; Veronese, N.; Vernuccio, L.; Catanese, G.; Inzerillo, F.; Salemi, G.; Barbagallo, M. Nutrition, physical activity, and other lifestyle factors in the prevention of cognitive decline and dementia. *Nutrients* **2021**, *13*, 4080. [CrossRef]
11. Palmer, K.; Vetrano, D.L.; Marengoni, A.; Tummolo, A.M.; Villani, E.R.; Acampora, N.; Bernabei, R.; Onder, G. Mediterranean diet, food consumption and risk of late-life depression: The Mugello study. *J. Nutr. Health Aging* **2018**, *22*, 569–574. [CrossRef]
12. Jafari, R.S.; Behrouz, V. Nordic diet and its benefits in neurological function: A systematic review of observational and intervention studies. *Front. Nutr.* **2023**, *10*, 1215358. [CrossRef]
13. Plassmann, H.; Schelski, D.S.; Simon, M.C.; Koban, L. How we decide what to eat: Toward an interdisciplinary model of gut-brain interactions. *Wiley Interdiscip. Rev. Cogn. Sci.* **2022**, *13*, e1562. [CrossRef] [PubMed]
14. García-Cabrerizo, R.; Carbia, C.; O'Riordan, K.J.; Schellekens, H.; Cryan, J.F. Microbiota-gut-brain axis as a regulator of reward processes. *J. Neurochem.* **2021**, *157*, 1495–1524. [CrossRef]
15. Long-Smith, C.; O'Riordan, K.J.; Clarke, G.; Stanton, C.; Dinan, T.G.; Cryan, J.F. Microbiota-gut-brain axis: New therapeutic opportunities. *Annu. Rev. Pharmacol.* **2020**, *60*, 477–502. [CrossRef] [PubMed]
16. Gupta, V.K.; Kim, M.; Bakshi, U.; Cunningham, K.Y.; Davis, J.M.; Lazaridis, K.N.; Nelson, H.; Chia, N.; Sung, J. A predictive index for health status using species-level gut microbiome profiling. *Nat. Commun.* **2020**, *11*, 4635. [CrossRef] [PubMed]
17. Iovino, M.; Messana, T.; Marucci, S.; Triggiani, D.; Giagulli, V.A.; Guastamacchia, E.; Piazzolla, G.; De Pergola, G.; Lisco, G.; Triggiani, V. The neurohypophyseal hormone oxytocin and eating behaviors: A narrative review. *Hormones* **2024**, *23*, 15–23. [CrossRef]
18. Godos, J.; Currenti, W.; Angelino, D.; Mena, P.; Castellano, S.; Caraci, F.; Galvano, F.; Del Rio, D.; Ferri, R.; Grosso, G. Diet and mental health: Review of the recent updates on molecular mechanisms. *Antioxidants* **2020**, *9*, 346. [CrossRef]
19. Pano, O.; Martínez-Lapiscina, E.H.; Sayón-Orea, C.; Martinez-Gonzalez, M.A.; Martinez, J.A.; Sanchez-Villegas, A. Healthy diet, depression and quality of life: A narrative review of biological mechanisms and primary prevention opportunities. *World J. Psychiatry* **2021**, *11*, 997–1016. [CrossRef]
20. Hauck, C.; Cook, B.; Ellrott, T. Food addiction.; eating addiction and eating disorders. *Proc. Nutr. Soc.* **2020**, *79*, 103–112. [CrossRef]
21. Robertson, S.; Strodl, E. Metacognitive therapy for binge eating disorder: A case series study. *Clin. Psychol.* **2020**, *24*, 143–154. [CrossRef]
22. Tecuta, L.; Schumann, R.; Ballardini, D.; Tomba, E. The Need to Control Thoughts in Eating Disorder Outpatients: A Longitudinal Study on Its Modification and Association with Eating Disorder Symptom Improvement. *J. Clin. Med.* **2022**, *11*, 2205. [CrossRef] [PubMed]
23. Gean, E.G.; Ayers, C.K.; Winchell, K.A.; Freeman, M.; Press, A.M.; Paynter, R.; Kansagara, D.; Nugent, S.M. Biological measures and diagnostic tools for Gulf War Illness—A systematic review. *Life Sci.* **2021**, *275*, 119360. [CrossRef] [PubMed]

24. Nugent, S.M.; Freeman, M.; Ayers, C.K.; Winchell, K.A.; Press, A.M.; O'Neil, M.E.; Paynter, R.; Kansagara, D. A Systematic Review of Therapeutic Interventions and Management Strategies for Gulf War Illness. *Mil. Med.* **2021**, *186*, e169–e178. [CrossRef]
25. Abraham, D.A.; Undela, K.; Narasimhan, U.; Rajanandh, M.G. Effect of L-Carnosine in children with autism spectrum disorders: A systematic review and meta-analysis of randomised controlled trials. *Amino Acids.* **2021**, *53*, 575–585. [CrossRef]
26. Zambrelli, E.; Lividini, A.; Spadavecchia, S.; Turner, K.; Canevini, M.P. Effects of Supplementation with Antioxidant Agents on Sleep in Autism Spectrum Disorder: A Review. *Front. Psychiatry* **2021**, *12*, 689277. [CrossRef]
27. Abraham, D.A.; Narasimhan, U.; Mahalingam, V.T.; Krishnan, M.; Ganesan, R.M.; Goh, K.W.; Tan, C.S.; Ming, L.C.; Ardianto, C. Estimation of Plasma Concentration of L-Carnosine and its Correlation with Core Symptoms of Autism Spectrum Disorder Children: A Pilot Clinical Trial. *Front. Biosci. (Landmark Ed.)* **2024**, *29*, 365. [CrossRef] [PubMed]
28. Nawrot, J.; Gornowicz-Porowska, J.; Budzianowski, J.; Nowak, G.; Schroeder, G.; Kurczewska, J. Medicinal Herbs in the Relief of Neurological, Cardiovascular, and Respiratory Symptoms after COVID-19 Infection A Literature Review. *Cells* **2022**, *11*, 1897. [CrossRef]
29. Hack, B.; Penna, E.M.; Talik, T.; Chandrashekhar, R.; Millard-Stafford, M. Effect of Guarana (*Paullinia cupana*) on Cognitive Performance: A Systematic Review and Meta-Analysis. *Nutrients* **2023**, *15*, 434. [CrossRef]
30. Jagim, A.R.; Harty, P.S.; Tinsley, G.M.; Kerksick, C.M.; Gonzalez, A.M.; Kreider, R.B.; Arent, S.M.; Jager, R.; Smith-Ryan, A.E.; Stout, J.R.; et al. International society of sports nutrition position stand: Energy drinks and energy shots. *J. Int. Soc. Sports Nutr.* **2023**, *20*, 2171314. [CrossRef]
31. de Araujo, D.P.; Pereira, P.T.V.T.; Fontes, A.J.C.; Marques, K.D.S.; de Moraes, É.B.; Guerra, R.N.M.; Garcia, J.B.S. The use of guarana (*Paullinia cupana*) as a dietary supplement for fatigue in cancer patients: A systematic review with a meta-analysis. *Support. Care Cancer* **2021**, *29*, 7171–7182. [CrossRef] [PubMed]
32. Peixoto, H.; Roxo, M.; Röhrig, T.; Richling, E.; Wang, X.; Wink, M. Anti-Aging and Antioxidant Potential of *Paullinia cupana* var. sorbilis: Findings in Caenorhabditis elegans Indicate a New Utilization for Roasted Seeds of Guarana. *Medicines* **2017**, *4*, 61. [CrossRef]
33. Felin, F.D.; Maia-Ribeiro, E.A.; Felin, C.D.; Bonotto, N.A.C.; Turra, B.O.; Roggia, I.; Azzolin, V.F.; Teixeira, C.F.; Mastella, M.H.; de Freitas, C.R.; et al. Amazonian Guarana- and Açai-Conjugated Extracts Improve Scratched Fibroblast Healing and *Eisenia fetida* Surgical Tail Amputation by Modulating Oxidative Metabolism. *Oxid. Med. Cell. Longev.* **2022**, *2022*, 3094362. [CrossRef]
34. Silvestrini, G.I.; Marino, F.; Cosentino, M. Effects of a commercial product containing guaraná on psychological well-being, anxiety and mood: A single-blind, placebo-controlled study in healthy subjects. *J. Negat. Results Biomed.* **2013**, *12*, 9. [CrossRef]
35. Park, J.W.; Park, B.J.; Lee, J.S.; Lee, E.J.; Ahn, Y.C.; Son, C.G. Systematic review of fatigue severity in ME/CFS patients: Insights from randomized controlled trials. *J. Transl. Med.* **2024**, *22*, 529. [CrossRef]
36. Cochrane, M.; Mitchell, E.; Hollingworth, W.; Crawley, E.; Trépel, D. Cost-effectiveness of Interventions for Chronic Fatigue Syndrome or Myalgic Encephalomyelitis: A Systematic Review of Economic Evaluations. *Appl. Health Econ. Health Policy* **2021**, *19*, 473–486. [CrossRef]
37. Moore, Y.; Serafimova, T.; Anderson, N.; King, H.; Richards, A.; Brigden, A.; Sinai, P.; Higgins, J.; Ascough, C.; Clery, P.; et al. Recovery from chronic fatigue syndrome: A systematic review-heterogeneity of definition limits study comparison. *Arch. Dis. Child.* **2021**, *106*, 1087–1094. [CrossRef]
38. Begagić, E.; Bečulić, H.; Džidić-Krivić, A.; Kadić Vukas, S.; Hadžić, S.; Mekić-Abazović, A.; Šegalo, S.; Papić, E.; Muchai Echengi, E.; Pugonja, R.; et al. Understanding the Significance of Hypoxia-Inducible Factors (HIFs) in Glioblastoma: A Systematic Review. *Cancers* **2024**, *16*, 2089. [CrossRef] [PubMed]
39. Botha, H.; Farah, C.S.; Koo, K.; Cirillo, N.; McCullough, M.; Paolini, R.; Celentano, A. The Role of Glucose Transporters in Oral Squamous Cell Carcinoma. *Biomolecules* **2021**, *11*, 1070. [CrossRef] [PubMed]
40. Cazzato, G.; Colagrande, A.; Cimmino, A.; Abbatepaolo, C.; Bellitti, E.; Romita, P.; Lospalluti, L.; Foti, C.; Arezzo, F.; Loizzi, V.; et al. GLUT1, GLUT3 Expression and 18FDG-PET/CT in Human Malignant Melanoma: What Relationship Exists? New Insights and Perspectives. *Cells* **2021**, *10*, 3090. [CrossRef]
41. Vovdenko, S.; Morozov, A.; Ali, S.; Kogan, E.; Bezrukov, E. Role of monocarboxylate transporters and glucose transporters in prostate cancer. *Urol. J.* **2023**, *90*, 491–498. [CrossRef] [PubMed]
42. Conte, F.; Sam, J.E.; Lefeber, D.J.; Passier, R. Metabolic Cardiomyopathies and Cardiac Defects in Inherited Disorders of Carbohydrate Metabolism: A Systematic Review. *Int. J. Mol. Sci.* **2023**, *24*, 8632. [CrossRef] [PubMed]
43. Wong, S.; Le, G.H.; Mansur, R.; Rosenblat, J.D.; Kwan, A.T.H.; Teopiz, K.M.; McIntyre, R.S. Effects of ketamine on metabolic parameters in depressive disorders: A systematic review. *J. Affect. Disord.* **2024**, *367*, 164–173. [CrossRef] [PubMed]
44. Kyrtata, N.; Emsley, H.C.A.; Sparasci, O.; Parkes, L.M.; Dickie, B.R. A Systematic Review of Glucose Transport Alterations in Alzheimer's Disease. *Front. Neurosci.* **2021**, *15*, 626636. [CrossRef]

45. Walton, C.C.; Keegan, R.J.; Martin, M.; Hallock, H. The potential role for cognitive training in sport: More research needed. *Front. Psychol.* **2018**, *9*, 1121. [CrossRef]
46. Subalatha, M.; Dhanush, R.; Amutha, S.; Ponpandi, M. A narrative review on the role of cognition, nutrition and energy availability in athletes of competitive sports to combat RED-S. *PeerJ* **2025**, *13*, e18849. [CrossRef]

nutrients

MDPI

Brief Report

Oral Supplementation of L-Carnosine Attenuates Acute-Stress-Induced Corticosterone Release and Mitigates Anxiety in CD157 Knockout Mice

Takahiro Tsuji [1,2,3,*,†], Kazumi Furuhara [1,†], Erchu Guo [1,4], Yijing Wu [1,5], Jing Zhong [6], Haruhiro Higashida [1], Yasuhiko Yamamoto [4] and Chiharu Tsuji [1,7,*]

1 Research Center for Child Mental Development, Kanazawa University, Kanazawa 920-8640, Japan; furururukz.999@gmail.com (K.F.); guoerchu123@gmail.com (E.G.); yaya763687757@163.com (Y.W.); haruhiro@med.kanazawa-u.ac.jp (H.H.)
2 Department of Ophthalmology, Faculty of Medical Sciences, University of Fukui, Fukui 910-1193, Japan
3 Life Science Innovation Center, University of Fukui, Fukui 910-1193, Japan
4 Departments of Biochemistry and Molecular Vascular Biology, Kanazawa University Graduate School of Medical Sciences, Kanazawa 920-8640, Japan; yasuyama@med.kanazawa-u.ac.jp
5 School of Pharmacy, Guangxi University of Chinese Medicine, Nanning 530011, China
6 Physiological Department, Guangxi University of Chinese Medicine, Nanning 530011, China; zhongjing1212@163.com
7 Department of Socioneurosciences, United Graduate School of Child Development, Osaka University, Kanazawa University, Hamamatsu University School of Medicine, Chiba University and University of Fukui, Kanazawa Campus, Kanazawa 920-8640, Japan
* Correspondence: tsuji-t@fukui-u.ac.jp (T.T.); ctsuji@kanazawa-u.ac.jp (C.T.)
† These authors contributed equally to this work.

Abstract: Corticosterone, an end product of the hypothalamic–pituitary–adrenal (HPA) axis, is a crucial stress hormone. A dysregulated HPA axis and corticosterone release play pivotal roles in the onset and persistence of symptoms of stress-related psychiatric disorders, such as anxiety. The intake of nutrients, probiotics, and prebiotic supplements decreases blood corticosterone levels. The dipeptide L-carnosine is composed of beta-alanine and L-histidine and is commercially available as a nutritional supplement for recovery from fatigue. L-carnosine is involved in stress-induced corticosterone responses and anxiety behaviors in rodents. Here, we assessed the effect of L-carnosine in CD157 knockout (KO) mice, a murine model of autism spectrum disorder (ASD). The uptake of L-carnosine suppressed the increase in plasma corticosterone levels in response to acute stress and attenuated anxiety-like behaviors in CD157 KO mice. These results suggest that L-carnosine supplementation may relieve anxiety by suppressing excessive stress responses in individuals with ASD.

Keywords: L-carnosine; CD157; autism spectrum disorder; corticosterone; anxiety; stress

Citation: Tsuji, T.; Furuhara, K.; Guo, E.; Wu, Y.; Zhong, J.; Higashida, H.; Yamamoto, Y.; Tsuji, C. Oral Supplementation of L-Carnosine Attenuates Acute-Stress-Induced Corticosterone Release and Mitigates Anxiety in CD157 Knockout Mice. *Nutrients* **2024**, *16*, 2821. https://doi.org/10.3390/nu16172821

Academic Editor: Asim K. Duttaroy

Received: 18 July 2024
Revised: 10 August 2024
Accepted: 14 August 2024
Published: 23 August 2024

1. Introduction

Organisms adapt to stress by stimulating the hypothalamic-pituitary-adrenal (HPA) axis to cope with environmental changes. The adrenal glands secrete corticosterone, the primary glucocorticoid in humans, which increases pulse and blood pressure, raises blood sugar levels, and suppresses excessive immune responses. However, excessive corticosterone levels weaken the prefrontal cortex and cause neuronal death in the hippocampus, leading to anxiety, depression, and other neurological and psychiatric disorders. Therefore, attempts have been made to reduce surplus corticosterone levels [1].

Several nutrients, probiotics, and prebiotics are potential therapeutic agents for mitigating excessive stress responses [2]. L-carnosine is an imidazole dipeptide composed of beta-alanine and L-histidine, and its concentration is very high in the skeletal muscle and brain of mammals. It can cross the blood–brain barrier or can be synthesized from the beta-alanine and histidine in the brain. In practice, L-carnosine has been marketed as a nutritional supplement for its anti-aging and fatigue-relieving properties and ameliorating effects on lifestyle-related diseases (e.g., diabetes, hypertension, and atherosclerosis) through its antioxidant and pH-buffering properties [3,4]. In the brain, it has beneficial effects on various neuropsychiatric disorders such as ischemic stroke, cognitive impairment [5,6], autism spectrum syndrome [7], schizophrenia [8,9], Alzheimer's disease and dementia [10,11], attention deficit hyperactivity disorder [12], and Gulf War syndrome [13]. L-carnosine is involved in stress-induced corticosterone responses and anxiety behaviors in rodents. L-carnosine-administered mice subjected to restraint stress showed suppressed elevation of plasma corticosterone levels compared to that in the control Kunming mice [14,15].

Bone marrow stromal cell antigen (BST-1), also known as CD157, was first cloned as a glycosyl phosphatidylinositol-anchored protein involved in the growth of pre-B cells [16]. CD157/BST-1 is a glycosyl phosphatidylinositol-anchored membrane protein that functions as an ADP ribosyl cyclase, and the loss of CD157 expression in mice results in anxiety-like behaviors and social behavioral deficits. It is a paralog of CD38 that catalyzes cyclic ADP-ribose to regulate intracellular Ca^{2+} [17]. CD157/BST-1 is constitutively expressed in the myeloid cells of peripheral blood mononuclear cells and regulates the humoral immune response [18]. Moreover, CD157/BST-1 is associated with neuropsychiatric disorders, such as Parkinson's disease, autism spectrum disorder (ASD), rapid eye movement sleep behavior disorder, major depressive disorder, restless leg syndrome/Willis–Ekbom disease, and Alzheimer's disease [19]. Although the physiological role of CD157 in the brain remains largely unexplored, an association between CD157/BST1 and ASD has been reported [20,21]. Homozygous CD157 knockout (CD157 KO) mice display social behavioral impairments and anxiety-related and depression-like behaviors, which can be restored by treatment with antidepressants or oxytocin [22–24]. These findings suggest that CD157 KO mice may be useful as a model of ASD with regard to modeling the behaviors associated with ASD symptoms. We previously observed that the chronic administration of L-carnosine ameliorates social behavioral deficits, which is a core symptom of ASD, in CD157 KO mice [25]. However, the effects of L-carnosine on other comorbid symptoms of ASD, such as anxiety-related behaviors and altered stress responses, have not yet been investigated in CD157 KO mice. In this study, we examined the effect of chronically administered L-carnosine on the corticosterone response induced by acute stress and anxiety-like behavior in CD157 KO mice.

2. Materials and Methods

2.1. Animals

C57BL6/N wild-type (WT) mice were obtained from Japan SLC Inc. (Hamamatsu, Japan) via Sankyo Laboratory Service Corporation (Toyama, Japan). CD157 KO mice were developed as previously described [18]. Homozygous CD157 KO mice were used in this study. WT and CD157 KO mice were housed at the Institute for Experimental Animals, Advanced Science Research Center, Kanazawa University, under standard conditions (22 °C; 12-h light/dark cycle, lights on at 8:45 a.m.) in standard mouse cages (300 × 160 × 110 mm) with sawdust bedding and access to food and water ad libitum. Mice weaned at 21–28 days of age were housed in same-sex groups of three to five animals until 11 weeks of age. Male mice were single-housed for 14 days before acute stress and behavioral tests were conducted. Carnosine-treated mice were maintained on a steady dose of L-carnosine (Phytopharma Co., Ltd., Yokohama, Japan) diluted in drinking water (0.09 g/100 mL) from weaning until the behavioral test. Water intake and body weight were measured during the experiment. This study was conducted in accordance with the Fundamental Guidelines for Proper Conduct of Animal Experiment and Related Activities in Academic Research Institutions under the jurisdiction of the Ministry of Education, Culture, Sports, Science and Technology of Japan. The protocol was approved by the Committee on Animal Experimentation of Kanazawa University (AP-143261, 11 April 2022). We divided the mice into three groups, wild-type (WT) as control, CD157 KO mice with or without L-carnosine administration (KO-Car or KO-Water). The number of mice used in this study is described in the text and figures.

2.2. Acute Stress

Forced swimming was performed as previously described [22]. Briefly, mice were placed individually in a cylinder (height 25 cm, diameter 15 cm) filled up to a 10 cm depth with water (25 ± 1 °C) for 6 min. A restraint stress study was performed by placing the mice in a 50 mL polypropylene conical tube (Eppendorf, Hamburg, Germany) with air holes for 10 min.

2.3. Plasma Sampling and Enzymatic Detection of Corticosterone

Male mice were anesthetized immediately after acute stress by an intraperitoneal injection of pentobarbital (35 mg/kg). Blood samples (0.8–1 mL) were collected by cardiac puncture, and 8–10 µL of 0.1 g/mL ethylenediaminetetraacetic acid was added. The samples were centrifuged at 1600× g for 15 min at 4 °C. Plasma samples (200–400 µL/mouse) were collected and stored at −80 °C until use.

2.4. Enzyme Immunoassay of Corticosterone

Immunoreactivity of plasma corticosterone was analyzed using a corticosterone ELISA kit (Cayman Chemical, Ann Arbor, MI USA), following the manufacturer's instructions. The plasma samples (5 µL) were thawed and diluted to 1:80 in assay buffer. Fifty microliters of the sample was used for the assay. Blood samples were assayed without protein extraction, as previously described [24]. The assay had two linear ranges covering a concentration range of 30–1000 pg/mL. The inter- and intra-assay coefficients of variation were <5%.

2.5. Elevated Plus Maze

The mice in the home cage were placed in the experiment room for at least one hour for habituation. Duration of elevated plus maze was five minutes. Behavior was measured using digital video system and ANY-maze software v. 6.35 (Sloelting Co., Wood Dale, IL, USA).

2.6. Statistical Analysis

Statistical analysis was performed using Prism v.8 (GraphPad Software Inc., San Diego, CA, USA). The data are presented as mean ± standard deviation in the text. The induction of corticosterone in the plasma after the stress tests was compared with the baseline plasma corticosterone levels in each group using an unpaired t-test. One-way analysis of variance (ANOVA) was used to assess the differences in plasma corticosterone levels among groups. Subsequently, Bonferroni's post hoc multiple comparison test was performed. Since we did not observe any effect of L-carnosine on plasma corticosterone levels in WT mice, no further behavioral examination of WT mice was conducted. For the behavioral examination, an unpaired t-test was conducted to compare each index between the KO-Water, KO-Car, and WT-Water groups.

3. Results

L-Carnosine Mitigated Forced Swimming or Restraint-Stress-Induced Elevation in Plasma Corticosterone Levels

Acute stress increases plasma corticosterone levels. The effects of L-carnosine intake on the plasma corticosterone levels after forced swimming were examined in the WT (WT-W) and CD157 KO mice with (KO-C) and without (KO-W) chronic L-carnosine intake. While the basal corticosterone levels did not change between the groups (Figure 1a, 5.3 ± 3.4 ng/µL (n = 8), 8.4 ± 4.8 ng/µL (n = 10), and 10.1 ± 7.4 ng/µL (n = 6) for WT-W, KO-W, and KO-C, respectively), forced swimming stress increased the plasma corticosterone levels in all groups (control vs. forced swimming, $p < 0.0001$ in all four groups, unpaired t-test, Figure 1b, 57.6 ± 11.1 ng/µL (n = 8), 74.8 ± 12.2 ng/µL (n = 11), and

57.8 ± 16.5 ng/μL (n = 9) for WT-W, KO-W, and KO-C, respectively). The corticosterone levels in the KO-W mice were higher than those in the WT mice, whereas the corticosterone levels in the KO-C mice were similar to those in WT-W mice. One-way ANOVA revealed a significant difference in corticosterone levels between the groups (F [2,25] = 5.420, p = 0.011), and post hoc analysis with Bonferroni's multiple comparisons test revealed significant differences in the corticosterone levels between the WT-W and KO-W groups and between the KO-W and KO-C groups (WT-W vs. KO-W, p = 0.032; KO-W vs. KO-C, p = 0.028).

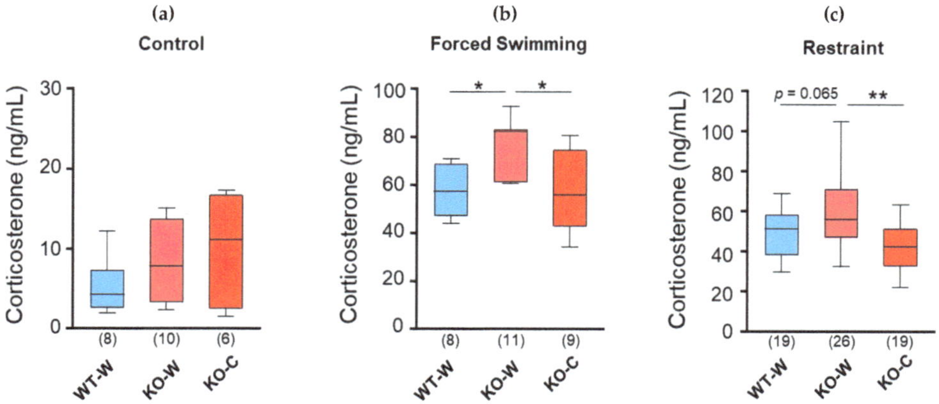

Figure 1. Plasma corticosterone level after acute stress in WT and CD157KO group with or without treatment of carnosine. (**a**) The plasma corticosterone without any stress as control. (**b**) The plasma corticosterone level after 6 min of forced swimming. (**c**) The plasma corticosterone levels after 6 min of restrained stress. Numbers of animals are shown in bars. Bars are represented in median and interquartile ranges in each group. * $p \leq 0.05$, ** $p \leq 0.01$.

Next, we examined the effect of L-carnosine on restraint stress. A single bout of restraint stress caused an increase in plasma corticosterone levels from the baseline values (Figure 1a) in all groups (p < 0.0001 in each group, unpaired t-test, Figure 1c, 49.2 ± 11.8 ng/μL (n = 19), 60.0 ± 18.7 ng/μL (n = 26), and 42.9 ± 12.1 ng/μL (n = 19) for WT-W, KO-W, and KO-C, respectively). The corticosterone levels in the KO-W mice were higher than those in the WT-W mice, whereas the corticosterone levels in the KO-C mice were similar to those in the WT-W mice. One-way ANOVA revealed a significant difference in the corticosterone levels between groups (F [2,61] = 7.375, p = 0.001), and post hoc analysis with Bonferroni's multiple comparisons test revealed a tendency to a significant difference between WT-W and KO-W mice (p = 0.065) and a highly significant difference between KO-W and KO-C mice (p = 0.001). These results showed that the CD157 KO mice were more responsive than the WT mice to acute physical stress and that the oral supplementation with L-carnosine of CD157 KO mice mitigated the acute-stress-induced increases in blood corticosterone levels.

We examined whether L-carnosine uptake ameliorated anxiety-like behavior in CD157 KO mice. Anxiety was assessed using the elevated plus maze assay. The number of entries in the open arm decreased in the KO-W mice compared to that in the WT-W mice (p = 0.067, unpaired t-test) but increased in the KO-C mice compared to that in the KO-W mice (p = 0.061, unpaired t-test, Figure 2a, 5.0 ± 5.1 (n = 15), 1.9 ± 2.4 ng/μL (n = 12), and 4.5 ± 3.8 (n = 13) for WT-W, KO-W, and KO-C, respectively). The time spent in the open arms by the KO-W mice was shorter than that of the WT-W and KO-C mice (p = 0.033 and 0.0073, unpaired t-test, respectively), and these were at a similar level between KO-C and WT-W mice (p = 0.85, unpaired t-test, Figure 2b, 56.2 ± 69.2 s (n = 15), 10.2 ± 14.5 s (n = 12) and 39.6 ± 31.6 s (n = 13), WT-W, KO-W and KO-C, respectively). Although one-way ANOVA revealed a significant difference between groups (F [2,37] = 3.242, p =0.050), post hoc analysis with Bonferroni's multiple comparisons test showed a significant difference in the corresponding test values only between the WT-W and KO-W mice ($p = 0.0468$). On the other hand, the time spent in the closed arm was not different among any of the groups ($p = 0.49$, WT-W vs. KO-W, and $p = 0.79$, KO-W vs. KO-C, unpaired t-test, Figure 2b, 137.9 ± 97.3 s ($n = 15$), 163.3 ± 93.0 s ($n = 12$), and 154.6 ± 71.0 s ($n = 13$) for WT-W, KO-W, and KO-C, respectively). These results demonstrated that L-carnosine ameliorated anxiety-like behavior in ASD mice.

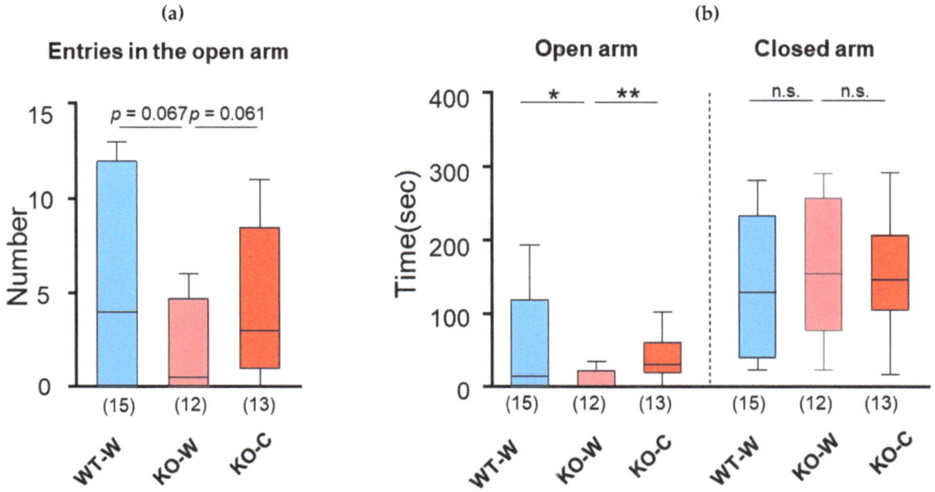

Figure 2. Elevated plus maze test. (**a**) Numbers of entries in the open arms. (**b**) Time in the open arm or the closed arm. Numbers of animals are shown in bars. Bars are represented in median and interquartile ranges in each group. * $p \leq 0.05$. ** $p \leq 0.01$. n.s.: not significant.

4. Discussion

Acute stress significantly increased corticosterone release in CD157 KO mice, whereas CD157 KO mice that were chronically administered L-carnosine showed corticosterone levels similar to those of WT mice. Furthermore, L-carnosine treatment reduced anxiety-like behaviors in CD157 KO mice.

We previously reported that L-carnosine uptake improves social recognition behavior deficits in CD157 KO mice, probably through the activation of oxytocin neurons in the hypothalamus and increased secretion of oxytocin [25]. Therefore, L-carnosine may reduce corticosterone secretion through the activation of the oxytocinergic pathway. Exposure to various physiological and psychological stressors (immobilization, shaking, social defeat, forced swimming, or intracerebroventricular infusion of corticotropin-releasing factor [CRF]) can activate oxytocin neurons and facilitate the release of oxytocin in rodents [26,27]. Oxytocin innervates CRF neurons in the paraventricular nucleus to inhibit their activation, thereby inhibiting CRF secretion [27]. Exogenous oxytocin reduces CRF secretion and mitigates physical and mental responses to acute stress [28–30]. Furthermore, oxytocin neurons modulate CRF neurons and project to the vagus nerve and solitary bundle nuclei, thereby stimulating the parasympathetic neurons and directly relieving stress [31]. Therefore, the administration of L-carnosine may relieve acute physical stress by decreasing corticosterone secretion through the oxytocinergic pathway.

Anxiety disorders occur frequently among individuals with ASD, with a meta-analysis estimating that approximately 40% of ASD youths havingat least one comorbid DSM-IV anxiety disorder [32]. Children with ASD have higher anxiety levels than typically developing children, and anxiety levels increase with intelligence quotient and age [33]. According to another meta-analysis, in autistic adults, although the prevalence rate is inconsistent depending on study design, the estimated current prevalence rate of anxiety is high, up to 27% [34]. Numerous studies have investigated cortisol responsiveness under physiological and/or psychosocial stress. Studies examining cortisol diurnal rhythms and cycles (cortisol arousal response, diurnal decline, and variability) indicate that relatively low-functioning individuals with autism show values different from those of typically developing individuals but do not consistently show similar changes in high-functioning individuals with autism [35]. In physically stressful environments, such as blood drawing, and mock magnetic resonance imaging scan, individuals with ASD respond more excessively to stressors than typically developed children. Furthermore, regarding psychosocial stressors, high reactivity has been observed in the playground during interactions with unfamiliar peers or short separations from a guardian [35]. Therefore, the hypersecretion of cortisol can be predicted for some psychological or non-psychological stress in people with autism. Our study suggests that the chronic intake of L-carnosine may reduce the dysregulated responsiveness of the HPA axis and help dampen the stress response in individuals with ASD.

One limitation of our study is that we only explored the effect of oral supplementation of L-carnosine from weaning to adulthood. Adolescence may be a sensitive time window for improving neuronal circuitry deficits. The environmental enrichment experienced during adolescence in rodents could restore the behavioral and emotional deficits induced by aversive experiences during the early postnatal age. Therefore, further investigations are necessary regarding the duration and time window of L-carnosine supplementation for understanding the underlying role of L-carnosine in anxiolytic effects and stress responses. Another limitation is that we used the ELISA assay to measure corticosterone level. Value obtained from ELISA assay may have certain biases due to sample matrix effects and cross-reactivity with other hormones. However, a correlation has been shown between LC-MS/MS and ELISA, although it could be disturbed in patients taking a corticosteroid synthesis inhibitor such as metyrapone or some steroid compounds [36]. Therefore, we used the ELISA assay in this study, which is generally admitted as a practical method for quantification.

5. Conclusions

This is the first study to demonstrate the anxiolytic effect of L-carnosine and the suppression of stress-induced corticosterone secretion by L-carnosine in an ASD mouse model. We found that L-carnosine supplementation may relieve anxiety by suppressing stress-induced hyperresponsivity, which appears in a subgroup of individuals with ASD.

Author Contributions: Conceptualization, T.T. and C.T.; methodology, T.T. and C.T.; validation, T.T., C.T., H.H. Y.Y. and J.Z.; formal analysis, C.T. and K.F.; investigation, C.T., K.F., E.G. and Y.W.; resources, H.H.; writing—original draft preparation, T.T. and C.T.; writing—review and editing, T.T., C.T., H.H. Y.Y. and J.Z.; funding acquisition, T.T. and C.T. All authors have read and agreed to the published version of the manuscript.

Funding: This research was funded by the Japan Society for the Promotion of Science KAKENHI, grant numbers JP 22K07346 (T.T.), 21J40098JP, and 24K10677 (C.T.); a grant from the Life Science Innovation Center, University of Fukui, number LSI 23103 (T.T.); and the Initiative for Realizing Diversity in the Research Environment, MEXT (C.T.). Also, funded by Tokai Bussan Co., Ltd. (C.T.). and partially supported by the Moonshot Research and Development Program, grant number JPMJMS2297 from Japan Science and Technology Agency, JST (C.T.).

Institutional Review Board Statement: The animal study protocol was approved by the Committee on Animal Experimentation of Kanazawa University (AP-143261, 11 April 2022).

Informed Consent Statement: Not applicable.

Data Availability Statement: The original contributions presented in the study are included in the article, further inquiries can be directed to the corresponding authors.

Conflicts of Interest: This study was funded by Tokai Bussan Co., Ltd. (C.T.). The other authors declare that this research was conducted in the absence of any commercial or financial relationships that could be construed as potential conflicts of interest.

References

1. Patel, V.K.; Vaishnaw, A.; Shirbhate, E.; Kore, R.; Singh, V.; Veerasamy, R.; Rajak, H. Cortisol as a Target for Treating Mental Disorders: A Promising Avenue for Therapy. *Mini Rev. Med. Chem.* **2024**, *24*, 588–600. [CrossRef]
2. Toyoda, A. Nutritional interventions for promoting stress resilience: Recent progress using psychosocial stress models of rodents. *Anim. Sci. J.* **2020**, *91*, e13478. [CrossRef]
3. Kohen, R.; Yamamoto, Y.; Cundy, K.C.; Ames, B.N. Antioxidant activity of carnosine, homocarnosine, and anserine present in muscle and brain. *Proc. Natl. Acad. Sci. USA* **1988**, *85*, 3175–3179. [CrossRef]
4. Davey, C.L. The significance of carnosine and anserine in striated skeletal muscle. *Arch. Biochem. Biophys.* **1960**, *89*, 303–308. [CrossRef]
5. Baek, S.H.; Noh, A.R.; Kim, K.A.; Akram, M.; Shin, Y.J.; Kim, E.S.; Yu, S.W.; Majid, A.; Bae, O.N. Modulation of mitochondrial function and autophagy mediates carnosine neuroprotection against ischemic brain damage. *Stroke* **2014**, *45*, 2438–2443. [CrossRef] [PubMed]
6. Hisatsune, T.; Kaneko, J.; Kurashige, H.; Cao, Y.; Satsu, H.; Totsuka, M.; Katakura, Y.; Imabayashi, E.; Matsuda, H. Effect of Anserine/Carnosine Supplementation on Verbal Episodic Memory in Elderly People. *J. Alzheimers Dis.* **2016**, *50*, 149–159. [CrossRef]
7. Abraham, D.A.; Undela, K.; Narasimhan, U.; Rajanandh, M.G. Effect of L-Carnosine in children with autism spectrum disorders: A systematic review and meta-analysis of randomised controlled trials. *Amino Acids* **2021**, *53*, 575–585. [CrossRef] [PubMed]
8. Ghajar, A.; Khoaie-Ardakani, M.R.; Shahmoradi, Z.; Alavi, A.R.; Afarideh, M.; Shalbafan, M.R.; Ghazizadeh-Hashemi, M.; Akhondzadeh, S. L-carnosine as an add-on to risperidone for treatment of negative symptoms in patients with stable schizophrenia: A double-blind, randomized placebo-controlled trial. *Psychiatry Res.* **2018**, *262*, 94–101. [CrossRef]
9. Tharoor, H.; Maran, S.; Chandan, A.K.; Pari, M.; Rao, S.; Durairaj, J. Cognitive and negative symptoms in schizophrenia with L-Carnosine adjuvant therapy—A randomized double-blind placebo-controlled study. *Pharmacol. Res. Perspect.* **2023**, *11*, e01074. [CrossRef]
10. Ding, Q.; Tanigawa, K.; Kaneko, J.; Totsuka, M.; Katakura, Y.; Imabayashi, E.; Matsuda, H.; Hisatsune, T. Anserine/Carnosine Supplementation Preserves Blood Flow in the Prefrontal Brain of Elderly People Carrying APOE e4. *Aging Dis.* **2018**, *9*, 334–345. [CrossRef] [PubMed]
11. Masuoka, N.; Yoshimine, C.; Hori, M.; Tanaka, M.; Asada, T.; Abe, K.; Hisatsune, T. Effects of Anserine/Carnosine Supplementation on Mild Cognitive Impairment with APOE4. *Nutrients* **2019**, *11*, 1626. [CrossRef] [PubMed]
12. Ghajar, A.; Aghajan-Nashtaei, F.; Afarideh, M.; Mohammadi, M.R.; Akhondzadeh, S. l-Carnosine as Adjunctive Therapy in Children and Adolescents with Attention-Deficit/Hyperactivity Disorder: A Randomized, Double-Blind, Placebo-Controlled Clinical Trial. *J. Child. Adolesc. Psychopharmacol.* **2018**, *28*, 331–338. [CrossRef]
13. Baraniuk, J.N.; El-Amin, S.; Corey, R.; Rayhan, R.; Timbol, C. Carnosine treatment for gulf war illness: A randomized controlled trial. *Glob. J. Health Sci.* **2013**, *5*, 69–81. [CrossRef]
14. Li, Y.F.; He, R.R.; Tsoi, B.; Li, X.D.; Li, W.X.; Abe, K.; Kurihara, H. Anti-stress effects of carnosine on restraint-evoked immunocompromise in mice through spleen lymphocyte number maintenance. *PLoS ONE* **2012**, *7*, e33190. [CrossRef]
15. Tsoi, B.; He, R.R.; Yang, D.H.; Li, Y.F.; Li, X.D.; Li, W.X.; Abe, K.; Kurihara, H. Carnosine ameliorates stress-induced glucose metabolism disorder in restrained mice. *J. Pharmacol. Sci.* **2011**, *117*, 223–229. [CrossRef]
16. Kaisho, T.; Ishikawa, J.; Oritani, K.; Inazawa, J.; Tomizawa, H.; Muraoka, O.; Ochi, T.; Hirano, T. BST-1, a surface molecule of bone marrow stromal cell lines that facilitates pre-B-cell growth. *Proc. Natl. Acad. Sci. USA* **1994**, *91*, 5325–5329. [CrossRef]
17. Malavasi, F.; Deaglio, S.; Funaro, A.; Ferrero, E.; Horenstein, A.L.; Ortolan, E.; Vaisitti, T.; Aydin, S. Evolution and function of the ADP ribosyl cyclase/CD38 gene family in physiology and pathology. *Physiol. Rev.* **2008**, *88*, 841–886. [CrossRef]
18. Ishihara, K.; Hirano, T. BST-1/CD157 regulates the humoral immune responses in vivo. *Chem. Immunol.* **2000**, *75*, 235–255. [CrossRef] [PubMed]
19. Yokoyama, S. Genetic polymorphisms of bone marrow stromal cell antigen-1 (BST-1/CD157): Implications for immune/inflammatory dysfunction in neuropsychiatric disorders. *Front. Immunol.* **2023**, *14*, 1197265. [CrossRef]
20. Yokoyama, S.; Al Mahmuda, N.; Munesue, T.; Hayashi, K.; Yagi, K.; Yamagishi, M.; Higashida, H. Association Study between the CD157/BST1 Gene and Autism Spectrum Disorders in a Japanese Population. *Brain Sci.* **2015**, *5*, 188–200. [CrossRef]
21. Mo, W.; Liu, J.; Zhang, Z.; Yu, H.; Yang, A.; Qu, F.; Hu, P.; Liu, Z.; Hu, F. A study of single nucleotide polymorphisms in CD157, AIM2 and JARID2 genes in Han Chinese children with autism spectrum disorder. *Nord. J. Psychiatry* **2018**, *72*, 179–183. [CrossRef] [PubMed]
22. Lopatina, O.; Yoshihara, T.; Nishimura, T.; Zhong, J.; Akther, S.; Fakhrul, A.A.; Liang, M.; Higashida, C.; Sumi, K.; Furuhara, K.; et al. Anxiety- and depression-like behavior in mice lacking the CD157/BST1 gene, a risk factor for Parkinson's disease. *Front. Behav. Neurosci.* **2014**, *8*, 133. [CrossRef]
23. Mizuno, A.; Cherepanov, S.M.; Kikuchi, Y.; Fakhrul, A.A.; Akther, S.; Deguchi, K.; Yoshihara, T.; Ishihara, K.; Shuto, S.; Higashida, H. Lipo-oxytocin-1, a Novel Oxytocin Analog Conjugated with Two Palmitoyl Groups, Has Long-Lasting Effects on Anxiety-Related Behavior and Social Avoidance in CD157 Knockout Mice. *Brain Sci.* **2015**, *5*, 3–13. [CrossRef]
24. Kasai, S.; Yoshihara, T.; Lopatina, O.; Ishihara, K.; Higashida, H. Selegiline Ameliorates Depression-Like Behavior in Mice Lacking the CD157/BST1 Gene, a Risk Factor for Parkinson's Disease. *Front. Behav. Neurosci.* **2017**, *11*, 75. [CrossRef]

25. Tsuji, T.; Furuhara, K.; Gerasimenko, M.; Shabalova, A.; Cherepanov, S.M.; Minami, K.; Higashida, H.; Tsuji, C. Oral Supplementation with L-Carnosine Attenuates Social Recognition Deficits in CD157KO Mice via Oxytocin Release. *Nutrients* **2022**, *14*, 803. [CrossRef]
26. Engelmann, M.; Ebner, K.; Landgraf, R.; Holsboer, F.; Wotjak, C.T. Emotional stress triggers intrahypothalamic but not peripheral release of oxytocin in male rats. *J. Neuroendocrinol.* **1999**, *11*, 867–872. [CrossRef] [PubMed]
27. Winter, J.; Jurek, B. The interplay between oxytocin and the CRF system: Regulation of the stress response. *Cell Tissue Res.* **2019**, *375*, 85–91. [CrossRef] [PubMed]
28. Windle, R.J.; Shanks, N.; Lightman, S.L.; Ingram, C.D. Central oxytocin administration reduces stress-induced corticosterone release and anxiety behavior in rats. *Endocrinology* **1997**, *138*, 2829–2834. [CrossRef] [PubMed]
29. Parker, K.J.; Buckmaster, C.L.; Schatzberg, A.F.; Lyons, D.M. Intranasal oxytocin administration attenuates the ACTH stress response in monkeys. *Psychoneuroendocrinology* **2005**, *30*, 924–929. [CrossRef]
30. Windle, R.J.; Kershaw, Y.M.; Shanks, N.; Wood, S.A.; Lightman, S.L.; Ingram, C.D. Oxytocin attenuates stress-induced c-fos mRNA expression in specific forebrain regions associated with modulation of hypothalamo-pituitary-adrenal activity. *J. Neurosci.* **2004**, *24*, 2974–2982. [CrossRef]
31. Karelina, K.; Norman, G.J. Oxytocin Influence on NTS: Beyond Homeostatic Regulation. *J. Neurosci.* **2009**, *29*, 4687–4689. [CrossRef] [PubMed]
32. van Steensel, F.J.; Bogels, S.M.; Perrin, S. Anxiety disorders in children and adolescents with autistic spectrum disorders: A meta-analysis. *Clin. Child. Fam. Psychol. Rev.* **2011**, *14*, 302–317. [CrossRef]
33. van Steensel, F.J.A.; Heeman, E.J. Anxiety Levels in Children with Autism Spectrum Disorder: A Meta-Analysis. *J. Child Fam. Stud.* **2017**, *26*, 1753–1767. [CrossRef] [PubMed]
34. Hollocks, M.J.; Lerh, J.W.; Magiati, I.; Meiser-Stedman, R.; Brugha, T.S. Anxiety and depression in adults with autism spectrum disorder: A systematic review and meta-analysis. *Psychol. Med.* **2019**, *49*, 559–572. [CrossRef] [PubMed]
35. Taylor, J.L.; Corbett, B.A. A review of rhythm and responsiveness of cortisol in individuals with autism spectrum disorders. *Psychoneuroendocrinology* **2014**, *49*, 207–228. [CrossRef] [PubMed]
36. Casals, G.; Hanzu, F.A. Cortisol Measurements in Cushing's Syndrome: Immunoassay or Mass Spectrometry? *Ann. Lab. Med.* **2020**, *40*, 285–296. [CrossRef]

nutrients

MDPI

Review

The Effect of Transcranial Direct Current Stimulation (tDCS) on Anorexia Nervosa: A Narrative Review

James Chmiel [1,*], Anna Gladka [2] and Jerzy Leszek [2]

[1] Institute of Neurofeedback and tDCS Poland, 70-393 Szczecin, Poland
[2] Department and Clinic of Psychiatry, Wrocław Medical University, 54-235 Wrocław, Poland
* Correspondence: jameschmiel1@gmail.com

Abstract: (1) Introduction: Anorexia nervosa (AN) is a severe, debilitating disease with high incidence and high mortality. The methods of treatment used so far are moderately effective. Evidence from neuroimaging studies helps to design modern methods of therapy. One of them is transcranial direct current stimulation (tDCS), a non-invasive brain neuromodulation technique. (2) Methods: The purpose of this narrative review is to bring together all studies investigating the use of tDCS in the treatment of AN and to evaluate its effect and efficiency. Searches were conducted in the Pubmed/Medline, Research Gate, and Cochrane databases. (3) Results: The literature search resulted in five articles. These studies provide preliminary evidence that tDCS has the potential to alter eating behaviour, body weight, and food intake. Additionally, tDCS reduced symptoms of depression. Throughout all trials, stimulation targeted the left dorsolateral prefrontal cortex (DLPFC). Although the number of studies included is limited, attempts were made to elucidate the potential mechanisms underlying tDCS action in individuals with AN. Recommendations for future tDCS research in AN were issued. (4) Conclusions: The included studies have shown that tDCS stimulation of the left DLPFC has a positive effect on AN clinical symptoms and may improve them, as measured by various assessment measures. It is important to conduct more in-depth research on the potential benefits of using tDCS for treating AN. This should entail well-designed studies incorporating advanced neuroimaging techniques, such as fMRI. The aim is to gain a better understanding of how tDCS works in AN.

Keywords: tDCS; transcranial direct current stimulation; anorexia nervosa; non-invasive brain stimulation; neurostimulation; neuromodulation; eating disorder

Citation: Chmiel, J.; Gladka, A.; Leszek, J. The Effect of Transcranial Direct Current Stimulation (tDCS) on Anorexia Nervosa: A Narrative Review. *Nutrients* **2023**, *15*, 4455. https://doi.org/10.3390/nu15204455

Academic Editors: Roser Granero and Gemma Guillazo-Blanch

Received: 18 September 2023
Revised: 17 October 2023
Accepted: 18 October 2023
Published: 20 October 2023

1. Introduction

Anorexia nervosa (AN) is a common and severe mental illness with multifactorial etiopathogenesis [1]. It transcends geographical and socioeconomic boundaries, affecting individuals worldwide. AN patients exhibit an obsession with food, leading to drastic food intake restrictions and a refusal to maintain a healthy body weight, as evidenced by a BMI below 18.5 kg/m2 [2]. Common eating behaviours among individuals with AN include prolonged meal gaps, calorie counting, selective eating schedules, and avoidance of certain food types [3]. Predisposing factors for AN include features of excessive cognitive control, such as obsessive–compulsive personality disorder, perfectionism, and a distorted perceived image of body shape or weight [4]. Patients experience intense fear and preoccupation concerning weight gain and body image.

The prevalence of AN is associated with a high morbidity rate [5]. This eating disorder imposes a substantial burden on physical and psychosocial well-being, with prevalence rates reaching as high as 4% in adolescent girls and young adult women [6]. It is important to note that AN is less commonly observed in men [7,8], with a lifetime prevalence rate that might be up to 0.3% [9], though this does not diminish the burden on male patients [10]. In women, significant weight loss can lead to amenorrhea, which is characterised by the absence of menstrual periods [11]. The cause of this phenomenon is believed to be dysfunction of the hypothalamic–pituitary axis [12]. However, in 2013, the American Psychiatric Association revised the diagnostic criteria for AN. They eliminated the strict weight requirements and the necessity for amenorrhea as a condition for diagnosis. This change stemmed from the recognition that hormonal changes in AN can vary, and some women, despite having low weights and exhibiting all the psychological symptoms of the disorder, may still experience regular menstrual cycles [12].

The availability of effective AN treatment methods is limited [13]. Cognitive-behavioural, psychodynamic, and family therapies are considered the treatments of choice and show moderate effectiveness [11]. Pharmacological therapy also has a limited role [14,15]. Selective serotonin reuptake inhibitors (SSRIs) and neuroleptics represent the primary treatment options, but their effectiveness is limited.

The outcomes of treatment for AN and the long-term prognosis are generally unfavourable [16]. AN has one of the highest mortality rates among all mental illnesses [17], with rates reaching up to 5.9% when considering all causes of death [18]. Notably, only about half of the patients achieve full recovery, and approximately one-third experience partial remission [11,19].

The Diagnostic and Statistical Manual of Mental Disorders, Fifth Edition (DSM-5), distinguishes between two clinical subtypes of AN: restrictive (AN-r) and binge eating/purging (AN-bp) [11]. Individuals with AN-r restrict their food intake and increase their physical activity, whereas those with AN-bp, in addition to restricting food, regularly engage in episodes of binge eating and/or purging behaviours [20]. These subtypes are characterised by distinct behaviours and personality traits. People with AN-bp tend to exhibit a greater inclination towards seeking novelty, sensation seeking, and higher impulsivity. On the other hand, individuals with AN-r demonstrate a lower tendency to seek novelty and exhibit higher levels of perseverance [21]. The presence of comorbidities can also vary between the subtypes. Those with AN-bp are more likely to experience substance abuse disorders, affective disorders, depression [22,23], impulsive behaviour [24], and borderline personality disorder [25]. In contrast, avoidant personality disorder is more commonly observed in individuals with AN-r [25].

The neurobiological basis of AN involves several neurotransmitters, including dopamine, serotonin, and norepinephrine, which play crucial roles in the development and maintenance of the disorder.

Dopamine is involved in modulating rewards and affect, and its dysregulation has been linked to the development of obsessive or ritualistic behaviours, such as the food rituals often seen in individuals with AN [26]. People with AN may exhibit impaired reward functioning, presenting as abstemious, anhedonic, and temperate in various behaviours from childhood, even before the onset of AN symptoms [27]. Dopamine is central in processing rewards, including food [28], and research has revealed altered striatal dopamine function in individuals with AN, particularly in response to highly palatable foods [29], possibly explaining their aversion to food. Unlike those without AN who experience pleasure from food, individuals with AN find it aversive, which might partially explain their persistent pursuit of self-starvation. Dopaminergic dysfunction also affects reward processing in situations unrelated to food, leading to difficulties in identifying the positive or negative value of stimuli [28].

Serotonergic dysfunction has been identified in AN [30]. Serotonin, a neurotransmitter known for its role in mood [31] and appetite regulation [32], is implicated in the disorder as a potential biological marker for AN [30]. Studies have linked certain genetic factors, such as the S allele of the 5-HTTLPR polymorphism of the serotonin transporter gene, to eating disorders, particularly AN [33]. Caloric restriction has a significant impact on serotonin availability in the brain, as tryptophan, a precursor to serotonin, is absorbed through food intake [34]. A restricted diet limits tryptophan availability, leading to decreased serotonin synthesis and increased oversensitivity to serotonin in postsynaptic receptors [34]. This depletion of serotonin may explain the high levels of anxiety and dysphoria often reported by individuals with AN. The dysregulation of serotonin receptors, particularly 5-HT1A and 5-HT2A, contributes to the persistence of AN symptoms and may explain the limited effectiveness of SSRIs in treating the disorder [28].

Norepinephrine, a neurotransmitter involved in regulating sympathetic arousal and anxiety [35], is elevated in individuals with AN, leading to heightened anxiety, particularly related to food and weight [28]. Early stages of dieting counteract this anxiety by depleting norepinephrine precursors typically obtained through food intake. This reduction in anxiety through dieting reinforces the behaviour, leading to further weight loss and the entrenchment of AN symptoms. Aberrant activity in the noradrenergic system is associated with irregular patterns of activation in the insula, a brain region implicated in AN [28].

The neurobiological basis of AN can be detected with fMRI. In individuals with the AN-restricting subtype, several studies have reported impaired brain function and metabolism at rest [36–43]. This dysfunction, characterised by reduced regional cerebral blood flow and a reduced regional cerebral metabolic rate of glucose, is evident in three key brain regions: the cingulate cortex (including Brodmann areas 24 and 32) [37–39,41], the parietal cortex (including the inferior parietal lobule) [42,43], and the frontal cortex (including the dorsolateral prefrontal cortex) [36–39,42,43]. In the AN binge–purge subtype, studies have demonstrated functional and metabolic reductions at rest in the bilateral frontal cortex [36,39,44]. Interestingly, these reductions have been shown to normalise after recovery [40]. Additionally, bilateral reductions in parietal metabolism and function have been observed, which also return to normal following recovery [36,44,45]. Furthermore, two studies have reported bilateral metabolic and functional reductions in the cingulate cortex, which also normalise after recovery [39,41].

Due to the high mortality rate associated with AN and the moderate effectiveness of currently utilised treatment methods, there is an obligation for the development and implementation of novel therapeutic approaches. Considering that AN is typified by alterations in brain neurobiology, and given the fMRI evidence pointing to reduced activity in specific brain regions, the application of a non-invasive brain stimulation technique, such as transcranial direct current stimulation (tDCS), holds promise for potential utility and effectiveness.

tDCS is a brain stimulation tool that allows the stimulation of the cerebral cortex by means of two or more sponge electrodes with opposite polarities (anode and cathode), soaked in saline and applied to the scalp [46]. It is painless, well tolerated, and safe, with no or few side effects [47]. The stimulator is a battery-powered device that delivers a small amount of direct current (usually 0.5–2 mA), some of which reaches the brain. Brain modulation depends on the polarity of the applied current. tDCS allows two types of stimulation: anodal and cathodal [48,49]. During tDCS, a current flows between the electrodes, making its effects non-focal. However, modifying the electrode size can enhance its focus [50]. Stimulation durations typically range from 15 to 30 min, with 20 min being the most common protocol. Anodal tDCS depolarises neurons, making them more excitable and facilitating firing, whereas cathodal tDCS hyperpolarises neurons, inhibiting firing below the stimulation site. Usually, target neurons are less excitable, and their spontaneous activity decreases [51]. The neurobiological effects of tDCS can persist beyond the stimulation period when applied for at least three minutes [48]. If tDCS is administered for more than 10 min with a current of 1 to 2 mA, the changes remain stable for at least one hour [52]. A single session of tDCS, lasting up to 15 min, has an impact on cortical excitability for approximately 90 min. Repeated stimulation can further extend this effect. The prolonged influence of tDCS on cortical excitability is associated with synaptic modulation mechanisms, as indicated by studies conducted on humans [53] and animal models [54,55]. tDCS induces calcium-dependent glutamatergic synaptic plasticity. The secondary effects of tDCS, both anodal and cathodal, can be prevented by blocking the N-methyl-D-aspartate (NMDA) receptor, but they can be enhanced by appropriate receptor agonists [56,57]. Anodal and cathodal tDCS decreases GABAergic activity [58], which may serve as a mechanism to regulate tDCS-induced plasticity. tDCS affects the balance between cortical excitation and inhibition by modulating the levels of γ-aminobutyric acid (GABA), glutamate/glutamine, and BDNF [59]. Low calcium amplification of the postsynaptic neuron leads to long-term depression (LTD), whereas a high concentration results in long-term potentiation (LTP) [60].

tDCS is a non-invasive technique that has been extensively studied for its ability to modulate cortical activity in humans, affecting perceptual, cognitive, and behavioural functions. It has shown effectiveness in a wide range of neurological and psychiatric disorders. For example, neurodevelopmental disorders, including autism spectrum disorder (ASD), schizophrenia (SCZ), and attention deficit/hyperactivity disorder (ADHD), are all characterised by imbalances in excitatory (E) and inhibitory (I) neural activity. These imbalances can lead to cognitive deficits, behavioural problems, and other symptoms. GABA and glutamate are neurotransmitters that are crucial for regulating E/I balance. Changes in the levels and functioning of these neurotransmitters have been observed in individuals with neurodevelopmental disorders. tDCS can lead to long-term effects on neural plasticity and connectivity. It may modulate neurotransmitters like dopamine, acetylcholine, and serotonin and affect membrane ion channels. Changes in GABA and glutamate levels, as well as the balance between them, are associated with tDCS-induced plasticity. Studies suggest that tDCS has potential therapeutic benefits for neurodevelopmental disorders. It can help restore E/I balance, improve cognitive function, and alleviate symptoms like social deficits, hallucinations, inattention, and impulsivity [61]. To date, several reviews have examined the effectiveness of tDCS in the treatment of AN [62–66]. However, they covered all eating disorders, including bulimia, binge eating, and food craving. AN itself is a heterogeneous disorder, and even more so, individual eating disorders are heterogeneous. Conducting such a general overview of all eating disorders may bias the results.

This narrative review focuses specifically on the application of tDCS to alleviate AN symptoms. tDCS can influence neurofunctional reorganisation and behavioural changes by altering cortical excitability. Given that AN is also associated with underactivity of various brain areas, it is well suited for neuromodulatory treatment.

2. Methods

2.1. Data Sources and Search Strategy

For this narrative review, J.C. and A.G. performed an independent online search using predefined criteria. The search combined the keywords 'transcranial direct current stimulation' or 'tDCS' with 'anorexia' or 'anorexia nervosa.' We considered publications in the Pubmed/Medline and Research Gate databases, with an access date of May 2023 and publication dates ranging from January 2008 to December 2022.

2.2. Study Selection Criteria

The eligibility criteria included clinical trials conducted in English during the specified period, investigating the effects of tDCS on AN. The exclusion criteria encompassed articles that were not published in English, reviews, and studies that did not use standardised psychological questionnaires.

3. Results

The screening process is represented in a flow chart (Figure 1). Initially, 8537 records underwent screening, with 8518 being excluded based on the evaluation of their titles and abstracts, primarily due to their topic relevance. Through the search strategies carried out in the database, 19 studies were identified. Of these, 14 studies were excluded on the grounds of their publication type. Following a comprehensive analysis of study titles and abstracts, 5 articles were deemed eligible for inclusion.

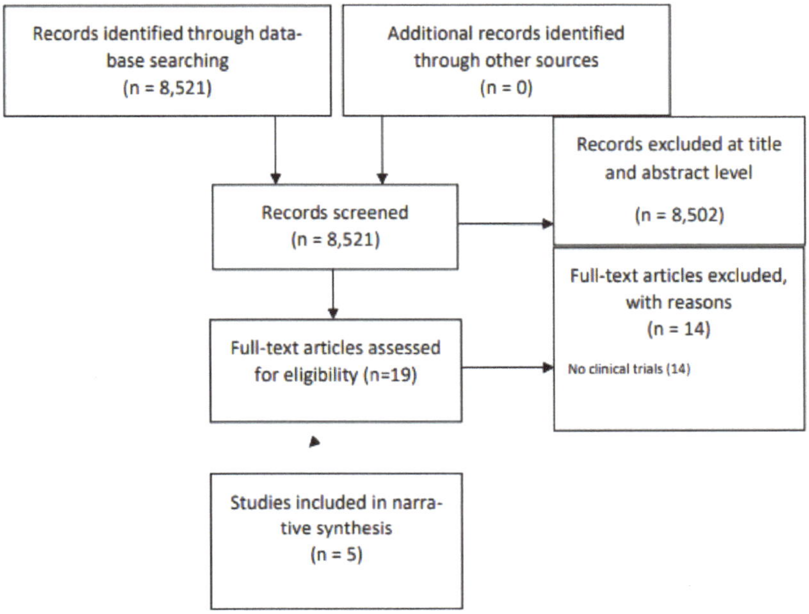

Figure 1. Flow chart depicting the different phases of the systematic review.

The studies that were found were published between 2014 and 2021. A total of 83 patients were enrolled (active tDCS = 50, sham tDCS = 21). One study was a randomised controlled trial (RCT), one study was single-blind and controlled, 2 studies were open-label, and one was a case report. Random assignment occurred in one study, and this particular study used sham stimulation for the control group. However, it is worth noting that the RCT study by Baumann et al. and the study by Costanzo et al. did not assess the blinding procedure.

3.1. Summary of Included Studies

The included studies are summarised in Table 1. In the study conducted by Khedr et al. [67], a total of seven patients participated in an open-label, single-arm experiment. Evaluations of tDCS effectiveness were carried out at three different time points: prior to tDCS sessions, immediately following the session, and one month later. Six patients used SSRIs during the study. The following measures were used: the Eating Disorder Inventory (EDI) to measure eating behaviour, the Eating Attitude Test (EAT-40) to measure symptoms of AN, and the Beck Depression Inventory (BDI) to measure symptoms of depression.

Baumann et al. [68] conducted a double-blind, randomised controlled trial to examine the effects of tDCS on eating behaviour, body weight, and depression in inpatients with AN. A total of 43 participants with AN were randomly assigned to receive either active tDCS (n = 22) or sham tDCS (n = 21). Outcome measures included the Eating Disorder Examination Questionnaire (EDE-Q) to measure eating psychopathology, the Zung Self-Rating Depression Scale (ZUNG) to measure depression, and Body Mass Index (BMI) to measure body weight. These assessments were conducted at four stages: (1) before tDCS treatment, (2) after tDCS treatment, (3) two weeks after the treatment, and (4) four weeks after the treatment. During treatment, patients took medication, mainly antidepressants and antipsychotics.

Table 1. Summary of main findings from articles included in the review.

Author, Citation	Population	Technical Specifications	Outcome Measurment	Main Results (Primary Outcomes Are Bolded)
Khedr et al. [67]	7 patients with AN (n = 7).	Anodal tDCS (2 mA) over the left dorsolateral prefrontal cortex (DLPFC) for 10 consecutive days (5 session/week), anodal tDCS for 25 min.	Eating Attitude Test (EAT), Eating Disorder Inventory (EDI) and Beck Depression Inventory (BDI). Pre-tDCS, post-tDCS, and one month later.	3 patients improved in all three rating scales post tDCS and after 1 month; 1 patient improved only in the BDI; 2 patients showed improvement at the end of session but returned to the baseline after one month. The 7th patient had no changes.
Baumann et al. [68]	43 inpatients with AN, active (n = 22) or sham (n = 21) tDCS.	2 mA anodal stimulation over the left DLPFC with the cathode over the right orbitofrontal region, 10–30 min sessions.	Eating Disorder Examination Questionnaire (EDE-Q), Zung Self-Rating Depression Scale (ZUNG), BMI; pre-tDCS, post-tDCS, and one month later.	No significant effect on complex psychopathology and weight recovery in patients with AN.
Costanzo et al. [69]	23 adolescents with AN, tDCS + therapy as usual (tDCS + (AU) n = 11) or a family-based therapy (FBT + AU n = 12).	1 mA, anodal electrode positioned over the left DLPFC and cathodal electrode over the right DLPFC; 20 min, 3 times a week for 6 weeks.	EDI-3, Bulimia (B), Global Psychological Maladjustment (GPM), Interpersonal Problems, BMI. Pre-, post-, one month, and 6 weeks after tDCS.	After 4 and 6 weeks, BMI increased in the tDCS group; in this group, a medium negative correlation was found between improvements in BMI, B and GPM.
Strumila et al. [70]	9 female patients with AN (n = 9).	Anodal 2 mA stimulation, anode on the left DLPFC, and cathode on the right DLPFC, 2 times per day for 25 min, 2 weeks.	Eating Disorder Inventory (EDI), Eating Disorder Examination Questionnaire (EDE-Q), Body Shape Questionnaire (BSQ-34), Beck Depression Inventory (BDI). Pre-, post-, and one month after tDCS.	Depression symptoms significantly decreased post and after 1 month. EDI decreased significantly post and 1 month after stimulation, EDE-Q questionnaire at 1 month was significantly lower.
Rząd et al. [71]	1 patient with AN (n = 1).	Anodal 2 mA stimulation, anode on the left DLPFC, and cathode on the right DLPFC, twice daily for 25 min for 2 weeks.	Fasting venous blood; Eating Attitudes Test, Rosenberg Self-Esteem scale, BDI, EDE-Q, Body Esteem Scale, Perceived Stress Scale. Pre-, post-, and 2 weeks after tDCS.	Improvement in anthropometric measurement, some blood parameters (e.g., ferritin), symptoms of depression and stress, and self-body image after two weeks

The aim of the study conducted by Costanzo et al. [69] was to investigate the potential of tDCS in modifying or resetting inter-hemispheric balance in adolescents with AN to restore control over eating behaviours. Twenty-three adolescents with AN participated in the study and received treatment as usual (AU), which included nutritional, pharmacological, and psychoeducational treatment. Additionally, they underwent either 18 sessions of tDCS combined with AU (tDCS + AU group, n = 11) or family-based therapy combined with AU (FBT + AU group, n = 12). All participants underwent clinical examinations to assess their mental health conditions. The evaluation of AN-related symptoms included measures such as the Eating Disorder Inventory (EDI-3), Eating Attitudes Test (EAT-26), and Body Uneasiness Test (BUT). Anxiety and depressive symptoms in the children were examined using the Multidimensional Anxiety Scale for Children (MASC) and the Children's Depression Inventory (CDI). BMI was also measured. Additionally, each participant received atypical antipsychotic medication, with aripiprazole being the specific drug used for treatment. Additionally, some individuals in the study were prescribed SSRIs (five in the tDCS group and nine in the FBT group), whereas a few received benzodiazepines (two in the tDCS group and one in the FBT group) as well.

Strumila et al. [70] conducted a pilot study to assess the effects of tDCS in a group of nine female patients with AN. During two weeks of stimulation, none of the participants underwent any specific re-feeding protocol or nutritional intervention, nor did they attend specialised psychological intervention groups. All the patients were prescribed a range of different types of psychiatric medication. The study measured the EDI, EDE-Q, Body Shape Questionnaire (BSQ-34), and BDI.

Rzad et al. [71] presented a case report involving the application of tDCS on an 18-year-old female participant. The study aimed to assess several aspects, including anthropometric measures, biological factors, and psychological aspects. Anthropometric measures were evaluated using a bioelectrical impedance analysis, and fasting venous blood samples were taken to analyze certain biological factors. The patient was taking sertraline (SSRI) during treatment. The study also featured a battery of psychological assessments, including the Eating Attitudes Test (EAT), the Rosenberg Self-Esteem Scale (RSS), the Beck Depression Inventory (BDI), the Eating Disorder Examination Questionnaire (EDE-Q), the Body Esteem Scale (BES), and the Perceived Stress Scale (PSS). Furthermore, Body Mass Index (BMI) was measured as part of the comprehensive evaluation.

3.2. Technical Aspects of tDCS in AN and Safety

The studies included in this review used different methodologies, which are discussed in detail based on the work of Thair et al. [72].

The most common electrode montage was bipolar, with both the anode and cathode electrodes directly placed on the brain and an equal current applied to both. In another study, a monopolar montage was employed, in which one electrode was positioned on the scalp and the other was positioned externally, for instance, on the arm.

All the studies included in this research employed anodal stimulation on the left dorsolateral prefrontal cortex (DLPFC). Four of the studies [68–71] followed the international 10–20 system to position the electrodes accurately. This method involves measuring the participant's head to identify specific regions of interest, and based on this, the anodal electrode was placed at F3. In one study [67], the left DLPFC was located by measuring the head 6 cm anterior to the left primary motor cortex along a parasagittal line. Regarding the reference (cathodal) electrode, its placement differed among the studies. In one study [67], the cathodal electrode was applied on the contralateral arm (extracephalic). Other studies once again employed the 10–20 system. In one study [68], the electrode was placed over the right orbitofrontal region (Fp2), and in three other studies [69–71], it was positioned over the right DLPFC (F4). The studies used different current intensities. One study [69] used 1 mA, whereas the others [67,68,70,71] used 2 mA. The duration of stimulation also varied. In some studies [67,70,71], it lasted 25 min. In one study [68], it lasted 30 min, and in another study [69], it lasted 20 min. Additionally, the frequency of stimulation differed among the studies. In two studies [67,68], tDCS sessions were administered daily for ten consecutive days, with five sessions per week. One study [69] utilised 18 sessions, three times a week, over a total of six weeks. In the case of two studies [70,71], they used 20 sessions, with two sessions per day for two weeks. Different sizes of electrodes were employed across the studies. One study [67] used a smaller anode (24 cm^2) and a larger cathode (100 cm^2). Similarly, another study [68] used an anode of 25 cm^2 and a cathode of 51 cm^2. In contrast, one study [69] used electrodes of the same size (25 cm^2). However, the size of the electrodes was not specified in two studies [70,71].

All five studies reported mild adverse effects associated with tDCS treatment. These effects included tingling, headaches, heaviness in the head, itching, and a scalp burning sensation. In the study by Khedr et al. [67], only transient local itching was reported by two patients, and no other adverse effects were observed. Costanzo et al. [69] found that the most common adverse effects were an itching sensation and burning sensation, reported by nine participants, especially during the initial seconds of stimulation. These sensations rapidly diminished with the addition of water with a sponge. Local redness was also reported by eight participants. Other effects, such as headaches and tingling, were reported by five participants.

In Strumila et al. [70] study, two-thirds of the participants experienced light redness and burning, which may be partially attributed to the skin fragility associated with AN.

Baumann et al. [68] reported various adverse effects, including a burning sensation (six patients), headache (four patients), tingling and itching (three patients), fatigue, acute mood changes, and pinching (two patients). One patient reported additional symptoms such as stitching, pressure in the head, blurred vision, scalp pain, hyperglycemia with the onset of diabetes mellitus type I, burning in the eyes, twitching of the eye, and a positive mood.

3.3. *Effects on Psychopathology and Eating Behaviour*

In the study by Khedr et al. [67], the first, third, and fourth patients showed improvement in the EDI. Among the subscales of the EDI, the most prominent changes were observed in body dissatisfaction, interpersonal distrust, interoceptive awareness, and ineffectiveness.

In the study by Baumann et al. [68], the primary analysis, based on ANOVA results, did not reveal any significant effects of tDCS on complex psychopathology and weight recovery in patients with AN as measured by the EDE-Q. However, the secondary analysis indicated a potential positive impact of tDCS treatment on questions 4 and 23 of the EDE-Q. In comparison to sham tDCS, active tDCS resulted in a significant improvement in self-evaluation based on body shape and a significant decrease in the need for excessive control over calorie intake during the four-week follow-up. It is important to note that these results did not survive multiple comparison correction.

In Costanzo et al.'s [69] study, both groups showed improvement across various EDI-3 subscales. Regardless of the group, a reduction in the mean scores was observed after treatment in the following areas: drive for thinness, body dissatisfaction, eating disorder risk, low self-esteem, personal alienation, interpersonal insecurity, interpersonal alienation, asceticism, ineffectiveness, interpersonal problems, and global psychological maladjustment (all $p < 0.05$). However, there was no noticeable improvement in the subscales of bulimia, interoceptive deficits, emotional dysregulation, perfectionism, fear of maturity, affective problems, and overcontrol (all $p > 0.10$). There was no improvement in BUT.

In the study by Strumila et al. [70], EDI scores decreased significantly, with a large effect size of 0.62. Additionally, the scores decreased significantly in the following subdimensions: inefficiency, perfectionism, distrust, interoceptive awareness, fear of maturity, and asceticism, with the mean effect size for all those items being around 0.45, indicating high efficacy. The remaining measures were not assessed immediately after the completion of the treatment.

In the study by Rzad et al. [71], improvement was observed in the RSS, EDE-Q, and BES scales.

3.4. *Effects on AN Symptoms*

In the study by Khedr et al. [67], the first, third, and fourth patients showed improvements in EAT.

In the study by Costanzo et al. [69], there was an improvement in EAT.

In the study by Rzad et al. [71], there was an improvement in EAT.

3.5. Effects on Depressive Symptoms

In the study by Khedr et al. [67], the first, third, and fourth patients improved in the BDI-II.

In the study by Baumann et al. [68], the researchers anticipated some improvement in the active group based on the ZUNG. However, upon the completion of the treatment (stage 2), the sham group exhibited better results in the total score and specific questions (5, 11, 12, 20) of the ZUNG ($p < 0.01$). When comparing the first and last stages, the sham group demonstrated a significant decrease for questions 10 and 16 ($p < 0.01$ and $p < 0.05$). In the study by Costanzo et al. [69], improvement in the CDI was demonstrated.

In the study by Strumila et al. [70], BDI depression scores were significantly reduced ($p < 0.01$, effect size 0.47).

In the study by Rzad et al. [71], depression scores for the BDI were reduced.

3.6. Effects on Anxiety

In the study by Costanzo et al. [69], regarding the MASC subscales, irrespective of the group, there was a decrease in the mean scores after treatment for physical symptoms and ADI (all $p < 0.05$), whereas there was no evident improvement in harm avoidance, social anxiety, and separation/panic (all $p > 0.10$).

In the study by Rzad et al. [71], stress scores (for simplicity, we placed them in the "anxiety" category) were lowered.

3.7. Effects on BMI

In the study by Baumann et al. [68], in both the sham and active groups, BMI values showed improvement, although not significantly. In Costanzo et al. [69] study, they found that BMI showed a significant improvement in the tDCS + AU group ($p < 0.001$), whereas in the FBT + AU group, there was no significant change in BMI after treatment when compared to the baseline ($p = 0.2$). The average percentage increase in BMI $[(T1 - T0)/T0 \times 100]$ was 13.3% (±9.4) in the tDCS + AU group, whereas in the FBT + AU group, it was only 4.2% (±5.7).

In the study by Rzad et al. [71], an improvement and an increase in BMI were achieved.

3.8. Effects on Other Measurements

In the study by Rzad et al. [71], following the two-week stimulation period, improvements were observed in anthropometric measurements and certain blood parameters, such as ferritin levels. Notably, no significant adverse changes in blood parameters were observed as a result of the intervention.

3.9. Durability of tDCS Effects

The studies had different follow-up periods. The studies by Khedr et al. [67], Costanzo et al. [69], and Strumila et al. [70] measured outcomes 1 month after intervention, the study by Baumann et al. [68] measured outcomes after 4 weeks, and the study by Rzad et al. [71] measured outcomes after 2 weeks.

In the study by Khedr et al. [67], the first, third, and fourth patients maintained improvements for all three scales one month after completing treatment.

In Costanzo et al.'s [69] study, when they followed up with the tDCS + AU group one month after the treatment had ended, they found that the positive effects for most of the psychological measures still remained (EAT-26, T0 vs. T2: $Z = 2.37$, $p = 0.02$; MASC, T0 vs. T2: $Z = 1.96$, $p = 0.05$; CDI, T0 vs. T2: $Z = 2.19$, $p = 0.04$). However, there was no significant change in the EDI-3 scores (T0 vs. T2: $Z = 1.33$, $p = 0.18$). Furthermore, there was no improvement in the BUT scores even after one month (T0 vs. T2: $Z = 0.56$, $p = 0.57$). The improvement was also maintained for BMI.

In the study by Strumila et al. [70], EDI scores were maintained one month after stimulation. There was also a notable decrease in the overall score of the EDE-Q, and this reduction had a substantial effect, with a magnitude of 0.42. Comparable outcomes were seen in the EDE-Q restraint and eating concern subcategories. Scores for the BSQ-34 and BDI also remained lower.

In the study by Rzad et al. [71], there was sustained improvement (and further improvement in scores) in EAT, RSS, BDI, EDE-Q, BES, PSS, and BMI two weeks after the completion of tDCS.

4. Discussion

Studies have consistently demonstrated that tDCS stimulation of the left DLPFC has a positive effect on AN clinical symptoms and may improve them, as measured with various assessment measures. In this section, we discuss the mechanisms of action of tDCS in AN and propose additional parameters that are worth investigating in future trials.

4.1. General Findings

There is an increased interest in the use of tDCS to modulate eating behaviour, leading to a diverse range of methodological approaches. Although these approaches are crucial for the initial exploration of tDCS effects on various populations and measures, it is important to establish a robust foundation of studies [64]. Most of the studies that were analysed are open-label studies or case studies, which means their results should be interpreted with caution. Nevertheless, these studies provide preliminary evidence that tDCS has the potential to alter eating behaviour, body weight, and food intake. Therefore, a recommendation can be made for further research and development of tDCS protocols that can be used in the treatment of AN.

All studies involved anodal stimulation of the left DLPFC, a region that is relevant to AN's pathophysiology. Current intensities varied from 1 mA for adolescents to 2 mA for adults, reflecting age-appropriate dosages. A lower current dose is usually used in children, but the stimulation is still effective. Stimulation frequency also varied. Once-daily stimulation is the standard approach and is the simplest to implement from an organisational perspective. However, in Strumila et al.'s [70] study, we can observe that, after twice-daily simulation during the one-month follow-up period, the improvement was not only maintained but also increased.

4.2. Impact on AN Symptoms, Psychopathology, and Eating Behaviours

The results from the included studies indicate that tDCS stimulation of the left DLPFC holds promise for influencing various aspects of AN symptoms, psychopathology, and eating behaviours. In the study by Khedr et al. [67], improvements were observed in EDI scores, specifically in areas such as body dissatisfaction, interpersonal distrust, interoceptive awareness, and ineffectiveness. These improvements were sustained one month after treatment. Only one patient who did not receive SSRIs showed no improvement. Additionally, the study reported improvements in the EAT, suggesting potential benefits in AN symptomatology, but only in combination with the use of SSRIs. Baumann et al. [68] reported mixed findings, with no significant effects on complex psychopathology and weight recovery as measured by the EDE-Q. However, a secondary analysis indicated potential positive impacts on specific aspects of body shape evaluation and the need for excessive calorie intake control, although these results did not survive multiple comparison correction. This suggests that tDCS may have nuanced effects on different aspects of AN. Costanzo et al.'s [69] study showed improvement across various EDI-3 subscales, indicating positive changes in aspects like drive for thinness, body dissatisfaction, and interpersonal issues. Both the tDCS + AU group and the family-based therapy + AU group showed improvements, emphasising the potential of tDCS as an adjunctive treatment. However, not all subscales showed improvement, highlighting the need for further research to pinpoint the specific areas where tDCS is most effective. Strumila et al.'s [70] study demonstrated significant reductions in EDI scores, indicating improvements in various aspects of psychopathology such as inefficiency, perfectionism, distrust, and fear of maturity. These changes were maintained one month after treatment. Rzad et al.'s [71] case report showed improvements in various psychological assessments, including the EAT, RSS, EDE-Q, BES, and PSS. These improvements suggest that tDCS may have a positive impact on a wide range of psychological factors associated with AN.

Overall, although these studies provide encouraging preliminary results, it is important to acknowledge the limitations of small sample sizes, open-label designs, and variations in tDCS protocols across studies. Further randomised controlled trials with larger sample sizes and standardised protocols are needed to confirm the efficacy of tDCS in AN treatment and to better understand the specific mechanisms underlying its effects. Additionally, future research should explore the potential long-term effects of tDCS treatment beyond the one-month follow-up period, as well as investigate the durability of improvements in AN symptoms and psychopathology over extended time frames. Moreover, the combination of tDCS with other therapeutic approaches, such as cognitive behavioural therapy or nutritional interventions, should be explored to determine if synergistic effects can be achieved in the treatment of AN.

4.3. Impact on BMI

Three of the included studies used BMI as outcomes and showed mixed results. In the study by Baumann et al. [68], both the active and sham tDCS groups showed improvement in BMI, although the improvement was not statistically significant. This suggests that tDCS may have a limited impact on BMI in this specific population, and additional factors such as nutritional interventions and psychotherapy may be necessary for significant weight gain. In the study by Costanzo et al. [69], the tDCS + AU group showed a significant improvement in BMI, with a notable average percentage increase. In contrast, the FBT + AU group did not exhibit a significant change in BMI after treatment. This suggests that tDCS, when combined with treatment as usual (AU), may have a beneficial effect on increasing BMI in adolescents with AN. In the case report by Rzad et al. [71], an improvement and increase in BMI were observed after tDCS treatment. Although this is a single case report, it still provides valuable insight into the potential of tDCS to positively influence BMI in AN. These mixed findings regarding the impact of tDCS on BMI highlight the complexity of AN treatment and the multifaceted nature of the disorder. It is possible that tDCS may have a more significant impact when combined with other therapeutic approaches, such as nutritional support and psychotherapy. Therefore, future research should explore the specific factors that contribute to changes in BMI in AN patients undergoing tDCS treatment.

4.4. Impact on Depression

Four studies investigated the effects of tDCS on depression in patients with AN, revealing mixed but predominantly positive results. In the studies conducted by Khedr et al. [67] and Rzad et al. [71], improvements in depression symptoms were observed following tDCS treatment. Khedr et al. reported that the first, second, third, and fourth patients in their study demonstrated improvements in BDI-II scores. This suggests that tDCS may have a positive effect on reducing depressive symptoms in AN patients but in combination with SSRIs.

In contrast, the study by Baumann et al. [68] presented more nuanced results. Although the researchers initially anticipated some improvement in the active tDCS group based on the ZUNG, they found that, upon the completion of the treatment, the sham group exhibited better results in the total score and specific questions of the ZUNG. Possible explanations for these findings include the presence of higher levels of MDD and higher doses of antidepressants, particularly mirtazapine, in the sham group, which could have influenced the results. Another possible interpretation is that, in individuals with AN, difficulties in experiencing and regulating emotions may arise as a result of the primary eating disorder pathology and could potentially intensify with age. Therefore, if the patients' core difficulties did not undergo sufficient changes, their moods may have remained unaffected.

Costanzo et al. [69] also demonstrated improvements in depressive symptoms using the CDI in their study of adolescents with AN who received tDCS treatment. This suggests that tDCS may have a positive impact on alleviating depressive symptoms in younger AN patients. Strumila et al. [70] reported significant reductions in BDI depression scores after tDCS treatment, indicating an improvement in depressive symptoms. This aligns with the findings from Khedr et al. [67] and Costanzo et al. [69].

4.5. Mechanisms of Action

In patients with AN, there is evidence of fronto-temporal hyperactivity in the right hemisphere (RH). The EEG study by Grunwald et al. [73] demonstrated hyperactivation in the RH of individuals with AN. Similarly, the positron emission tomography (PET) study conducted by Galusca et al. focused on serotonin activity around 5-HT1A receptors in people with AN, revealing an increased number of serotonergic junctions, particularly in the fronto-temporal regions of the RH [74,75].

Anodal tDCS, which has an excitatory effect, enhances the excitability of the left DLPFC and helps restore the interhemispheric balance by counteracting overactivity in the right DLPFC. Additionally, the effects of tDCS may extend to distant brain structures associated with the site of stimulation, which are also implicated in the underlying mechanisms of AN [67].

The pathogenesis of AN involves imbalances in serotonergic signaling in the ventral striatum, potentially related to the aversive aspects of the disorder [75,76]. Another theory proposes disruptions in reward pathways, as alterations in the dopamine system can affect reward circuitry, leading to anxiety and dysphoric moods [75,77]. Wagner et al. [78] discovered a dopamine imbalance in the ventral striatum of AN patients, characterised by decreased neuronal activity and hyperexcitability of the caudate nucleus.

In individuals with eating disorders, reward pathways are activated by disease-related stimuli but may not respond as strongly to typical rewarding stimuli. Excessive activation of the ventral striatum occurs in response to body-weight-related stimuli. Tanaka et al. [79] demonstrated that tDCS stimulation of the cortex can modulate dopamine release in the striatum. Cathodal tDCS, but not anodal tDCS, led to increased extracellular dopamine levels in the rat striatum for over 400 min. These findings suggest that tDCS may directly or indirectly impact the dopaminergic system in the basal ganglia, potentially affecting certain pathophysiological mechanisms of AN, including mesocortical dopaminergic pathways and increased food intake [75]. However, it remains unclear whether a current of such intensity can effectively reach deeper brain structures in humans.

In the study by Fonteneau et al. [80], bifrontal tDCS was applied to the human brain to investigate its effects on subcortical dopamine transmission during and immediately after stimulation. Right anodal and left cathodal tDCS resulted in a significant increase in extracellular dopamine transmission in the striatum, which is involved in the reward–motivation network. Mesolimbic dopaminergic projections in the striatum play a crucial role in guiding eating behaviour by modulating appetitive motivational processes. It has been suggested that disturbances in dopaminergic reward pathways contribute to the pathogenesis of AN [75,81,82].

The DLPFC plays a significant role in regulating emotions. By stimulating this region, the desire for dietary behaviours and calorie restrictions can be reduced. AN is characterised by excessive cognitive control, with the DLPFC being a key component of the cognitive control system. Even after recovery, individuals with a history of AN often exhibit heightened cognitive control over reward processing. Given these observations, inhibiting the left DLPFC has the potential to alleviate excessive cognitive control in AN [68].

tDCS has proven to be effective in reducing depressive symptoms in individuals with AN. This is not surprising, as tDCS has been commonly studied in depression treatment, and anodal stimulation of the left DLPFC has shown promise in depression therapy [83,84]. The underlying hypothesis behind using tDCS for depression is that it targets dysfunctions in various cortical and subcortical regions, including the prefrontal cortex [85], amygdala [86], and hippocampus [87]. Depressed individuals often have imbalances in brain activity, with increased activity in the right cortex and decreased activity in the left cortex. tDCS works by enhancing activity in the left DLPFC while reducing activity in the right cortex, aiming to address the neurophysiological imbalances associated with depression [88]. Moreover, tDCS may have an impact on dopamine secretion in the striatum. Some studies have indicated that applying tDCS to the left DLPFC increases dopamine secretion [89,90], which is significant because depression has been linked to dopaminergic dysfunction [91–93]. This positive effect on dopamine production could contribute to alleviating depression symptoms in AN. However, more neuroimaging studies are needed to confirm prefrontal dysfunction in AN patients and the specific effect of tDCS on this area of the brain. Nonetheless, the potential of tDCS as a non-invasive and promising treatment for depression in AN warrants further exploration and investigation.

4.6. Safety and Acceptance

tDCS is safe and acceptable for patients. The main risks are associated with the device (burn and skin irritation), interference with the psychiatric treatment, and adverse effects on cognitive performance. Regarding AN, there have been limited safety and acceptability studies [66].

4.7. Ethical Issues

The ethical considerations for tDCS arise from the application of the therapy to a population of very vulnerable and physically frail patients with severe and persistent AN. In this case, their ability to make healthy decisions is limited. Ethicists studying tDCS have also raised concerns that tDCS could be perceived as a form of "mind control" that increases patients' dependence and helplessness and reduces their sense of authenticity [94,95]. The scant literature to date examining the views of patients treated with tDCS shows that they are capable of understanding the issues of benefits and risks to their authenticity [65].

4.8. Review Limitations and Risk of Bias

It should be emphasised that the research was analysed in the form of a narrative review. This raises some concerns about the lack of objectivity. Due to the small number of studies, it is not possible to conduct a meta-analysis. However, this is the first review of research focused solely on AN. Previous work, as mentioned earlier, has also included other eating disorders and positively assessed the impact of tDCS. Eating disorders are heterogeneous, so generalising the effects and effectiveness of treatments for all disorders raises significant concerns about biased results. Reviews should cover only one disorder. Another limitation of this review is the potential impact of psychotropic medication in the included studies, which may have introduced bias into the results. According to Normann et al. [96], SSRIs can enhance the response to tDCS. In healthy individuals, the chronic intake of SSRIs increased facilitative plasticity in the visual cortex, converting inhibitory plasticity to facilitation [96]. Citalopram, an SSRI, was found to enhance and prolong the facilitation induced by anodal tDCS while converting cathodal tDCS-induced inhibition into facilitation [97]. Therefore, patients in the study by Khedr et al. [67] who were taking SSRIs might have had an enhanced response to tDCS and a more pronounced treatment effect. Conversely, drugs that interfere with dopaminergic signaling, such as antipsychotics, are believed to have a negative impact on tDCS plasticity [69,98]. Aripiprazole, the medication used by all participants in Costanzo et al.'s [69] study, is a partial agonist of the D2 receptor and differs from other antipsychotics that act as pure antagonists [99]. Aripiprazole may specifically enhance the hypothesised effect of tDCS in regulating the tonic dopamine (DA) component in the striatum, as it inhibits the phasic component while preserving the release of the tonic DA component to some extent [69,100].

4.9. Future Directions

The evidence to date suggests that, although tDCS has potential for the treatment of people with AN, much of this potential is yet to be discovered. There is still significant heterogeneity in response to treatment. The optimisation of protocols, patient selection, treatment goals, and intervention parameters remains to be explored. Optimising the protocols will require extensive research to address issues such as frequency, duration, intensity of stimulation, and target selection. Given that AN is a heterogeneous disorder, finding a single "optimal" protocol is unlikely. Using personalised interventions to target specific subgroups of patients will be a valuable option. It is crucial to gain a deeper understanding of neural, neurocognitive, and biological correlations, markers, and outcome predictors, as they can help provide personalised treatments and individualised protocols. Work is underway to develop a rationale for the use of neuromodulatory therapies based on evolving neural models of eating disorders. These advances and increased knowledge about neural networks and their interconnections may lead to the emergence of new hypotheses regarding the etiology and treatment of AN [65]. Trials involving multimodal neuroimaging, neurocognitive tasks, and clinical measures should be conducted [64]. Future trials should include larger samples to be sufficiently powerful.

Individuals with AN frequently suffer from comorbidities, with depression being the most common. As noted in a review [62], the mood component in the research raises a methodological problem: the simultaneous improvement of body weight and mood in people with AN makes it impossible to identify a specific effect on AN. The measurement of depressive symptoms with a subgroup analysis of non-depressed patients could help solve this problem [62].

The review [62] highlights an important factor that should be taken into account, which is the variability of brain states associated with the metabolic status. In individuals with AN, the nutritional status can exert a more pronounced impact on brain functioning compared to other mental disorders. The nutritional status has been found to influence treatment responses, particularly in relation to antidepressants, which are less effective in underweight patients [101]. Consequently, nutritional status may play a role in determining the response or non-response to treatment and can potentially confound the effectiveness of neuromodulation techniques.

tDCS technology continues to evolve and increasingly enables more precise targeting of treatment, probing deeper areas of the brain, using shorter and more powerful protocols, and stimulating multiple brain regions simultaneously. According to new evidence, these types of interventions may work synergistically when used with various forms of cognitive training, but this has not yet been explored in AN [102].

5. Conclusions

In conclusion, the small evidence base so far suggests that tDCS has a positive effect on AN symptoms and is an effective and safe tool in the treatment of AN, and its tolerance is high. However, there are many knowledge gaps regarding the optimisation of protocols and mechanisms of action. Additionally, the use of tDCS in conjunction with another intervention or alone raises questions. As advances in knowledge better elucidate the brain mechanisms of AN, there will be an opportunity to make better use of tDCS. To establish a stronger evidence base and validate the therapeutic efficacy in this disorder, further randomised controlled trials (RCTs) are imperative.

Author Contributions: Conceptualisation, J.C. and J.L.; methodology, J.C. and J.L.; writing—original draft preparation, J.C., A.G. and J.L. writing—review and editing, J.C., A.G. and J.L.; supervision, J.L. All authors have read and agreed to the published version of the manuscript.

Funding: This research received no external funding.

Institutional Review Board Statement: Not applicable.

Informed Consent Statement: Not applicable.

Data Availability Statement: No new data were created or analysed in this study. Data sharing is not applicable to this article.

Conflicts of Interest: The authors declare no conflict of interest.

References

1. Hudson, J.I.; Hiripi, E.; Pope, H.G., Jr.; Kessler, J. The prevalence and correlates of eating disorders in the National Comorbidity Survey Replication. *Biol. Psychiatry* **2007**, *61*, 348–358. [CrossRef]
2. Zhu, Y.; Hu, X.; Wang, J.; Chen, J.; Guo, Q.; Li, C.; Enck, P. Processing of food, body and emotional stimuli in anorexia nervosa: A systematic review and meta-analysis of functional magnetic resonance imaging studies. *Eur. Eat. Disord. Rev.* **2012**, *20*, 439–450. [CrossRef] [PubMed]
3. Kaye, W.H.; Fudge, J.L.; Paulus, M. New insights into symptoms and neurocircuit function of anorexia nervosa. *Nat. Rev. Neurosci.* **2009**, *10*, 573–584. [CrossRef] [PubMed]
4. Johnson, J.G.; Cohen, P.; Kasen, S.; Brook, J.S. Personality disorder traits evident by early adulthood and risk for eating and weight problems during middle adulthood. *Int. J. Eat. Disord.* **2006**, *39*, 184–192. [CrossRef]
5. Arcelus, J.; Mitchell, A.J.; Wales, J.; Nielsen, S. Mortality rates in patients with anorexia nervosa and other eating disorders: A meta-analysis of 36 studies. *Arch. Gen. Psychiatry* **2011**, *68*, 724–731. [CrossRef]
6. Smink, F.R.; van Hoeken, D.; Hoek, H.W. Epidemiology, course, and outcome of eating disorders. *Curr. Opin. Psychiatry* **2013**, *26*, 543–548. [CrossRef]
7. Su, T.; Gong, J.; Tang, G.; Qiu, S.; Chen, P.; Chen, G.; Wang, J.; Huang, L.; Wang, Y. Structural and functional brain alterations in anorexia nervosa: A multimodal meta-analysis of neuroimaging studies. *Hum. Brain Mapp.* **2021**, *42*, 5154–5169. [CrossRef] [PubMed]
8. Fairburn, C.G.; Harrison, P.J. Eating disorders. *Lancet* **2003**, *361*, 407–416. [CrossRef]
9. van Eeden, A.E.; van Hoeken, D.; Hoek, H.W. Incidence, prevalence and mortality of anorexia nervosa and bulimia nervosa. *Curr. Opin. Psychiatry* **2021**, *34*, 515–524. [CrossRef]
10. Murray, S.B.; Nagata, J.M.; Griffiths, S.; Calzo, J.P.; Brown, T.A.; Mitchison, D.; Blashill, A.J.; Mond, J.M. The enigma of male eating disorders: A critical review and synthesis. *Clin. Psychol. Rev.* **2017**, *57*, 1–11. [CrossRef]
11. Esposito, R.; Cieri, F.; di Giannantonio, M.; Tartaro, A. The role of body image and self-perception in anorexia nervosa: The neuroimaging perspective. *J. Neuropsychol.* **2018**, *12*, 41–52. [CrossRef]
12. Schorr, M.; Miller, K.K. The endocrine manifestations of anorexia nervosa: Mechanisms and management. *Nat. Rev. Endocrinol.* **2017**, *13*, 174–186. [CrossRef] [PubMed]
13. Zipfel, S.; Giel, K.E.; Bulik, C.M.; Hay, P.; Schmidt, U. Anorexia nervosa: Aetiology, assessment, and treatment. *Lancet Psychiatry* **2015**, *2*, 1099–1111. [CrossRef] [PubMed]
14. Gustavsson, A.; Svensson, M.; Jacobi, F.; Allgulander, C.; Alonso, J.; Beghi, E.; Dodel, R.; Ekman, M.; Faravelli, C.; Fratiglioni, L.; et al. Cost of disorders of the brain in Europe 2010. *Eur. Neuropsychopharmacol.* **2011**, *21*, 718–779. [CrossRef] [PubMed]
15. Garner, D.; Desmond, M.; Desai, J.; Lockert, J. The disconnect between treatment outcome data and reimbursement for the treatment of anorexia nervosa. *Int. J. Physiatry* **2016**, *2*, 1–6. [CrossRef]
16. Steinhausen, H.C. The outcome of anorexia nervosa in the 20th century. *Am. J. Psychiatry* **2002**, *159*, 1284–1293. [CrossRef]
17. Zipfel, S.; Lowe, B.; Reas, D.L.; Deter, H.C.; Herzog, W. Long-term prognosis in anorexia nervosa: Lessons from a 21-year follow-up study. *Lancet* **2000**, *355*, 721–722. [CrossRef]
18. Sullivan, P.F. Mortality in anorexia nervosa. *Am. J. Psychiatry* **1995**, *152*, 1073–1074.
19. Phillipou, A.; Rossell, S.L.; Castle, D.J. The neurobiology of anorexia nervosa: A systematic review. *Aust. N. Z. J. Psychiatry* **2014**, *48*, 128–152. [CrossRef]
20. Murao, E.; Sugihara, G.; Isobe, M.; Noda, T.; Kawabata, M.; Matsukawa, N.; Takahashi, H.; Murai, T.; Noma, S. Differences in neural responses to reward and punishment processing between anorexia nervosa subtypes: An fMRI study. *Psychiatry Clin. Neurosci.* **2017**, *71*, 647–658. [CrossRef]
21. Cassin, S.E.; von Ranson, K.M. Personality and eating disorders: A decade in review. *Clin. Psychol. Rev.* **2005**, *25*, 895–916. [CrossRef] [PubMed]
22. Herzog, D.B.; Keller, M.B.; Sacks, N.R.; Yeh, C.J.; Lavori, P.W. Psychiatric comorbidity in treatment-seeking anorexics and bulimics. *J. Am. Acad. Child Adolesc. Psychiatry* **1992**, *31*, 810–818. [CrossRef] [PubMed]
23. Fouladi, F.; Mitchell, J.E.; Crosby, R.D.; Engel, S.G.; Crow, S.; Hill, L.; Le Grange, D.; Powers, P.; Steffen, K.J. Prevalence of Alcohol and Other Substance Use in Patients with Eating Disorders. *Eur. Eat. Disord. Rev.* **2015**, *23*, 531–536. [CrossRef]
24. Nagata, T.; Kawarada, Y.; Kiriike, N.; Iketani, T. Multi-impulsivity of Japanese patients with eating disorders: Primary and secondary impulsivity. *Psychiatry Res.* **2000**, *94*, 239–250. [CrossRef] [PubMed]
25. Diaz-Marsa, M.; Carrasco, J.L.; Saiz, J. A study of temperament and personality in anorexia and bulimia nervosa. *J. Personal. Disord.* **2000**, *14*, 352–359. [CrossRef]
26. Kaye, W.H. Neurobiology of anorexia and bulimia nervosa. *Physiol. Behav.* **2008**, *94*, 121–135. [CrossRef]
27. Frank, G.; Bailer, U.F.; Henry, S.; Drevets, W.; Meltzer, C.C.; Price, J.C.; Mathis, C.A.; Wagner, A.; Hoge, J.; Ziolko, S.; et al. Increased dopamine D2/D3 receptor binding after recovery from anorexia nervosa measured by positron emission tomography and [^{11}C]raclopride. *Biol. Psychiatry* **2005**, *58*, 908–912. [CrossRef]
28. Higgins, A. The Neurobiology of Anorexia Nervosa. In *Anorexia and Bulimia Nervosa*; IntechOpen: London, UK, 2019.
29. Avena, N.M.; Bocarsly, M.E. Dysregulation of brain reward systems in eating disorders: Neurochemical information from animal models of binge eating, bulimia nervosa, and anorexia nervosa. *Neuropharmacology* **2012**, *63*, 87–96. [CrossRef]

30. Riva, G. Neurobiology of Anorexia Nervosa: Serotonin Dysfunctions Link Self-Starvation with Body Image Disturbances through an Impaired Body Memory. *Front. Hum. Neurosci.* **2016**, *10*, 600. [CrossRef]
31. Jenkins, T.A.; Nguyen, J.C.; Polglaze, K.E.; Bertrand, P.P. Influence of Tryptophan and Serotonin on Mood and Cognition with a Possible Role of the Gut-Brain Axis. *Nutrients* **2016**, *8*, 56. [CrossRef]
32. Yabut, J.M.; Crane, J.D.; Green, A.E.; Keating, D.J.; Khan, W.I.; Steinberg, G.R. Emerging Roles for Serotonin in Regulating Metabolism: New Implications for an Ancient Molecule. *Endocr. Rev.* **2019**, *40*, 1092–1107. [CrossRef] [PubMed]
33. Calati, R.; De Ronchi, D.; Bellini, M.; Serretti, A. The 5-HTTLPR polymorphism and eating disorders: A meta-analysis. *Int. J. Eat. Disord.* **2011**, *44*, 191–199. [CrossRef]
34. Haleem, D.J. Serotonin neurotransmission in anorexia nervosa. *Behav. Pharmacol.* **2012**, *23*, 478–495. [CrossRef] [PubMed]
35. Isingrini, E.; Perret, L.; Rainer, Q.; Amilhon, B.; Guma, E.; Tanti, A.; Martin, G.; Robinson, J.; Moquin, L.; Marti, F.; et al. Resilience to chronic stress is mediated by noradrenergic regulation of dopamine neurons. *Nat. Neurosci.* **2016**, *19*, 560–563. [CrossRef] [PubMed]
36. Delvenne, V.; Lotstra, F.; Goldman, S.; Biver, F.; De Maertelaer, V.; Appelboom-Fondu, J.; Schoutens, A.; Bidaut, L.M.; Luxen, A.; Mendelwicz, J. Brain hypometabolism of glucose in anorexia nervosa: A PET scan study. *Biol. Psychiatry* **1995**, *37*, 161–169. [CrossRef] [PubMed]
37. Kojima, S.; Nagai, N.; Nakabeppu, Y.; Muranaga, T.; Deguchi, D.; Nakajo, M.; Masuda, A.; Nozoe, S.I.; Naruo, T. Comparison of regional cerebral blood flow in patients with anorexia nervosa before and after weight gain. *Psychiatry Res.* **2005**, *140*, 251–258. [CrossRef]
38. Naruo, T.; Nakabeppu, Y.; Deguchi, D.; Nagai, N.; Tsutsui, J.; Nakajo, M.; Nozoe, S.I. Decreases in blood perfusion of the anterior cingulate gyri in anorexia nervosa restricters assessed by SPECT image analysis. *BMC Psychiatry* **2001**, *1*, 2. [CrossRef]
39. Takano, A.; Shiga, T.; Kitagawa, N.; Koyama, T.; Katoh, C.; Tsukamoto, E.; Tamaki, N. Abnormal neuronal network in anorexia nervosa studied with I-123-IMP SPECT. *Psychiatry Res.* **2001**, *107*, 45–50. [CrossRef]
40. Frank, G.K.; Bailer, U.F.; Meltzer, C.C.; Price, J.C.; Mathis, C.A.; Wagner, A.; Becker, C.; Kaye, W.H. Regional cerebral blood flow after recovery from anorexia or bulimia nervosa. *Int. J. Eat. Disord.* **2007**, *40*, 488–492. [CrossRef]
41. Yonezawa, H.; Otagaki, Y.; Miyake, Y.; Okamoto, Y.; Yamawaki, S. No differences are seen in the regional cerebral blood flow in the restricting type of anorexia nervosa compared with the binge eating/purging type. *Psychiatry Clin. Neurosci.* **2008**, *62*, 26–33. [CrossRef]
42. Beato-Fernández, L.; Rodríguez-Cano, T.; García-Vilches, I.; García-Vicente, A.; Poblete-García, V.; Castrejon, A.S.; Toro, J. Changes in regional cerebral blood flow after body image exposure in eating disorders. *Psychiatry Res.* **2009**, *171*, 129–137. [CrossRef] [PubMed]
43. Wagner, A.; Ruf, M.; Braus, D.F.; Schmidt, M.H. Neuronal activity changes and body image distortion in anorexia nervosa. *Neuroreport* **2003**, *14*, 2193–2197. [CrossRef] [PubMed]
44. Kuruoglu, A.C.; Kapucu, O.; Atasever, T.; Arikan, Z.; Işik, E.; Unlü, M. Technetium-99m-HMPAO brain SPECT in anorexia nervosa. *J. Nucl. Med.* **1998**, *39*, 304–306.
45. Pietrini, F.; Castellini, G.; Ricca, V.; Polito, C.; Pupi, A.; Faravelli, C. Functional neuroimaging in anorexia nervosa: A clinical approach. *Eur. Psychiatry* **2011**, *26*, 176–182. [CrossRef]
46. Been, G.; Ngo, T.T.; Miller, S.M.; Fitzgerald, P.B. The use of tDCS and CVS as methods of non-invasive brain stimulation. *Brain Res. Rev.* **2007**, *56*, 346–361. [CrossRef] [PubMed]
47. Frank, E.; Wilfurth, S.; Landgrebe, M.; Eichhammer, P.; Hajak, G.; Langguth, B. Anodal skin lesions after treatment with transcranial direct current stimulation. *Brain Stimul.* **2010**, *3*, 58–59. [CrossRef]
48. Nitsche, M.A.; Paulus, W. Excitability changes induced in the human motor cortex by weak transcranial direct current stimulation. *J. Physiol.* **2000**, *527*, 633–639. [CrossRef]
49. Lang, N.; Siebner, H.R.; Ward, N.S.; Lee, L.; Nitsche, M.A.; Paulus, W.; Rothwell, J.C.; Lemon, R.N.; Frackowiak, R.S. How does transcranial DC stimulation of the primary motor cortex alter regional neuronal activity in the human brain? *Eur. J. Neurosci.* **2005**, *22*, 495–504. [CrossRef]
50. Nitsche, M.A.; Doemkes, S.; Karaköse, T.; Antal, A.; Liebetanz, D.; Lang, N.; Tergau, F.; Paulus, W. Shaping the effects of transcranial direct current stimulation of the human motor cortex. *J. Neurophysiol.* **2007**, *97*, 3109–3117. [CrossRef]
51. Bikson, M.; Grossman, P.; Thomas, C.; Zannou, A.L.; Jiang, J.; Adnan, T.; Mourdoukoutas, A.P.; Kronberg, G.; Truong, D.; Boggio, P.; et al. Safety of Transcranial Direct Current Stimulation: Evidence Based Update. *Brain Stimul.* **2016**, *9*, 641–661. [CrossRef]
52. Nitsche, M.A.; Paulus, W. Sustained excitability elevations induced by transcranial DC motor cortex stimulation in humans. *Neurology* **2001**, *57*, 1899–1901. [CrossRef]
53. Nitsche, M.A.; Koschack, J.; Pohlers, H.; Hullemann, S.; Paulus, W.; Happe, S. Effects of frontal transcranial direct current stimulation on emotional state and processing in healthy humans. *Front. Psychol.* **2012**, *3*, 58. [CrossRef]
54. Fritsch, B.; Reis, J.; Martinowich, K.; Schambra, H.M.; Ji, Y.; Cohen, L.G.; Lu, B. Direct current stimulation promotes BDNF-dependent synaptic plasticity: Potential implications for motor learning. *Neuron* **2010**, *66*, 198–204. [CrossRef]
55. Kronberg, G.; Bridi, M.; Abel, T.; Bikson, M.; Parra, L.C. Direct current stimulation modulates LTP and LTD: Activity dependence and dendritic effects. *Brain Stimul.* **2017**, *10*, 51–58. [CrossRef]

56. Nitsche, M.A.; Liebetanz, D.; Schlitterlau, A.; Henschke, U.; Fricke, K.; Frommann, K.; Lang, N.; Henning, S.; Paulus, W.; Tergau, F. GABAergic modulation of DC stimulation-induced motor cortex excitability shifts in humans. *Eur. J. Neurosci.* **2004**, *19*, 2720–2726. [CrossRef]
57. Nitsche, M.A.; Seeber, A.; Frommann, K.; Klein, C.C.; Rochford, C.; Nitsche, M.S.; Fricke, K.; Liebetanz, D.; Lang, N.; Antal, A.; et al. Modulating parameters of excitability during and after transcranial direct current stimulationof the human motor cortex. *J. Physiol.* **2005**, *568 Pt 1*, 291–303. [CrossRef]
58. Stagg, C.J.; Best, J.G.; Stephenson, M.C.; O'Shea, J.; Wylezinska, M.; Kincses, Z.T.; Morris, P.G.; Matthews, P.M.; Johansen-Berg, H. Polarity-sensitive modulation of cortical neurotransmitters by transcranial stimulation. *J. Neurosci.* **2009**, *29*, 5202–5206. [CrossRef]
59. Reed, T.; Cohen Kadosh, R. Transcranial electrical stimulation (tES) mechanisms and its effects on cortical excitability and connectivity. *J. Inherit. Metab. Dis.* **2018**, *41*, 1123–1130. [CrossRef]
60. Lisman, J.E. Three Ca^{2+} levels affect plasticity differently: The LTP zone, the LTD zone and no man's land. *J. Physiol.* **2001**, *532 Pt 2*, 28. [CrossRef]
61. Sousa, B.; Martins, J.; Castelo-Branco, M.; Gonçalves, J. Transcranial Direct Current Stimulation as an Approach to Mitigate Neurodevelopmental Disorders Affecting Excitation/Inhibition Balance: Focus on Autism Spectrum Disorder, Schizophrenia, and Attention Deficit/Hyperactivity Disorder. *J. Clin. Med.* **2022**, *11*, 2839. [CrossRef]
62. Duriez, P.; Bou Khalil, R.; Chamoun, Y.; Maatoug, R.; Strumila, R.; Seneque, M.; Gorwood, P.; Courtet, P.; Guillaume, S. Brain Stimulation in Eating Disorders: State of the Art and Future Perspectives. *J. Clin. Med.* **2020**, *9*, 2358. [CrossRef]
63. Beaumont, J.D.; Smith, N.C.; Starr, D.; Davis, D.; Dalton, M.; Nowicky, A.; Russell, M.; Barwood, M.J. Modulating eating behavior with transcranial direct current stimulation (tDCS): A systematic literature review on the impact of eating behavior traits. *Obes. Rev.* **2022**, *23*, e13364. [CrossRef] [PubMed]
64. Gallop, L.; Flynn, M.; Campbell, I.C.; Schmidt, U. Neuromodulation and Eating Disorders. *Curr. Psychiatry Rep.* **2022**, *24*, 61–69. [CrossRef]
65. Dalton, B.; Bartholdy, S.; Campbell, I.C.; Schmidt, U. Neurostimulation in Clinical and Sub-clinical Eating Disorders: A Systematic Update of the Literature. *Curr. Neuropharmacol.* **2018**, *16*, 1174–1192. [CrossRef]
66. Hall, P.A.; Vincent, C.M.; Burhan, A.M. Non-invasive brain stimulation for food cravings, consumption, and disorders of eating: A review of methods, findings and controversies. *Appetite* **2018**, *124*, 78–88. [CrossRef] [PubMed]
67. Khedr, E.M.; Elfetoh, N.A.; Ali, A.M.; Noamany, M. Anodal transcranial direct current stimulation over the dorsolateral prefrontal cortex improves anorexia nervosa: A pilot study. *Restor. Neurol. Neurosci.* **2014**, *32*, 789–797. [CrossRef] [PubMed]
68. Baumann, S.; Mareš, T.; Albrecht, J.; Anders, M.; Vochosková, K.; Hill, M.; Bulant, J.; Yamamotová, A.; Štastný, O.; Novák, T.; et al. Effects of Transcranial Direct Current Stimulation Treatment for Anorexia Nervosa. *Front. Psychiatry* **2021**, *12*, 717255. [CrossRef]
69. Costanzo, F.; Menghini, D.; Maritato, A.; Castiglioni, M.C.; Mereu, A.; Varuzza, C.; Zanna, V.; Vicari, S. New Treatment Perspectives in Adolescents with Anorexia Nervosa: The Efficacy of Non-invasive Brain-Directed Treatment. *Front. Behav. Neurosci.* **2018**, *12*, 133. [CrossRef] [PubMed]
70. Strumila, R.; Thiebaut, S.; Jaussent, I.; Seneque, M.; Attal, J.; Courtet, P.; Guillaume, S. Safety and efficacy of transcranial direct current stimulation (tDCS) in the treatment of Anorexia Nervosa. The open-label STAR study. *Brain Stimul.* **2019**, *12*, 1325–1327. [CrossRef]
71. Rząd, Z.; Szewczyk, P.; Rog, J.; Karakula-Juchnowicz, H. Efficiency of Transcranial Direct Current Stimulation (tDCS) in Anorexia Nervosa Treatment-Case Report. *Curr. Probl. Psychiatry* **2022**, *23*, 111–117. [CrossRef]
72. Thair, H.; Holloway, A.L.; Newport, R.; Smith, A.D. Transcranial Direct Current Stimulation (tDCS): A Beginner's Guide for Design and Implementation. *Front. Neurosci.* **2017**, *11*, 641. [CrossRef]
73. Grunwald, M.; Weiss, T.; Assmann, B.; Ettrich, C. Stable asymmetric interhemispheric theta power in patients with anorexia nervosa during haptic perception even after weight gain: A longitudinal study. *J. Clin. Exp. Neuropsychol.* **2004**, *26*, 608–620. [CrossRef] [PubMed]
74. Galusca, B.; Costes, N.; Zito, N.G.; Peyron, R.; Bossu, C.; Lang, F.; Estour, B. Organic background of restrictive-type anorexia nervosa suggested by increased serotonin1A receptor binding in right frontotemporal cortex of both lean and recovered patients:18F. MPPF PET scan study. *Biol. Psychiatry* **2008**, *64*, 1009–1013. [CrossRef]
75. Pellón Mendoza, A.R.; Castaño Castaño, S. Application of Direct Transcranial Current as Non-Invasive Therapy in Eating Disorders: An Intervention Proposal. *MLS Psychol. Res.* **2020**, *3*, 79–98. [CrossRef]
76. Taghva, A.; Corrigan, J.D.; Rezai, A.R. Obesity and brain addiction circuitry: Implications for deep brain stimulation. *Neurosurgery* **2012**, *71*, 224–238. [CrossRef] [PubMed]
77. Kaye, W.H.; Wierenga, C.E.; Bailer, U.F.; Simmons, A.N.; Wagner, A.; Bischoff-Grethe, A. Does a shared neurobiology for foods and drugs of abuse contribute to extremes of food ingestion in anorexia and bulimia nervosa? *Biol. Psychiatry* **2013**, *73*, 836–842. [CrossRef] [PubMed]
78. Wagner, A.; Aizenstein, H.; Venkatraman, V.K.; Fudge, J.; May, J.C.; Mazurkewicz, L.; Carter, C. Altered reward processing in women recovered from anorexia nervosa. *Am. J. Psychiatry* **2007**, *164*, 1842–1849. [CrossRef]
79. Tanaka, T.; Takano, Y.; Tanaka, S.; Hironaka, N.; Kobayashi, K.; Hanakawa, T.; Watanabe, K.; Honda, M. Transcranial direct-current stimulation increasesextracellular dopamine levels in the rat striatum. *Front. Syst. Neurosci.* **2013**, *7*, 6. [CrossRef]
80. Fonteneau, C.; Redoute, J.; Haesebaert, F.; Le Bars, D.; Costes, N.; Suaud-Chagny, M.F.; Brunelin, J. Frontal Transcranial Direct Current Stimulation Induces Dopamine Release in the Ventral Striatum in Human. *Cereb. Cortex* **2018**, *28*, 2636–2646. [CrossRef]

81. Casper, R.C. The "drive for activity" and "restlessness" in anorexia nervosa: Potential pathways. *J. Affect. Disord.* **2006**, *92*, 99–107. [CrossRef]
82. Alcaro, A.; Huber, R.; Panksepp, J. Behavioral functions of the mesolimbic dopaminergic system: An affective neuroethological perspective. *Brain Res. Rev.* **2007**, *56*, 283–321. [CrossRef] [PubMed]
83. Palm, U.; Hasan, A.; Strube, W.; Padberg, F. tDCS for the treatment of depression: A comprehensive review. *Eur. Arch. Psychiatry Clin. Neurosci.* **2016**, *266*, 681–694. [CrossRef]
84. Woodham, R.; Rimmer, R.M.; Mutz, J.; Fu, C.H.Y. Is tDCS a potential first line treatment for major depression? *Int. Rev. Psychiatry* **2021**, *33*, 250–265. [CrossRef] [PubMed]
85. Pizzagalli, D.A.; Roberts, A.C. Prefrontal cortex and depression. *Neuropsychopharmacology* **2022**, *47*, 225–246. [CrossRef] [PubMed]
86. Hamilton, J.P.; Siemer, M.; Gotlib, I.H. Amygdala volume in major depressive disorder: A meta-analysis of magnetic resonance imaging studies. *Mol. Psychiatry* **2008**, *13*, 993–1000. [CrossRef]
87. Sheline, Y.I. Depression and the hippocampus: Cause or effect? *Biol. Psychiatry* **2011**, *70*, 308–309. [CrossRef]
88. Brunoni, A.R.; Ferrucci, R.; Fregni, F.; Boggio, P.S.; Priori, A. Transcranial direct current stimulation for the treatment of major depressive disorder: A summary of preclinical, clinical and translational findings. *Prog. Neuro-Psychopharmacol. Biol. Psychiatry* **2012**, *39*, 9–16. [CrossRef]
89. Fukai, M.; Bunai, T.; Hirosawa, T.; Kikuchi, M.; Ito, S.; Minabe, Y.; Ouchi, Y. Endogenous dopamine release under transcranial direct-current stimulation governs enhanced attention: A study with positron emission tomography. *Transl. Psychiatry* **2019**, *9*, 115. [CrossRef]
90. Bunai, T.; Hirosawa, T.; Kikuchi, M.; Fukai, M.; Yokokura, M.; Ito, S.; Takata, Y.; Terada, T.; Ouchi, Y. tDCS-induced modulation of GABA concentration and dopamine release in the human brain: A combination study of magnetic resonance spectroscopy and positron emission tomography. *Brain Stimul.* **2021**, *14*, 154–160. [CrossRef]
91. Dunlop, B.W.; Nemeroff, C.B. The role of dopamine in the pathophysiology of depression. *Arch. Gen. Psychiatry* **2007**, *64*, 327–337. [CrossRef]
92. Belujon, P.; Grace, A.A. Dopamine System Dysregulation in Major Depressive Disorders. *Int. J. Neuropsychopharmacol.* **2017**, *20*, 1036–1046. [CrossRef] [PubMed]
93. Delva, N.C.; Stanwood, G.D. Dysregulation of brain dopamine systems in major depressive disorder. *Exp. Biol. Med.* **2021**, *246*, 1084–1093. [CrossRef]
94. Maslen, H.; Pugh, J.; Savulescu, J. The ethics of deep brain stimulation for the treatment of anorexia nervosa. *Neuroethics* **2015**, *8*, 215–230. [CrossRef] [PubMed]
95. Koivuniemi, A.; Otto, K. When "altering brain function" becomes "mind control". *Front. Syst. Neurosci.* **2014**, *8*, 202. [CrossRef] [PubMed]
96. Normann, C.; Schmitz, D.; Fürmaier, A.; Döing, C.; Bach, M. Long-term plasticity of visually evoked potentials in humans is altered in major depression. *Biol. Psychiatry* **2007**, *62*, 373–380. [CrossRef] [PubMed]
97. Nitsche, M.A.; Kuo, M.F.; Ralf Karrasch, R.; Wächter, B.; Liebetanz, D.; Paulus, W. Serotonin affects transcranial direct current-induced neuroplasticity in humans. *Biol. Psychiatry* **2009**, *66*, 503–508. [CrossRef]
98. Monte-Silva, K.; Kuo, M.F.; Thirugnanasambandam, N.; Liebetanz, D.; Paulus, W.; Nitsche, M.A. Dose-dependent inverted U-shaped effect of dopamine (D2-like) receptor activation on focal and nonfocal plasticity in humans. *J. Neurosci.* **2009**, *29*, 6124–6131. [CrossRef]
99. Tuplin, E.W.; Holahan, M.R. Aripiprazole, A Drug that Displays Partial Agonism and Functional Selectivity. *Curr. Neuropharmacol.* **2017**, *15*, 1192–1207. [CrossRef]
100. Hamamura, T.; Harada, T. Unique pharmacological profile of aripiprazole as the phasic component buster. *Psychopharmacology* **2007**, *191*, 741–743. [CrossRef]
101. Blanchet, C.; Guillaume, S.; Bat-Pitault, F.; Carles, M.E.; Clarke, J.; Dodin, V.; Duriez, P.; Gerardin, P.; Hanachi-Guidoum, M.; Iceta, S.; et al. Medication in AN: A Multidisciplinary Overview of Meta-Analyses and Systematic Reviews. *J. Clin. Med.* **2019**, *8*, 278. [CrossRef]
102. Burton, C.Z.; Garnett, E.O.; Capellari, E.; Chang, S.E.; Tso, I.F.; Hampstead, B.M.; Taylor, S.F. Combined Cognitive Training and Transcranial Direct Current Stimulation in Neuropsychiatric Disorders: A Systematic Review and Meta-analysis. *Biol. Psychiatry Cogn. Neurosci. Neuroimaging* **2023**, *8*, 151–161. [CrossRef] [PubMed]

nutrients

MDPI

Review

The Effectiveness of Transcranial Direct Current Stimulation (tDCS) in Binge Eating Disorder (BED)—Review and Insight into the Mechanisms of Action

James Chmiel [1,*], Donata Kurpas [2], Filip Rybakowski [3] and Jerzy Leszek [4]

1 Institute of Neurofeedback and tDCS Poland, 70-393 Szczecin, Poland
2 Department of Family and Pediatric Nursing, Faculty of Health Sciences, Wrocław Medical University, 51-618 Wrocław, Poland
3 Department and Clinic of Psychiatry, Poznan University of Medical Sciences, 61-701 Poznań, Poland
4 Department and Clinic of Psychiatry, Wrocław Medical University, 54-235 Wrocław, Poland
* Correspondence: chmielsoon@interia.eu

Abstract: Introduction: Binge eating disorder (BED) is the most common eating disorder among those contributing to the development of obesity, and thus acts as a significant burden on the lives and health of patients. It is characterized by complex neurobiology, which includes changes in brain activity and neurotransmitter secretion. Existing treatments are moderately effective, and so the search for new therapies that are effective and safe is ongoing. Aim and Methods: This review examines the use of transcranial direct current stimulation (tDCS) in the treatment of binge eating disorder. Searches were conducted on the PubMed/Medline, Research Gate, and Cochrane databases. Results: Six studies were found that matched the review topic. All of them used the anodal stimulation of the right dorsolateral prefrontal cortex (DLPFC) in BED patients. tDCS proved effective in reducing food cravings, the desire to binge eat, the number of binging episodes, and food intake. It also improved the outcomes of inhibitory control and the treatment of eating disorder psychopathology. The potential mechanisms of action of tDCS in BED are explained, limitations in current research are outlined, and recommendations for future research are provided. Conclusions: Preliminary evidence suggests that the anodal application of tDCS to the right DLPFC reduces the symptoms of BED. However, caution should be exercised in the broader use of tDCS in this context due to the small number of studies performed and the small number of patients included. Future studies should incorporate neuroimaging and neurophysiological measurements to elucidate the potential mechanisms of action of tDCS in BED.

Keywords: tDCS; transcranial direct current stimulation; binge eating disorder; non-invasive brain stimulation; neurostimulation; neuromodulation; eating disorder

Citation: Chmiel, J.; Kurpas, D.; Rybakowski, F.; Leszek, J. The Effectiveness of Transcranial Direct Current Stimulation (tDCS) in Binge Eating Disorder (BED)—Review and Insight into the Mechanisms of Action. *Nutrients* **2024**, *16*, 1521. https://doi.org/10.3390/nu16101521

Academic Editors: Roser Granero and Gemma Guillazo-Blanch

Received: 10 April 2024
Revised: 12 May 2024
Accepted: 16 May 2024
Published: 17 May 2024

1. Introduction

Binge eating disorder (BED) is the most common eating disorder (ED) and affects 3–5% of the US population [1]. It is included as a diagnostic entity in the Fifth Edition of the Diagnostic and Statistical Manual of Mental Disorders (DSM-5) [2,3]. It is characterized by recurrent ($\geq$1 per week for 3 months), short ($\leq$2 h) episodes of binge eating [4]. The affected person loses control and consumes a significant amount of food, eating far more than what he or she would eat under normal circumstances and times. During a binge eating episode, patients may eat large amounts of food. Even though they do not feel physically hungry or have metabolic needs [5], they eat faster than usual and until they feel the discomfort of over-satiation [6]. Binge eating episodes are associated with guilt and anxiety. Patients with BED often eat secretly, being ashamed of their behavior and lack of ability to control food intake [7].

A diagnosis of BED can be conducted when there are uncontrollable eating episodes lasting for 2 h, for at least 2 days a week for 6 months. At the same time, patients do not engage in compensatory behaviors typical of bulimia, such as inducing vomiting, using laxatives, and intense physical activity [8]. In the International Classification of Diseases and Related Health Problems, Tenth Edition (ICD-10), BED has been classified among Other Eating Disorders (F50.81) without any further diagnostic criteria [2]. New guidelines have been added in ICD-11 that allow binge eating and eating control to be assessed subjectively and objectively.

BED is the most common eating disorder, but its prevalence varies due to the different definitions of compulsive eating [8]. It is more common in women (3.5%) than in men (2%) [4,9]. The lifetime prevalence in young individuals is >1% [10]. A meta-analysis by Qian et al. [11] estimated the lifetime prevalence of BED at 2.22%. It is common in obese people (5% to 30%) [12,13], but a significant proportion of people with BED (17–30%) are of normal weight [14].

The coexistence of other psychiatric conditions often characterizes patients with BEDs. People with BED have a distorted image of their body and its weight [8] and worry more about their shape than people who do not have BED [15,16]. According to Grilo [17], 67% of patients with BED have at least one additional mental disorder during their lifetime. They are more likely to suffer from depression [8], anxiety [18], substance-use disorders [19], and other mental disorders [20]. A meta-analysis by Friborg et al. [21] of nine studies estimated the prevalence of personality disorders in people with BED to stand at 29%. The most common were avoidant personality disorder (12%) and obsessive–compulsive and borderline disorders (10%). People with BED are more likely to seek treatment for mood and anxiety disorders than for BED [22]. Undiagnosed BED means that the treatment of mental disorders may be suboptimal, as prescribed antidepressants often increase appetite, thus worsening inappropriate eating behavior [23]. People with BED have sleep disorders [24], heightened risk of metabolic syndrome [25] and fibromyalgia [20], an increased incidence of irritable bowel syndrome, earlier menarche, neck–shoulder pain, lower back pain, chronic muscular pain, impairment due to physical health [24], and attention deficit hyperactivity disorder (ADHD) [10]. Obesity is a common disease coexisting with BED and both diseases increase the risk of dyslipidemia, diabetes, and hypertension [25]. Further data suggest that the functioning of the reproductive and cardiovascular systems may also be impaired in people with BED [26]. In terms of risk factors, alcohol abuse, the worsening of depressive symptoms, taking medication for psychiatric reasons, and low self-esteem all increase the likelihood of developing BED [27].

The treatment of BED is aimed at reducing the frequency of binge eating and eating-related cognitive disorders, lowering BMI and improving metabolic health (in patients with obesity), and improving mental health (in patients with mental disorders) [4]. The methods used for this include cognitive behavioral therapy (CBT) [28], pharmacological therapy [29], or a combination of both methods [4]. The APA recommends a combined approach of CBT and treatment with selective serotonin reuptake inhibitors [4].

2. Neurobiology of BED

The neurobiology of BED is similar to that seen in substance abuse disorders [5]. Like drugs, food activates brain reward pathways [30,31]. Food cues induce the same neural plasticity and gene expression in the mesolimbic–cortical reward pathway and in the brain regions responsible for learning and memory [5,32]. Research on the neurotransmitters involved in BED has focused on neurotransmission in the endogenous opioid and dopaminergic systems because of their functions in motivation, cognitive control [33], and the rewarding of eating behavior [34]. Endogenous opioids in the nucleus accumbens have been linked to the hedonic properties of food and are dysregulated in individuals with BED [35]. Eating sweet foods increases opioid receptor binding in the reward system [5,36]. Opioid receptor binding in the insular cortex is reduced in people with BED [37]. In a rat study, the intake of sweet liquids was associated with increased mu-1 opioid receptor binding in the hippocampus, cingulate cortex, locus coeruleus, and accumbens shell [38].

Regarding dopamine, eating disorders have been linked to dopaminergic dysregulation in the central nervous system [39,40]. Eating tasty food activates dopaminergic neurons in the nucleus accumbens (NAc), ventral striatum, and other reward centers [32]. The development of BED has been linked to repeated stimulation of this system to alleviate the psychological effects of stress [41]. Further evidence of BED-induced changes in dopaminergic pathways supports the fact that binge eating is addictive. In a rat study, binge eating increased dopamine binding in the nucleus accumbens and striatum [42]. In another study, rats fed on palatable food showed decreased dopamine D2 binding in the striatum [39]. In the Colantuoni et al. [38] study, rats addicted to drinking sugary solutions showed increased dopamine D1 receptor binding in the NAc and decreased D2 receptor binding in the dorsal striatum. Overall, palatable food consumption likely increases reward sensitivity and obesity, and decreases dopamine release. However, the development of behaviors leading to food addiction may be mediated by an imbalance associated with reduced dopamine D2 receptor levels coupled with relatively higher levels of dopamine D1 receptor signaling in the dorsolateral striatum [34]. Detailed information on the neurobiology of BED is included in [5,6,34].

As shown above, BED is associated with many changes in the brain, which primarily affect the reward systems. Current treatments are moderately effective and interventions targeting the brain directly are needed. One of them may be transcranial direct current stimulation (tDCS), a non-invasive technique that has already been proven to work in terms of reducing food cravings and drug cravings.

3. Transcranial Direct Current Stimulation (tDCS)

tDCS involves the application of low-intensity electrical currents to the scalp in roder to modulate brain activity [43]. The technique has gained increasing attention in recent years due to its potential therapeutic applications in various neurological and psychiatric disorders and its potential to enhance cognitive function in healthy individuals. During tDCS, two or more electrodes are placed onto the scalp, and a low-intensity direct current is applied to modulate the activity of underlying neural circuits [44]. The anode is typically placed over the brain region intended for stimulation, while the cathode is placed onto a remote area. The current flow between the electrodes leads to changes in the membrane potential of neurons in the underlying brain tissue, which can modulate their firing rate and synaptic plasticity [45]. The effects of tDCS on brain activity are thought to be mediated by changes in the excitability of cortical neurons, synaptic plasticity, and neuroplasticity. The exact mechanisms of action are still the subject of ongoing research, but it is thought that tDCS may enhance or suppress the activity of specific neural networks depending on the location and polarity of the electrodes.

Several reviews have investigated the effectiveness of tDCS in EDs, including BED, with promising results [46–50]. However, these investigations have included all EDs, which may lead to misleading conclusions about the effectiveness of BED alone. In addition, there have recently been new clinical trials in BED that have not been included. Therefore, the purpose of this review is to analyze all studies investigating the effectiveness of tDCS in the treatment of BED, to examine the effects of stimulation on various aspects of BED and cognitive constructs, to try to elucidate potential mechanisms, to propose new therapy targets, and to investigate safety. Moreover, a review of research on the use of tDCS in BED may be useful because, as previously mentioned, the neurobiology of BED is similar to that of substance addiction. Several reviews have shown that tDCS is effective in treating nicotine [51] and alcohol use disorder [52]. It is therefore worth comparing the effectiveness of tDCS between substance addiction and BED.

4. Methods

4.1. Data Sources and Search Strategy

For this review, J. Ch., D. K., F. R., and J. L. performed an independent online search using predefined criteria. The following combined keywords were used: "transcranial direct current stimulation" OR "tDCS" AND "binge eating disorder" OR "BED". We considered publications in the PubMed/Medline, Research Gate, and Cochrane databases, with an access date of March 2024 and publication dates ranging from January 2000 to March 2024.

4.2. Study Selection Criteria

Eligibility criteria included clinical trials conducted in English that were published from 2008 to 2024. We considered studies investigating the effects of tDCS on binge eating disorder. The exclusion criteria encompassed articles that still needed to be published in English and reviews.

4.3. Screening Process

Multiple screening processes were implemented to guarantee the inclusion of pertinent research and the rejection of those that did not satisfy the predetermined criteria. Independent reviewers J. Ch., D. K., F. R., and J. L. thoroughly examined the titles and abstracts during the first screening process.

4.3.1. Title and Abstract Screening

To find studies that would fit the inclusion requirements, each reviewer evaluated the titles and abstracts of the records they could find independently. The relevance to transcranial direct current stimulation and its impact on binge eating disorder were the main screening criteria used during this phase.

4.3.2. Full-Text Assessment

After screening for titles and abstracts, the chosen papers were subjected to a thorough full-text evaluation. To ascertain if the full articles satisfied the comprehensive eligibility requirements, reviewers focused on adding clinical trials to the study that were carried out in English and released between January 2000 and March 2024.

5. Results

The screening process is illustrated in a flow chart (Figure 1). All told, 46 studies were found using the search techniques used in the databases. Based on the assessment of their titles and abstracts, 35 papers were eliminated. The reasons for this included the exclusion of study reviews (n = 14), the removal of duplicates (n = 8), and the lack of testing for tDCS in binge eating disorder (n = 13). A total of 11 papers were then found and subjected to a thorough full-text evaluation. Five of these studies were disqualified because the effect of tDCS on binge eating disorder was not measured. After thoroughly examining the texts, six articles were found to be suitable for inclusion.

The studies found were published between 2016 and 2023. A total of 165 patients were enrolled. Two studies were proofs of concept [53,54] and four studies were RCTs [55–58]. Random assignment occurred in five studies [54–58]. All studies used sham stimulation for the control group. In four studies [53,55–57], patients and experimenters were blinded; in the study by Burgess et al. [54], only patients were blinded. A current of 1 or 2 mA was used. As for the montage of the electrodes, a unipolar montage was the most common, in which one electrode was placed on the scalp and the other was placed extracranially on the left deltoid muscle [53,54,56–58]. In the one remaining study [55], both electrodes were placed over the brain and the same current was passed through the anode and cathode.

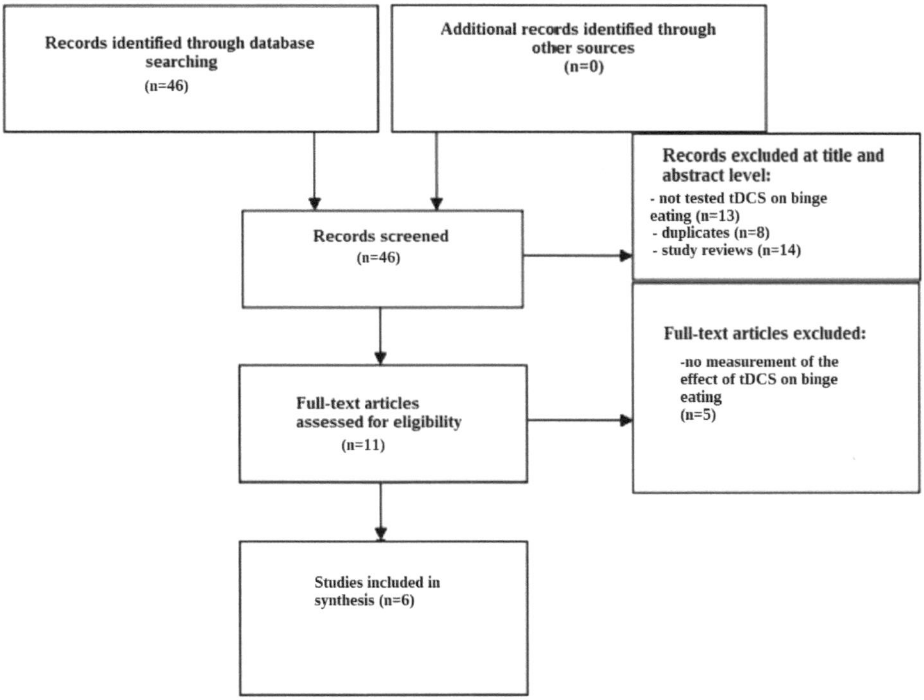

Figure 1. Flow chart depicting the different phases of the systematic review.

5.1. Summary of Included Studies

The studies included are summarized in Table 1. A crossover design, double-blind, randomized, and placebo-controlled proof-of-concept study by Max et al. [53] examined the impact of food-modified antisaccade tasks and the right dlPFC anodal tDCS on response inhibition in a BED-diagnosed sample. Participants diagnosed with BED included both normal-weight and obese adults. Sixteen subjects participated in the 1 mA condition, and 15 subjects participated in the 2 mA condition. Participants received either real tDCS or sham tDCS, which were given in a random order. tDCS was delivered for 20 min. Using the international 10–20 electrode placement system, the cathode was positioned in an extracephalic manner on the left deltoid muscle and the anode was positioned above F4 (right DLPFC). Response inhibition was measured by an antisaccade task, which required the suppression of dominant responses (i.e., saccade) towards a newly appearing picture in the visual field. The self-reported frequency of binge eating episodes was used to measure binge eating frequency.

In a proof-of-concept study by Burgess et al. [54], 30 adults with BED or subthreshold BED and obesity participated. Participants received one session of real or sham tDCS (20 min, 2 mA). The cathode was positioned over the left DLPFC (F3), and the anode was positioned over the right DLPFC (F4). The outcome measures used were Binge Eating Scale (BES), employed to measure binge eating frequency; the Dutch Eating Behavior Questionnaire-Restraint Subscale (DEBQ-R), used to measure food intake; and the Palatable Eating Motives Scale (PEMS), used to measure food craving and desire to binge eat.

Table 1. Summary of main findings from articles included in the review.

Author, Citation	Population	Used Test	Interventions	Stimulation Site	Current Intensity	Duration (min)	Main Findings in Treatment Group
Max et al. [53]	31 participants: 1 mA condition (n = 16), 2 mA condition (n = 15)	Self-reported frequency of binge eating episodes, antisaccades task	1 session of real or sham tDCS	Anode on right DLPFC (F4), cathode on the left deltoid muscle	1 mA or 2 mA	20	- A significant decrease in self-reported binge eating episodes over time was observed only in the group that had 2 mA stimulation, and there was no change in the group that had 1 mA stimulation. - All patients improved over the three measurement points concerning error rate and the latencies of correct antisaccades. The stimulation did not affect error rates, but the group that had 2 mA stimulation improved with faster latencies of correct antisaccades compared to sham stimulation, and the group that went through 1 mA stimulation showed slower latencies.

Table 1. *Cont.*

Author, Citation	Population	Used Test	Interventions	Stimulation Site	Current Intensity	Duration (min)	Main Findings in Treatment Group
Burgess et al. [54]	30 participants	Binge Eating Scale (BES), Dutch Eating Behavior Questionnaire-Restraint Subscale (DEBQ-R), Palatable Eating Motives Scale (PEMS)	1 session of real or sham tDCS	Anode on the right DLPFC (F4), cathode on the left DLPFC (F3)	2 mA	20 min	- There was no effect of tDCS on binge eating frequency. - tDCS significantly reduced food intake, as measured by DEBQ-R. Participants ate fewer total kcals in the lab after tDCS (614.50 ± 55.5) versus after sham (689.54 ± 60.8) treatment, with an 11% reduction. After tDCS treatment, participants ate 324.72 ± 30.5 kcals of the preferred food versus the 393.52 ± 36.3 kcals eaten after sham treatment, and there was a 17.5% reduction. - tDCS significantly reduced food craving, as measured by PEMS. The decreased intake of palatable food for Reward Enhancement motives accounted for 20% of the variance in terms of reducing food craving. Additionally, tDCS significantly reduced the desire to binge eat, which was also measured by PEMS. An r-ANOVA showed that tDCS reduced desire to binge eat on the day of the stimulation, roughly 5–6 h post-stimulation, in men only.

Table 1. *Cont.*

Author, Citation	Population	Used Test	Interventions	Stimulation Site	Current Intensity	Duration (min)	Main Findings in Treatment Group
Gordon et al. [55]	15 participants: real tDCS (n = 6), sham tDCS (n = 9)	Not reported, frequency of binge eating	6 sessions	Anode on the right DLPFC (F4), cathode on the left DLPFC (F3)	2 mA	Not reported	- A reduction in binge eating episodes was observed by six participants (ABM and real tDCS n = 2; ABM and sham tDCS n = 4), ranging from 'a little bit' to a 'huge difference'.
Giel et al. [56]	41 participants	Eating Disorder Examination (EDE), used to assess inhibitory control capacity, measured the course of the error rate (%) of the food-related eye-tracking task from the beginning of the training (T1) over each training session until immediately after the training (T7) compared to baseline (T0) values and the results of the Three-Factor Eating Questionnaire (TFEQ).	6 sessions	Anode on the right DLPFC (F4), no reference electrode data	2 mA	20 min	- In the real tDCS group, the BE frequency was reduced from 18.6 to 4.4 (T8) and to 3.8 (T9). - The results showed significant improvement in inhibitory control over the training period and showed a significant effect at T7 as compared to T0 in both study arms. - The results in TFEQ showed that this measure decreased from 10.6 (T0) to 9.3 (T7 and T8) after real tDCS.

Table 1. *Cont.*

Author, Citation	Population	Used Test	Interventions	Stimulation Site	Current Intensity	Duration (min)	Main Findings in Treatment Group
Beaumont et al. [57]	17 participants	Appetite visual analogue scale (VAS), the Food Craving Questionnaire-State (FCQ-S), the Leeds Food Preference Questionnaire (LFPQ), Control of Eating Questionnaire (CoEQ)	2 sessions, real or sham tDCS	Anode on the right DLPFC (F4), cathode on the occipital zero point (Oz)	2 mA	20 min	- VAS hunger levels following active tDCS treatment grew to meet those of post-sham stimulation, indicating a substantial change from pre- to post-tDCS (F(1, 15) = 6.796, p = 0.020, = 0.312, BF10 = 0.188). This effect was no longer significant (F(1, 30) = 0.610, p = 0.441, = 0.020, BF10 = 0.680) when baseline hunger was taken into account. - When comparing measures of fullness (F(1, 15) = 1.282, p = 0.275, = 0.079, BF10 = 0.040), prospective consumption (F(1, 15) = 2.606, p = 0.127, = 0.148, BF10 = 0.063), and desire to eat (F(1, 15) = 1.452, p = 0.247, = 0.088, BF10 = 0.054), there were no significant differences observed between the active and sham tDCS. Bayes factors suggested moderate-to-strong evidence in favor of the null hypothesis.

Table 1. *Cont.*

Author, Citation	Population	Used Test	Interventions	Stimulation Site	Current Intensity	Duration (min)	Main Findings in Treatment Group
Beaumont et al. [57]	17 participants	Appetite visual analogue scale (VAS), the Food Craving Questionnaire-State (FCQ-S), the Leeds Food Preference Questionnaire (LFPQ), Control of Eating Questionnaire (CoEQ)	2 sessions, real or sham tDCS	Anode on the right DLPFC (F4), cathode on the occipital zero point (Oz)	2 mA	20 min	- Regarding LFPQ, all assessments showed no significant impacts, with the exception of explicit desire and preference for HFSW foods. The preference for HFSW foods rose after active tDCS and fell after sham tDCS for both explicit like and desire. ANCOVA was used to assess if the difference in baseline hunger was the cause of these substantial effects; when hunger was taken into account, the difference between pre- and post-tDCS phases ceased to be significant. - Regarding FCQ-S, scores for food cravings after active versus sham procedures did not differ. In the CoEQ assessment, results for savory food cravings were close to significant (active 45.3 ± 17.9 mm, sham 49.4 ± 20.6 mm) (t(13) = 2.128, $p = 0.053$), indicating that savory food cravings decrease when active procedures are followed.
Max et al. [58]	31 participants: real tDCS (n = 15), sham tDCS (n = 16)	Food Craving Questionnaire-State (FCQ-S), Eating Disorder Examination (EDE)	6 sessions	Anode on the right DLPFC (F4), cathode was positioned extracephalic on the left deltoid muscle	2 mA	20	- The number of binge eating episodes decreased (from 17.35 to 6.26). - The total FCQ score improved (from 38.26 to 37.97). - The EDE score improved (from 2.61 to 2.04).

The aim of the randomized controlled trial of Gordon et al. [55] was to explore participants' experience of approach bias modification training (ABM) with tDCS for BED. ABM is a cognitive intervention method that aims to mitigate automatic cognitive bias towards substance use or unhealthy behaviors by retraining the brain's automatic response tendencies. Fifteen participants received six sessions of concurrent ABM training with either real (n = 6) or sham (n = 9) tDCS. The current intensity was 2 mA, the anode was applied to the right DLPFC (F4), and the cathode was applied to the left DLPFC (F3). The duration of the intervention was not reported, and the outcome measurements needed to be provided. The primary outcome was the frequency of binge eating.

The study of Giel et al. [56] sought to show the clinical use and viability of a tDCS-enhanced inhibitory control training program in efforts to lower BE episodes, performing a monocentric clinical phase II double-blind randomized trial with two parallel arms. Six sessions of food-related inhibitory control training were randomly paired with 2 mA real or sham tDCS of the right DLPFC for forty-one adult outpatients with full-syndrome BED. No reference electrode data were used. The tDCS session lasted for 20 min. The primary outcome was the difference in BE frequency between the baseline values and those from four weeks after treatment termination (T8; primary) and twelve weeks later (T9; secondary). The binge eating frequency was measured by the Eating Disorder Examination (EDE). To assess inhibitory control capacity, we measured the course of the error rate (%) of the food-related eye-tracking task from the beginning of the training (T1) over each training session until immediately after the training (T7) as compared to the baseline values (T0). Feelings of hunger were measured by the Three-Factor Eating Questionnaire (TFEQ).

In the study of Beaumont et al. [57], two sessions of double-blind, randomized, counterbalanced anodal, and sham tDCS were completed over the right dorsolateral prefrontal cortex at a frequency of 2 mA for 20 min by seventeen females with mild-to-moderate binge eating behavior. Prior to the study, the participants' weights were consistent for three months, with most of them (n = 9) being healthy weights; two were classed as obese, while six were overweight. The cathode was placed over the occipital zero point (Oz). Pre- and post-tDCS measures included the subjective appetite visual analogue scale (VAS), which measured hunger; the Food Craving Questionnaire-State (FCQ-S), measuring food craving; the Leeds Food Preference Questionnaire (LFPQ), measuring subjective desire or craving for foods; and Control of Eating Questionnaire (CoEQ), measuring craving.

A computer-based inhibitory control training program augmented by tDCS was examined in a randomized controlled experiment by Max et al. [58] at a 6-week follow-up. Patients were assessed in terms of eating behavior, general impulsivity, food cravings, and eating disorder psychopathology in both evaluations using an experimental virtual reality paradigm. Some 31 participants took part in the study (active tDCS n = 15, sham tDCS n = 16). The anode was placed on the right DLPFC (F4), and the cathode was positioned extracephalic on the left deltoid muscle. We carried out 6 sessions at an intensity of 2 mA. tDCS sessions lasted for 20 min. The Food Craving Questionnaire-State (FCQ-S) was used to measure craving. General eating disorder psychopathology and binge eating frequency were measured via Eating Disorder Examination (EDE).

5.2. Effects on Binge Eating Episodes and Frequency

In [53], a significant decrease in self-reported binge eating episodes over time was observed, but only in the group that had 2 mA stimulation, and there was no change in the group that had 1 mA stimulation.

In [54], a Wilcoxon signed-rank test indicated that there was no effect of tDCS on binge eating frequency, as measured by BES.

In [55], six participants observed a reduction in binge eating episodes (ABM and real tDCS n = 2; ABM and sham tDCS n = 4), ranging from 'a little bit' to a 'huge difference'.

In [56], BE frequency in the real tDCS group was reduced from 18.6 to 4.4 (T8) and to 3.8 (T9).

In [58], the number of binge eating episodes decreased (from 17.35 to 6.26).

5.3. Effects on Inhibitory Control (Response Inhibition)

In [53], all patients improved over the three measurement points concerning the error rate and latencies of correct antisaccades. The stimulation did not affect error rates, but the group that had 2 mA stimulation improved with faster latencies of correct antisaccades compared to sham stimulation, and the group that had 1 mA stimulation showed slower latencies.

In [56], the results showed a significant improvement over the training period and showed a significant effect at T7 as compared to T0 in both study arms.

5.4. Effects on Food Intake

In the study of Burgess et al. [54], tDCS significantly reduced food intake, as measured by DEBQ-R. Participants ate fewer total kcals in the lab after tDCS (614.50 $\pm$ 55.5) versus after sham (689.54 $\pm$ 60.8), with an 11% reduction. After tDCS, participants ate 324.72 $\pm$ 30.5 kcals of the preferred food versus 393.52 $\pm$ 36.3 kcals after sham, a 17.5% reduction.

5.5. Effects on Food Craving, Hunger and Desire to Binge Eat

In [53], tDCS significantly reduced food craving, as measured by PEMS. The decreased the intake of palatable food due to Reward Enhancement motives accounted for 20% of the variance in the reductions in food craving. Additionally, tDCS significantly reduced the desire to binge eat, which is also measured by PEMS. An r-ANOVA showed that tDCS reduced desire to binge eat on the day of the stimulation, roughly 5–6 h post-stimulation, in men only.

In [56], the results of the TFEQ showed that this measure decreased from 10.6 (T0) to 9.3 (T7 and T8) after real tDCS.

In [57], studying the appetite visual analogue scale (VAS), hunger levels following active tDCS treatment grew to meet those of post-sham stimulation, indicating a substantial change from pre-to post-tDCS (F(1, 15) = 6.796, p = 0.020, = 0.312, BF10 = 0.188). This effect was no longer significant (F(1, 30) = 0.610, p = 0.441, = 0.020, BF10 = 0.680) when baseline hunger was taken into account. When comparing measures of fullness (F(1, 15) = 1.282, p = 0.275, = 0.079, BF10 = 0.040), prospective consumption (F(1, 15) = 2.606, p = 0.127, = 0.148, BF10 = 0.063), and desire to eat (F(1, 15) = 1.452, p = 0.247, = 0.088, BF10 = 0.054), no significant differences were observed between the active and sham tDCS. Bayes factors suggested that there was moderate-to-strong evidence in favor of the null hypothesis. Regarding LFPQ, all the assessments showed no significant impacts, except for explicit desire and a preference for HFSW foods. The preference for HFSW foods rose after active tDCS and fell after sham tDCS for both explicit like and desire. ANCOVA was used to assess if the difference in baseline hunger was the cause of these substantial effects; when hunger was considered, the difference between pre- and post-tDCS ceased to be significant. Regarding FCQ-S, scores for food cravings after active versus sham procedures did not differ. In the CoEQ results, savory food cravings were close to significant (active 45.3 $\pm$ 17.9 mm, sham 49.4 $\pm$ 20.6 mm) (t(13) = 2.128, p = 0.053), indicating that savory food cravings decrease when active procedures are followed.

In [58], the total FCQ score improved (from 38.26 to 37.97).

5.6. Effects on Eating Disorder Psychopathology

The EDE score improved in [58] (from 2.61 to 2.04).

6. Discussion

This review includes a wide range of research that uses tDCS to examine how it affects food intake, food intake episodes, inhibitory control, and related psychopathological features in people with binge eating disorder. Despite having different methods, the trials provide important information about the potential of tDCS as an adjuvant therapy strategy for BED.

6.1. Impact of tDCS on Binge Eating Episodes and Frequency

The diverse outcomes observed across the studies underscore the nuanced impact of tDCS on binge eating episodes. While Burgess et al. [54] found no significant effect on binge eating frequency, Max et al. [53] reported a marked reduction in self-reported episodes, particularly in the group receiving 2 mA stimulation. Gordon et al. [55] noted fewer binge eating episodes in individuals undergoing approach bias modification training with real tDCS. Contrarily, real tDCS led to significant reductions in binge eating frequency in the studies by Giel et al. [56] and Max et al. [58]. The discrepancy in findings may be attributed to the inclusion of individuals with subthreshold BED in the study by Burgess et al. [54], possibly diluting the impact on binge eating episodes. Overall, stimulation of the right DLPFC at 2 mA appears to be effective in decreasing the frequency of BED episodes, suggesting the potential utility of adjunct interventions, such as approach bias modification training, to augment the effects of tDCS synergistically.

6.2. Impact of tDCS on Inhibitory Control (Response Inhibition)

Across studies, improvements in inhibitory control, particularly in response inhibition tasks, were consistently observed. Max et al. [53] reported faster latencies of accurate antisaccades with 2 mA stimulation, indicative of enhanced inhibitory control. Similarly, Giel et al. [56] noted a significant improvement in both study arms during the training phase. These findings suggest that the stimulation of the right DLPFC at 2 mA may enhance inhibitory control in individuals with BED, with discernible effects after a single session.

6.3. Impact of tDCS on Food Intake

tDCS demonstrated a significant impact on food intake, as evidenced by decreased consumption following stimulation. Burgess et al. [54] reported a substantial decrease in overall food intake and calories from preferred meals after treatment with active tDCS compared to sham, with effects evident after a single session. Song et al.'s [59] meta-analysis suggests that a greater number of tDCS sessions may further enhance the reduction in food intake, warranting exploration in future studies in order to optimize treatment efficacy.

6.4. Impact of tDCS on Food Craving, Hunger, and Desire to Binge Eat

The evidence suggests that there are varying outcomes regarding the effects of tDCS on hunger, food cravings, and binge eating tendencies. Burgess et al. [54] reported a notable decrease in food cravings and binge eating inclination following tDCS, contrasting with the findings Giel et al. [56] in terms of reduced TFEQ scores post-real tDCS. Notably, Beaumont et al. [57] highlighted the moderating role of baseline hunger levels on the effects of active tDCS, indicating potential variability in individual responses. Moreover, individuals with elevated BMI and BED tend to exhibit heightened food craving [60–62], underlining the necessity for future studies to stratify participants based on similar BMI values and confirmed clinical BED to account for potential differences in the effects of tDCS across different BED severity levels. Sex-specific differences were evident, with men showing greater susceptibility to tDCS-induced reductions in food cravings and binge eating desires compared to women, as observed by Ray et al. [63]. Additionally, Ray et al. [64] highlighted the influence of expectations on hunger reduction and eating behavior, indicating that individuals who believed they received active tDCS experienced more significant improvements in hunger and eating compared to those who believed they received sham tDCS, regardless of the actual stimulation received. It is worth emphasizing that persons with elevated BMI and BED display higher food craving [60–62]. Therefore, will be necessary in future studies to create groups with similar BMI values and with confirmed clinical BED, because the impact of tDCS on people with different degrees of BED (subBED or no BED) and on people with different BMI may be different. Men were more susceptible to the effects of tDCS on food cravings and the desire to binge eat than women, suggesting that the effect on craving reduction may be sex-specific. Ray et al. [63] also reported on the impacts of sex, showing that only women with low attentional impulsivity saw a decrease in food cravings. Expectations also influence the impact of tDCS on reducing hunger and eating. In the study of Ray et al. [64] into obese people, it was shown that people who claimed (regardless of the actual type of stimulation) that they had participated in active tDCS achieved better results in terms of reducing hunger and eating than people who claimed that they were in the sham tDCS group.

6.5. Impact of tDCS on Eating Disorder Psychopathology

tDCS exhibited promising effects on the psychopathology of eating disorders, as reflected by the improvements in Eating Disorder Examination scores post-stimulation noted by Max et al. [58]. This suggests the broader applicability of tDCS in terms of addressing various facets of BED beyond specific behaviors, highlighting its potential as a comprehensive treatment approach.

7. Mechanisms of Action of tDCS in Binge Eating Disorder

Defined, if somewhat overlapping, brain areas and neurocircuitry control food-related appetite, decision making, executive function, and impulsivity. For instance, the triggering of food hunger involves a vast brain network that includes the amygdala [65], lateral hypothalamus [66], ventral striatum (nucleus accumbens) [67], and ventral tegmental region [68]. On the other hand, goal-directed and habitual decision making is primarily coordinated by the dorsal striatum, which is further subdivided into the dorsomedial striatum (caudate) and the dorsolateral striatum (putamen) [69]. The primary neurological basis of executive function is the prefrontal cortex, particularly the lateral prefrontal cortex [70]. Although the precise anatomical correlates of impulsivity remain unknown, it is thought that several brain areas, including the striatum, temporal pole, insula, anterior cingulate cortex, prefrontal cortex, and hippocampus, are implicated [69]. Due to its widely distributed receptors in the brain regions and neurocircuitry, implicated in food craving [71], decision making [72], executive function [73], and impulsivity [74], as well as its functional associations with these risk factors, the neurotransmitter dopamine has garnered increasing attention in the field of binge eating.

Mesolimbic circuits are formed by dopamine neurons in the ventral tegmental area [75] sending projections to the ventral striatum [69], the primary brain region related to food cravings [69]. Motivation has long been linked to the mesolimbic dopaminergic system [76]. The commencement of food consumption is facilitated by the hyperactive mesolimbic dopaminergic system, which in the context of eating habits increases incentive salience or cravings for food-related rewards [77,78].

The evidence from most studies indicates that people with BED have reduced dopamine levels and reduced dopamine activity [69]. The concept that a hypodopaminergic condition causes binge eating is in line with reward-related models or theories that address drug addiction (dopamine desensitization theory) [79], obesity (dynamic vulnerability model) [80], and alcohol-use disorder (three-stage model) [81]. The reward surfeit and reward deficit hypotheses are two competing dopamine-related ideas that are discussed in the literature on obesity [69]. The former suggests that eating high-energy foods enhances reward responsiveness, or dopamine signaling, which in turn raises the risk of obesity; the latter suggests that the opposite occurs [69].

It has been shown that applying tDCS to the frontal areas causes the release of dopamine into the striatum [82,83]. This proves the effects of tDCS on the dopaminergic system and the reward system. Since BED is highly correlated with substance-use disorder [84], and because both conditions share common neurobiological underpinnings related to interruptions in the dopaminergic pathways, tDCS may offer a potential avenue for intervention. Considering the dopamine desensitization theory of drug addiction [79], tDCS could be explored as a tool to modulate dopamine release during different stages of BED. By targeting the striatum, which is associated with reward processing, tDCS may influence dopamine release and help to regulate the reward-related mechanisms implicated in both binge eating and substance use and may potentially counteract the decreased dopamine release and downregulated responses associated with chronic binge eating. Similarly, in alignment with the three-stage model of alcohol dependence, tDCS might be applied to target the ventral striatum during the binge/intoxication stage. This could potentially mitigate the positive reinforcement processes that contribute to the initial transition into addiction. Additionally, tDCS might be explored in addressing compromised dopamine functions during the withdrawal/negative affect stage, potentially reducing sensitivity to rewards and tolerance.

The prefrontal cortex is the primary regulator of inhibitory control over behavior [85]. Dysregulations and lower baseline activity in PFC areas have been identified in persons with BED [86]. In addition, there are deficiencies in inhibitory control [87], especially in the medial prefrontal cortex (mPFC) [87], and we see increased activation in response to food signals [88]. Two competing systems are conceptualized: a "STOP" system that is damaged in compulsive eating and a "GO" system that is sensitized in obsessive eating [89]. The "GO" system's brain activity may have been modulated by tDCS when applied to the right DLPFC. Through focusing on the hyper-responsive regions linked to food cues, tDCS may have regulated or diminished the heightened reactivity to stimuli that cause cravings in people with BED. In the case of compulsive eating, this modulation may have improved inhibitory control and decreased impulsivity by creating a better balance between the "GO" and "STOP" systems.

8. Limitations and Prospects for Further Research

Although the results from the studies included in this review are promising, there are several factors that should be considered in the design of future studies of tDCS in BED.

8.1. Heterogeneity in Methodologies

There is significant methodological variation across the included research, which makes it difficult to combine data and reach firm conclusions. Methodological diversity is influenced, for example, by variations in the tDCS application with respect to reference electrode montage. Furthermore, the lack of a consistent framework for outcome measurements contributes to methodological variability, with some studies emphasizing psychopathological aspects or inhibitory control while focusing mostly on self-reported bouts of binge eating.

8.2. Lack of Consistency in Outcome Measures

The studies included in this review demonstrate significant inconsistency in the choice of outcome measures, making it more difficult to develop a coherent picture of how tDCS affects BED. The lack of consistent evaluations amongst studies makes it more difficult to synthesize the data and restricts how broadly the conclusions can be applied. While some studies use measures of inhibitory control or psychopathological characteristics linked to BED, others concentrate mostly on self-reported BED episodes. For example, heterogeneity is introduced into the assessment of the frequency, food intake, food cravings, and desire to binge eat when a variety of tools are used, such as the Binge Eating Scale (BES), Eating Disorder Examination (EDE), Dutch Eating Behavior Questionnaire-Restraint Subscale (DEBQ-R), and Palatable Eating Motives Scale (PEMS). Future studies should place a high priority on adopting standardized outcome measures in order to resolve this discrepancy and guarantee a thorough and coherent assessment of the effects of tDCS on BED. The development of a consensus regarding the essential evaluation instruments associated with binge eating behavior, inhibitory control, and psychopathological characteristics would improve the validity and applicability of results. Furthermore, establishing a common set of outcome measures for tDCS trials in BED will help with meta-analyses and lead to a more sophisticated comprehension of the intervention's effects.

8.3. Limited Sample Sizes and Diversity

The inclusion of very small sample sizes, which may jeopardize the findings' robustness and generalizability, as a common issue seen in the examined studies. Some studies had small sample sizes, casting doubt on their statistical power and capacity to identify meaningful effects. The results' external validity was further limited by the variation in participant characteristics, such as age, gender, and body mass index (BMI). Several studies were primarily focused on demographic groups, such as samples that were primarily female or those within a particular BMI range. This limited the applicability of the findings to a larger community of people with BED. The lack of varied participant profiles restricted our ability to comprehend the potential effects of tDCS on various BED population subgroups. Future studies should put an emphasis on using larger and more varied sample sizes to solve these constraints. Using more participants with a greater range of ages, different gender identities, and varied BMI categories will improve the study's external validity and enable a more thorough investigation of the effects of tDCS on various subpopulations. A more nuanced assessment of the intervention's effectiveness and its potential relevance to a variety of demographic groups impacted by BED will be made possible by using robust and inclusive sampling methodologies.

8.4. Lack of Long-Term Follow-Up

The majority of the examined studies' have the conspicuous disadvantage of reliance on comparatively brief follow-up evaluations, which raises questions regarding the long-term sustainability and durability of the benefits of tDCS on BED. Numerous studies that were part of this evaluation evaluated results from just after the intervention, providing little information about how long-lasting the apparent gains will be. Our comprehension of the long-term effects of tDCS on binge eating behavior, inhibitory control, and psychopathological traits linked to BED is hampered by the lack of strong long-term follow-up data. Since BED is frequently accompanied by chronicity, assessing tDCS's potential as a long-term therapeutic intervention requires an understanding of its long-term impacts. Future studies should include thorough long-term follow-up evaluations to track the trajectory of the effects of tDCS over a prolonged period in order to address this shortcoming. This will offer insightful information about sustaining treatment benefits, preventing relapses, and maintaining the general stability of the noted improvements. Including extensive follow-up periods in longitudinal studies will enhance our comprehension of the temporal dynamics of the effects of tDCS in BED patients.

8.5. Potential Sex-Specific Effects

tDCS may have sex-specific impacts on the outcomes of BED according to a significant finding from the evaluated research. While most studies offer insightful information on the general effectiveness of tDCS, there is growing evidence that suggests gender may have a role in how tDCS affects food cravings and the urge to binge eat. Research by Burgess et al. [54] and Ray et al. [63] demonstrates that men and women respond differently to tDCS, with men exhibiting a more marked decrease in food cravings and the urge to binge eat. This suggests that the effects of tDCS may be modulated differently depending on a person's sex, highlighting the need for more research and greater comprehension of gender-related variations in treatment outcomes. Future studies should use gender-specific stratified analyses to address this possible sex specificity and separate the complex effects of tDCS in BED patients who are male and female. Investigations should also look into any underlying causes of these sex-specific variances, such as hormone changes or psychological issues. The refinement of treatment techniques and customization of therapies based on individual characteristics will come from a more thorough study of the interaction between tDCS, sex, and BED outcomes.

8.6. Influence of Expectations

The impact of participant expectations on the results of tDCS in BED is another feature highlighted by the evaluated studies. Several studies, such as the work of Ray et al. [64], indicate that participant expectations may have a major influence on how well tDCS reduces appetite and eating habits. Regardless of the actual type of stimulation, Ray et al. [64] showed that people who thought they were receiving active tDCS performed better in terms of lowering appetite and eating than people who thought they were in the sham tDCS group. This emphasizes how crucial it is to take psychological aspects like participant expectations into account when analyzing the results of tDCS. Future studies should include techniques to rigorously regulate and evaluate participant expectations to address the impact of expectations. This could entail applying placebo-controlled designs, evaluating participant perceptions of the kind of stimulation they received, and investigating the relationship between expectations and tDCS results. Comprehending the influence of expectations on results will lead to a more sophisticated analysis of tDCS effectiveness in BED and help design individualized treatment plans that consider psychological aspects.

8.7. Influence of Genetics

The effect of tDCS on appetite may depend on genetics, as shown by a study by Fassini et al. [90]. In this study, DLPFC stimulation was performed in 38 obese women. participants were categorized based on the existence or lack of a Met allele (associated with decreased COMT enzyme activity). The findings demonstrated that whereas the acitivity of Met carriers tDCS saw the greatest drop in appetite over time, non-Met carriers receiving active tDCS maintained high levels of apetite. Therefore, future studies should perform genetic testing for the presence of the Met allele to check whether the reduction in appetite in BED patients depends on the participants' genetic variant. When selecting appropriate genetic polymorphisms associated with BED, we recommend using the review by Manfredi et al. [91].

8.8. Considering Comorbidities as Confounding Factors

As stated in the introduction, BED is often accompanied by comorbidities that may complicate treatment outcomes. Future studies on tDCS in BED should use detailed psychiatric diagnostics of patients to determine their psychiatric condition and include or exclude patients with a given disease to control for its impact on treatment outcomes.

8.9. Incorporation of Neurophysiological and Neuroimaging Measurements

Little is known about the mechanisms of action of tDCS in BED. In addition to the behavioral measurements used so far, future studies need to use new measurement methods, such as electroencephalography (EEG), functional magnetic resonance imaging (fMRI), and positron emission tomography (PET).

8.10. Methodological Limitations of This Review

In the methods section, we utilized approaches that are typically associated with systematic reviews to enhance the rigor and quality of our study. However, it is important to note that our review does not strictly adhere to the criteria outlined by the PRISMA guidelines for systematic reviews and meta-analyses. While our methodology draws on elements commonly found in systematic reviews, our study is distinct in its scope and methodology.

9. Conclusions

There is growing interest in the use of tDCS in eating disorders, including binge eating disorder. The evidence to date supports the effectiveness of stimulation in improving symptoms of BED, such as food craving, food intake, number of binge eating episodes, and inhibitory control. However, conclusions should be treated with caution. There is little research on tDCS in BED, and the total sample of patients is also small. Further RCTs are needed, with sufficiently large and homogeneous patient samples, to establish the use of this treatment.

Author Contributions: Conceptualization, J.C. and J.L.; methodology, J.C. and J.L.; writing—original draft preparation, J.C. writing—review and editing, J.C. and F.R.; supervision, J.L.; English corrections: D.K. All authors have read and agreed to the published version of the manuscript.

Funding: This research received no external funding.

Conflicts of Interest: The authors declare no conflict of interest.

References

1. Nagata, J.M.; Smith-Russack, Z.; Paul, A.; Saldana, G.A.; Shao, I.Y.; Al-Shoaibi, A.A.A.; Chaphekar, A.V.; Downey, A.E.; He, J.; Murray, S.B.; et al. The social epidemiology of binge-eating disorder and behaviors in early adolescents. *J. Eat. Disord.* **2023**, *11*, 182. [CrossRef]
2. Hilbert, A. Binge-Eating Disorder. *Psychiatr. Clin. N. Am.* **2019**, *42*, 33–43. [CrossRef] [PubMed]
3. American Psychiatric Association. *Diagnostic and Statistical Manual of Mental Disorders (DSM-5)*, 5th ed.; American Psychiatric Association: Washington, DC, USA, 2013.
4. Brownley, K.A.; Berkman, N.D.; Peat, C.M.; Lohr, K.N.; Cullen, K.E.; Bann, C.M.; Bulik, C.M. Binge-Eating Disorder in Adults: A Systematic Review and Meta-analysis. *Ann. Intern. Med.* **2016**, *165*, 409–420. [CrossRef]
5. Mathes, W.F.; Brownley, K.A.; Mo, X.; Bulik, C.M. The biology of binge eating. *Appetite* **2009**, *52*, 545–553. [CrossRef] [PubMed]
6. Guerdjikova, A.I.; Mori, N.; Casuto, L.S.; McElroy, S.L. Update on Binge Eating Disorder. *Med. Clin. N. Am.* **2019**, *103*, 669–680. [CrossRef]
7. Marzilli, E.; Cerniglia, L.; Cimino, S. A narrative review of binge eating disorder in adolescence: Prevalence, impact, and psychological treatment strategies. *Adolesc. Health Med. Ther.* **2018**, *9*, 17–30. [CrossRef]
8. Araujo, D.M.; Santos, G.F.; Nardi, A.E. Binge eating disorder and depression: A systematic review. *World J. Biol. Psychiatry* **2010**, *11 Pt 2*, 199–207. [CrossRef]
9. Hay, P.; Girosi, F.; Mond, J. Prevalence and sociodemographic correlates of DSM-5 eating disorders in the Australian population. *J. Eat. Disord.* **2015**, *3*, 19. [CrossRef] [PubMed]
10. Cossrow, N.; Pawaskar, M.; Witt, E.A.; Ming, E.E.; Victor, T.W.; Herman, B.K.; Wadden, T.A.; Erder, M.H. Estimating the prevalence of binge eating disorder in a community sample from the United States: Comparing DSM-IV-TR and DSM-5 criteria. *J. Clin. Psychiatry* **2016**, *77*, e968–e974. [CrossRef]
11. Qian, J.; Hu, Q.; Wan, Y.; Li, T.; Wu, M.; Ren, Z.; Yu, D. Prevalence of eating disorders in the general population: A systematic review. *Shanghai Arch. Psychiatry* **2013**, *25*, 212–223.
12. Spitzer, R.L.; Yanovski, S.; Wadden, T.; Wing, R.; Marcus, M.D.; Stunkard, A.; Devlin, M.; Mitchell, J.; Hasin, D.; Horne, R.L. Binge eating disorder: Its further validation in a multisite study. *Int. J. Eat. Disord.* **1993**, *13*, 137–153. [CrossRef] [PubMed]
13. Fairburn, C.G.; Cooper, Z.; Doll, H.A.; Norman, P.; O'Connor, M. The natural course of bulimia nervosa and binge eating disorder in young women. *Arch. Gen. Psychiatry* **2000**, *57*, 659–665. [CrossRef] [PubMed]
14. Goldschmidt, A.B.; Le Grange, D.; Powers, P.; Crow, S.J.; Hill, L.L.; Peterson, C.B.; Crosby, R.D.; Mitchell, J.E. Eating disorder symptomatology in normal-weight vs. obese individuals with binge eating disorder. *Obesity* **2011**, *19*, 1515–1518. [CrossRef] [PubMed]
15. Didie, E.R.; Fitzgibbon, M. Binge eating and psychological distress: Is the degree of obesity a factor? *Eat. Behav.* **2005**, *6*, 35–41. [CrossRef] [PubMed]
16. Lynch, W.C.; Heil, D.P.; Wagner, E.; Havens, M.D. Body dissatisfaction mediates the association between body mass index and risky weight control behaviors among White and Native American adolescent girls. *Appetite* **2008**, *51*, 210–213. [CrossRef]
17. Grilo, C.M. Why no cognitive body image feature such as overvaluation of shape/weight in the binge eating disorder diagnosis? *Int. J. Eat. Disord.* **2013**, *46*, 208–211. [CrossRef]
18. Rosenbaum, D.L.; White, K.S. The Role of Anxiety in Binge Eating Behavior: A Critical Examination of Theory and Empirical Literature. *Health Psychol. Res.* **2013**, *1*, e19. [CrossRef]
19. Blanco-Gandia, M.C.; Montagud-Romero, S.; Rodríguez-Arias, M. Binge eating and psychostimulant addiction. *World J. Psychiatry* **2021**, *11*, 517–529. [CrossRef]
20. Javaras, K.N.; Pope, H.G.; Lalonde, J.K.; Roberts, J.L.; Nillni, Y.I.; Laird, N.M.; Bulik, C.M.; Crow, S.J.; McElroy, S.L.; Walsh, B.T.; et al. Co-occurrence of binge eating disorder with psychiatric and medical disorders. *J. Clin. Psychiatry* **2008**, *69*, 266–273. [CrossRef]
21. Friborg, O.; Martinussen, M.; Kaiser, S.; Øvergård, K.T.; Martinsen, E.W.; Schmierer, P.; Rosenvinge, J.H. Personality disorders in eating disorder not otherwise specified and binge eating disorder: A meta-analysis of comorbidity studies. *J. Nerv. Ment. Dis.* **2014**, *202*, 119–125. [CrossRef]
22. Kessler, R.C.; Berglund, P.A.; Chiu, W.T.; Deitz, A.C.; Hudson, J.I.; Shahly, V.; Aguilar-Gaxiola, S.; Alonso, J.; Angermeyer, M.C.; Benjet, C.; et al. The prevalence and correlates of binge eating disorder in the World Health Organization World Mental Health Surveys. *Biol. Psychiatry* **2013**, *73*, 904–914. [CrossRef] [PubMed]

23. Citrome, L. Binge-Eating Disorder and Comorbid Conditions: Differential Diagnosis and Implications for Treatment. *J. Clin. Psychiatry* **2017**, *78* (Suppl. S1), 9–13. [CrossRef] [PubMed]
24. Bulik, C.M.; Reichborn-Kjennerud, T. Medical morbidity in binge eating disorder. *Int. J. Eat. Disord.* **2003**, *34* (Suppl. S1), S39–S46. [CrossRef]
25. Hudson, J.I.; Lalonde, J.K.; Coit, C.E.; Tsuang, M.T.; McElroy, S.L.; Crow, S.J.; Bulik, C.M.; Hudson, M.S.; Yanovski, J.A.; Rosenthal, N.R.; et al. Longitudinal study of the diagnosis of components of the metabolic syndrome in individuals with binge-eating disorder. *Am. J. Clin. Nutr.* **2010**, *91*, 1568–1573. [CrossRef] [PubMed]
26. Mitchell, J.E. Medical comorbidity and medical complications associated with binge-eating disorder. *Int. J. Eat. Disord.* **2016**, *49*, 319–323. [CrossRef] [PubMed]
27. Mitchell, J.E.; King, W.C.; Courcoulas, A.; Dakin, G.; Elder, K.; Engel, S.; Flum, D.; Kalarchian, M.; Khandelwal, S.; Pender, J.; et al. Eating behavior and eating disorders in adults before bariatric surgery. *Int. J. Eat. Disord.* **2015**, *48*, 215–222. [CrossRef] [PubMed]
28. Vocks, S.; Tuschen-Caffier, B.; Pietrowsky, R.; Rustenbach, S.J.; Kersting, A.; Herpertz, S. Meta-analysis of the effectiveness of psychological and pharmacological treatments for binge eating disorder. *Int. J. Eat. Disord.* **2010**, *43*, 205–217. [CrossRef] [PubMed]
29. Reas, D.L.; Grilo, C.M. Review and meta-analysis of pharmacotherapy for binge-eating disorder. *Obesity* **2008**, *16*, 2024–2038. [CrossRef]
30. Adam, T.C.; Epel, E.S. Stress, eating and the reward system. *Physiol. Behav.* **2007**, *91*, 449–458. [CrossRef]
31. Johnson, R.D. Opioid involvement in feeding behaviour and the pathogenesis of certain eating disorders. *Med. Hypotheses* **1995**, *45*, 491–497. [CrossRef]
32. Kelley, A.E.; Schiltz, C.A.; Landry, C.F. Neural systems recruited by drug- and food-related cues: Studies of gene activation in corticolimbic regions. *Physiol. Behav.* **2005**, *86*, 11–14. [CrossRef] [PubMed]
33. Heal, D.J.; Smith, S.L. Prospects for new drugs to treat binge-eating disorder: Insights from psychopathology and neuropharmacology. *J. Psychopharmacol.* **2022**, *36*, 680–703. [CrossRef]
34. Kessler, R.M.; Hutson, P.H.; Herman, B.K.; Potenza, M.N. The neurobiological basis of binge-eating disorder. *Neurosci. Biobehav. Rev.* **2016**, *63*, 223–238. [CrossRef] [PubMed]
35. Davis, C.A.; Levitan, R.D.; Reid, C.; Carter, J.C.; Kaplan, A.S.; Patte, K.A.; King, N.; Curtis, C.; Kennedy, J.L. Dopamine for "wanting" and opioids for "liking": A comparison of obese adults with and without binge eating. *Obesity* **2009**, *17*, 1220–1225. [CrossRef] [PubMed]
36. Kelley, A.E.; Bakshi, V.P.; Haber, S.N.; Steininger, T.L.; Will, M.J.; Zhang, M. Opioid modulation of taste hedonics within the ventral striatum. *Physiol. Behav.* **2002**, *76*, 365–377. [CrossRef] [PubMed]
37. Bencherif, B.; Guarda, A.S.; Colantuoni, C.; Ravert, H.T.; Dannals, R.F.; Frost, J.J. Regional mu-opioid receptor binding in insular cortex is decreased in bulimia nervosa and correlates inversely with fasting behavior. *J. Nucl. Med.* **2005**, *46*, 1349–1351. [PubMed]
38. Colantuoni, C.; Schwenker, J.; McCarthy, J.; Rada, P.; Ladenheim, B.; Cadet, J.L.; Schwartz, G.J.; Moran, T.H.; Hoebel, B.G. Excessive sugar intake alters binding to dopamine and mu- opioid receptors in the brain. *Neuroreport* **2001**, *12*, 3549–3552. [CrossRef] [PubMed]
39. Johnson, P.M.; Kenny, P.J. Dopamine D2 receptors in addiction- like reward dysfunction and compulsive eating in obese rats. *Nat. Neurosci.* **2010**, *13*, 635–641. [CrossRef] [PubMed]
40. Pothos, E.N.; Creese, I.; Hoebel, B.G. Restricted eating with weight loss selectively decreases extracellular dopamine in the nucleus accumbens and alters dopamine response to amphetamine, morphine, and food intake. *J. Neurosci.* **1995**, *15*, 6640–6650. [CrossRef]
41. Koob, G.F.; Le Moal, M. Addiction and the brain antireward system. *Annu. Rev. Psychol.* **2008**, *59*, 29–53. [CrossRef]
42. Avena, N.M.; Rada, P.; Hoebel, B.G. Evidence for sugar addiction: Behavioral and neurochemical effects of intermittent, excessive sugar intake. *Neurosci. Biobehav. Rev.* **2008**, *32*, 20–39. [CrossRef] [PubMed]
43. Nitsche, M.A.; Cohen, L.G.; Wassermann, E.M.; Priori, A.; Lang, N.; Antal, A.; Paulus, W.; Hummel, F.; Boggio, P.S.; Fregni, F.; et al. Transcranial direct current stimulation: State of the art 2008. *Brain Stimul.* **2008**, *1*, 206–223. [CrossRef] [PubMed]
44. Brunoni, A.R.; Nitsche, M.A.; Bolognini, N.; Bikson, M.; Wagner, T.; Merabet, L.; Edwards, D.J.; Valero-Cabre, A.; Rotenberg, A.; Pascual-Leone, A.; et al. Clinical research with transcranial direct current stimulation (tDCS): Challenges and future directions. *Brain Stimul.* **2012**, *5*, 175–195. [CrossRef] [PubMed]
45. Priori, A. Brain polarization in humans: A reappraisal of an old tool for prolonged non-invasive modulation of brain excitability. *Clin. Neurophysiol.* **2003**, *114*, 589–595. [CrossRef] [PubMed]
46. Duriez, P.; Bou Khalil, R.; Chamoun, Y.; Maatoug, R.; Strumila, R.; Seneque, M.; Gorwood, P.; Courtet, P.; Guillaume, S. Brain Stimulation in Eating Disorders: State of the Art and Future Perspectives. *J. Clin. Med.* **2020**, *9*, 2358. [CrossRef]
47. Beaumont, J.D.; Smith, N.C.; Starr, D.; Davis, D.; Dalton, M.; Nowicky, A.; Russell, M.; Barwood, M.J. Modulating eating behavior with transcranial direct current stimulation (tDCS): A systematic literature review on the impact of eating behavior traits. *Obes. Rev.* **2022**, *23*, e13364. [CrossRef]
48. Gallop, L.; Flynn, M.; Campbell, I.C.; Schmidt, U. Neuromodulation and Eating Disorders. *Curr. Psychiatry Rep.* **2022**, *24*, 61–69. [CrossRef] [PubMed]
49. Dalton, B.; Bartholdy, S.; Campbell, I.C.; Schmidt, U. Neurostimulation in Clinical and Sub-clinical Eating Disorders: A Systematic Update of the Literature. *Curr. Neuropharmacol.* **2018**, *16*, 1174–1192. [CrossRef]

50. Hall, P.A.; Vincent, C.M.; Burhan, A.M. Non-invasive brain stimulation for food cravings, consumption, and disorders of eating: A review of methods, findings and controversies. *Appetite* **2018**, *124*, 78–88. [CrossRef]
51. Kang, N.; Kim, R.K.; Kim, H.J. Effects of transcranial direct current stimulation on symptoms of nicotine dependence: A systematic review and meta-analysis. *Addict. Behav.* **2019**, *96*, 133–139. [CrossRef]
52. Kim, H.J.; Kang, N. Bilateral transcranial direct current stimulation attenuated symptoms of alcohol use disorder: A systematic review and meta-analysis. *Prog. Neuropsychopharmacol. Biol. Psychiatry* **2021**, *108*, 110160. [CrossRef] [PubMed]
53. Max, S.M.; Plewnia, C.; Zipfel, S.; Giel, K.E.; Schag, K. Combined antisaccade task and transcranial direct current stimulation to increase response inhibition in binge eating disorder. *Eur. Arch. Psychiatry Clin. Neurosci.* **2021**, *271*, 17–28. [CrossRef]
54. Burgess, E.E.; Sylvester, M.D.; Morse, K.E.; Amthor, F.R.; Mrug, S.; Lokken, K.L.; Osborn, M.K.; Soleymani, T.; Boggiano, M.M. Effects of transcranial direct current stimulation (tDCS) on binge eating disorder. *Int. J. Eat. Disord.* **2016**, *49*, 930–936. [CrossRef]
55. Gordon, G.; Williamson, G.; Gkofa, V.; Schmidt, U.; Brockmeyer, T.; Campbell, I. Participants' experience of approach bias modification training with transcranial Direct Current Stimulation as a combination treatment for binge eating disorder. *Eur. Eat. Disord. Rev.* **2021**, *29*, 969–984. [CrossRef]
56. Giel, K.E.; Schag, K.; Max, S.M.; Martus, P.; Zipfel, S.; Fallgatter, A.J.; Plewnia, C. Inhibitory Control Training Enhanced by Transcranial Direct Current Stimulation to Reduce Binge Eating Episodes: Findings from the Randomized Phase II ACCElect Trial. *Psychother. Psychosom.* **2023**, *92*, 101–112. [CrossRef]
57. Beaumont, J.D.; Dalton, M.; Davis, D.; Finlayson, G.; Nowicky, A.; Russell, M.; Barwood, M.J. No effect of prefrontal transcranial direct current stimulation (tDCS) on food craving, food reward and subjective appetite in females displaying mild-to-moderate binge-type behaviour. *Appetite* **2023**, *189*, 106997. [CrossRef] [PubMed]
58. Max, S.M.; Schag, K.; Giel, K.E.; Plewnia, C. Behavioural biases in the interaction with food objects in virtual reality and its clinical implication for binge eating disorder. *Eat. Weight. Disord.* **2023**, *28*, 46. [CrossRef]
59. Song, S.; Zilverstand, A.; Gui, W.; Li, H.J.; Zhou, X. Effects of single-session versus multi-session non-invasive brain stimulation on craving and consumption in individuals with drug addiction, eating disorders or obesity: A meta-analysis. *Brain Stimul.* **2019**, *12*, 606–618. [CrossRef] [PubMed]
60. Greeno, C.G.; Wing, R.R.; Shiffman, S. Binge antecedents in obese women with and without binge eating disorder. *J. Consult. Clin. Psychol.* **2000**, *68*, 95–102. [CrossRef]
61. Waters, A.; Hill, A.; Waller, G. Bulimics' responses to food cravings: Is binge-eating a product of hunger or emotional state? *Behav. Res. Ther.* **2001**, *39*, 877–886. [CrossRef]
62. White, M.A.; Grilo, C.M. Psychometric properties of the Food Craving Inventory among obese patients with binge eating disorder. *Eat. Behav.* **2005**, *6*, 239–245. [CrossRef] [PubMed]
63. Ray, M.K.; Sylvester, M.D.; Osborn, L.; Helms, J.; Turan, B.; Burgess, E.E.; Boggiano, M.M. The critical role of cognitive-based trait differences in transcranial direct current stimulation (tDCS) suppression of food craving and eating in frank obesity. *Appetite* **2017**, *116*, 568–574. [CrossRef] [PubMed]
64. Ray, M.K.; Sylvester, M.D.; Helton, A.; Pittman, B.R.; Wagstaff, L.E.; McRae, T.R.; Turan, B.; Fontaine, K.R.; Amthor, F.R.; Boggiano, M.M. The effect of expectation on transcranial direct current stimulation (tDCS) to suppress food craving and eating in individuals with overweight and obesity. *Appetite* **2019**, *136*, 1–7. [CrossRef]
65. Blechert, J.; Klackl, J.; Miedl, S.F.; Wilhelm, F.H. To eat or not to eat: Effects of food availability on reward system activity during food picture viewing. *Appetite* **2016**, *99*, 254–261. [CrossRef] [PubMed]
66. Talakoub, O.; Paiva, R.R.; Milosevic, M.; Hoexter, M.Q.; Franco, R.; Alho, E.; Navarro, J.; Pereira, J.F., Jr.; Popovic, M.R.; Savage, C.; et al. Lateral hypothalamic activity indicates hunger and satiety states in humans. *Ann. Clin. Transl. Neurol.* **2017**, *4*, 897–901. [CrossRef] [PubMed]
67. Contreras-Rodríguez, O.; Martín-Pérez, C.; Vilar-López, R.; Verdejo-Garcia, A. Ventral and Dorsal Striatum Networks in Obesity: Link to Food Craving and Weight Gain. *Biol. Psychiatry* **2017**, *81*, 789–796. [CrossRef]
68. Meye, F.J.; Adan, R.A. Feelings about food: The ventral tegmental area in food reward and emotional eating. *Trends Pharmacol. Sci.* **2014**, *35*, 31–40. [CrossRef]
69. Yu, Y.; Miller, R.; Groth, S.W. A literature review of dopamine in binge eating. *J. Eat. Disord.* **2022**, *10*, 11. [CrossRef] [PubMed]
70. Jones, D.T.; Graff-Radford, J. Executive Dysfunction and the Prefrontal Cortex. *Continuum* **2021**, *27*, 1586–1601. [CrossRef]
71. Volkow, N.D.; Wang, G.J.; Baler, R.D. Reward, dopamine and the control of food intake: Implications for obesity. *Trends Cogn. Sci.* **2011**, *15*, 37–46. [CrossRef]
72. Jenni, N.L.; Larkin, J.D.; Floresco, S.B. Prefrontal Dopamine D1 and D2 Receptors Regulate Dissociable Aspects of Decision Making via Distinct Ventral Striatal and Amygdalar Circuits. *J. Neurosci.* **2017**, *37*, 6200–6213. [CrossRef] [PubMed]
73. Logue, S.F.; Gould, T.J. The neural and genetic basis of executive function: Attention, cognitive flexibility, and response inhibition. *Pharmacol. Biochem. Behav.* **2014**, *123*, 45–54. [CrossRef] [PubMed]
74. London, E.D. Human Brain Imaging Links Dopaminergic Systems to Impulsivity. *Curr. Top. Behav. Neurosci.* **2020**, *47*, 53–71.
75. Settell, M.L.; Testini, P.; Cho, S.; Lee, J.H.; Blaha, C.D.; Jo, H.J.; Lee, K.H.; Min, H.K. Functional Circuitry Effect of Ventral Tegmental Area Deep Brain Stimulation: Imaging and Neurochemical Evidence of Mesocortical and Mesolimbic Pathway Modulation. *Front. Neurosci.* **2017**, *11*, 104. [CrossRef]
76. Alcaro, A.; Huber, R.; Panksepp, J. Behavioral functions of the mesolimbic dopaminergic system: An affective neuroethological perspective. *Brain Res. Rev.* **2007**, *56*, 283–321. [CrossRef]

77. Simon, J.J.; Skunde, M.; Hamze Sinno, M.; Brockmeyer, T.; Herpertz, S.C.; Bendszus, M.; Herzog, W.; Friederich, H.C. Impaired Cross-Talk between Mesolimbic Food Reward Processing and Metabolic Signaling Predicts Body Mass Index. *Front. Behav. Neurosci.* **2014**, *8*, 359.
78. Hebebrand, J.; Albayrak, Ö.; Adan, R.; Antel, J.; Dieguez, C.; de Jong, J.; Leng, G.; Menzies, J.; Mercer, J.G.; Murphy, M.; et al. "Eating addiction", rather than "food addiction", better captures addictive-like eating behavior. *Neurosci. Biobehav. Rev.* **2014**, *47*, 295–306. [CrossRef]
79. Berridge, K.C.; Robinson, T.E. Liking, wanting, and the incentive-sensitization theory of addiction. *Am. Psychol.* **2016**, *71*, 670–679. [CrossRef]
80. Stice, E.; Burger, K. Neural vulnerability factors for obesity. *Clin. Psychol. Rev.* **2019**, *68*, 38–53. [CrossRef] [PubMed]
81. Koob, G.F.; Volkow, N.D. Neurobiology of addiction: A neurocircuitry analysis. *Lancet Psychiatry* **2016**, *3*, 760–773. [CrossRef] [PubMed]
82. Fukai, M.; Bunai, T.; Hirosawa, T.; Kikuchi, M.; Ito, S.; Minabe, Y.; Ouchi, Y. Endogenous dopamine release under transcranial direct-current stimulation governs enhanced attention: A study with positron emission tomography. *Transl. Psychiatry* **2019**, *9*, 115. [CrossRef]
83. Bunai, T.; Hirosawa, T.; Kikuchi, M.; Fukai, M.; Yokokura, M.; Ito, S.; Takata, Y.; Terada, T.; Ouchi, Y. tDCS-induced modulation of GABA concentration and dopamine release in the human brain: A combination study of magnetic resonance spectroscopy and positron emission tomography. *Brain Stimul.* **2021**, *14*, 154–160. [CrossRef]
84. Schreiber, L.R.; Odlaug, B.L.; Grant, J.E. The overlap between binge eating disorder and substance use disorders: Diagnosis and neurobiology. *J. Behav. Addict.* **2013**, *2*, 191–198. [CrossRef]
85. Anderson, M.C.; Bunce, J.G.; Barbas, H. Prefrontal-hippocampal pathways underlying inhibitory control over memory. *Neurobiol. Learn. Mem.* **2016**, *134 Pt A*, 145–161. [CrossRef]
86. Volkow, N.D.; Wang, G.J.; Telang, F.; Fowler, J.S.; Thanos, P.K.; Logan, J.; Alexoff, D.; Ding, Y.-S.; Wong, C.; Ma, Y.; et al. Low dopamine striatal D2 receptors are associated with prefrontal metabolism in obese subjects: Possible contributing factors. *Neuroimage* **2008**, *42*, 1537–1543. [CrossRef]
87. Batterink, L.; Yokum, S.; Stice, E. Body mass correlates inversely with inhibitory control in response to food among adolescent girls: An fMRI study. *Neuroimage* **2010**, *52*, 1696–1703. [CrossRef]
88. Dimitropoulos, A.; Tkach, J.; Ho, A.; Kennedy, J. Greater corticolimbic activation to high-calorie food cues after eating in obese vs. normal-weight adults. *Appetite* **2012**, *58*, 303–312. [CrossRef]
89. Moore, C.F.; Sabino, V.; Koob, G.F.; Cottone, P. Neuroscience of Compulsive Eating Behavior. *Front. Neurosci.* **2017**, *11*, 469. [CrossRef] [PubMed]
90. Fassini, P.G.; Das, S.K.; Suen, V.M.M.; Magerowski, G.; Marchini, J.S.; da Silva, W.A., Jr.; Changyu, S.; Alonso-Alonso, M. Appetite effects of prefrontal stimulation depend on COMT Val158Met polymorphism: A randomized clinical trial. *Appetite* **2019**, *140*, 142–150. [CrossRef] [PubMed]
91. Manfredi, L.; Accoto, A.; Couyoumdjian, A.; Conversi, D. A Systematic Review of Genetic Polymorphisms Associated with Binge Eating Disorder. *Nutrients* **2021**, *13*, 848. [CrossRef] [PubMed]

nutrients

MDPI

Review

Neurodevelopment Is Dependent on Maternal Diet: Placenta and Brain Glucose Transporters GLUT1 and GLUT3

Tomoko Daida [1], Bo-Chul Shin [1], Carlos Cepeda [2] and Sherin U. Devaskar [1,*]

[1] Department of Pediatrics, Division of Neonatology and Developmental Biology and Neonatal Research Center, at the UCLA Children's Discovery and Innovation Institute, David Geffen School of Medicine at UCLA, Los Angeles, CA 90095, USA; tdaida@mednet.ucla.edu (T.D.); bshin@mednet.ucla.edu (B.-C.S.)

[2] Intellectual and Developmental Disabilities Research Center and Brain Research Institute, David Geffen School of Medicine at UCLA, Los Angeles, CA 90095, USA

* Correspondence: sdevaskar@mednet.ucla.edu

Abstract: Glucose is the primary energy source for most mammalian cells and its transport is affected by a family of facilitative glucose transporters (GLUTs) encoded by the SLC2 gene. GLUT1 and GLUT3, highly expressed isoforms in the blood–brain barrier and neuronal membranes, respectively, are associated with multiple neurodevelopmental disorders including epilepsy, dyslexia, ADHD, and autism spectrum disorder (ASD). Dietary therapies, such as the ketogenic diet, are widely accepted treatments for patients with the GLUT1 deficiency syndrome, while ameliorating certain symptoms associated with GLUT3 deficiency in animal models. A ketogenic diet, high-fat diet, and calorie/energy restriction during prenatal and postnatal stages can also alter the placental and brain GLUTs expression with long-term consequences on neurobehavior. This review focuses primarily on the role of diet/energy perturbations upon GLUT isoform-mediated emergence of neurodevelopmental and neurodegenerative disorders.

Keywords: glucose transporter; glucose transporter 3; maternal diet; postnatal diet; neurodevelopment; neurodevelopmental disorders; neurodegenerative disorders; Huntington's disease; brain; placenta

Citation: Daida, T.; Shin, B.-C.; Cepeda, C.; Devaskar, S.U. Neurodevelopment Is Dependent on Maternal Diet: Placenta and Brain Glucose Transporters GLUT1 and GLUT3. *Nutrients* **2024**, *16*, 2363. https://doi.org/10.3390/nu16142363

Academic Editor: Claude Billeaud

Received: 12 June 2024
Revised: 9 July 2024
Accepted: 19 July 2024
Published: 21 July 2024

1. Introduction

Glucose is the primary energy source for neuronal oxidative metabolism under normal physiological conditions in mammals. A family of facilitative glucose transporters (GLUTs) that transfer glucose down a concentration gradient play a critical role in transporting glucose across lipid bi-layered cellular membranes. In the brain, despite the existence of various other isoforms, GLUT1 and GLUT3 isoforms play a major role in fueling energy requirements [1]. GLUT1 is expressed mainly in the endothelial cells of the blood–brain barrier (BBB), astrocytic processes, and oligodendrocytes found in both gray and white matter [2]. In the endothelial cells of the BBB, GLUT1 is present at both the luminal and abluminal membranes of the endothelial cells, thereby transferring glucose from the blood within the capillaries to the brain interstitium [1]. On the other hand, GLUT3 is located predominantly in pre- and post-synaptic neuronal dendrites and other small neuronal processes, along with axons. In this location, GLUT3 mediates the transport of glucose into high-energy-demanding neurons [2,3]. This is accomplished due to the high affinity of GLUT3 compared to that of the other GLUT isoforms [4]. Owing to its expression in neurons and its abundance in the cortex and cerebellum, GLUT3, more than GLUT1, is considered critically essential for neurotransmission [3,5]. As glucose is the primary energy source for neuronal cells, any condition that lends itself to creating GLUT3 deficiency, as in the case of dietary restrictions, hypoxic–ischemia or significant hypoglycemia, can result in a panoply of neurodevelopmental disorders such as dyslexia, autism spectrum disorder (ASD), epilepsy, and attention-deficit/hyperactivity disorder (ADHD) [6–10]. In addition, there are other conditions that present later in life such as Huntington's disease (HD) and

Alzheimer's disease (AD), where GLUT3 deficiency is also encountered. In the presence of glucopenia, alternate fuels such as ketone bodies, lactate, and fatty acids are recruited to meet the energy demands of the brain. These substrates are deemed essential in the absence or deficiency of glucose but are not as efficient as glucose in supplying the required cellular energy. Ketones and lactate are transported via the family of monocarboxylate transporters (MCTs), with the MCT1 isoform expressed in the BBB and astrocytes, while MCT2 is found in neurons [11,12]. This is the mechanism behind the amelioration of certain conditions such as epilepsy when a ketogenic diet is introduced therapeutically [13].

GLUT1 and GLUT3 are also expressed as the main isoforms within the early developing embryo and placenta. In the early embryo, in the pre-implantation phase and blastocysts, GLUT1 has been observed primarily in the apical membranes of the trophectoderm and the cells of the inner cell mass [14]. In contrast, GLUT3 is limited in its expression mainly to the basal aspect of the trophectoderm [4]. Absence of either isoform interferes with normal embryonic development resulting in demise, while a deficiency is noted to cause cellular apoptosis [15–17]. In addition to these isoforms, GLUT8 has also been observed at this stage and results in a reduction in the litter size rather than complete demise of all embryos, when absent [18].

GLUT1 and GLUT3 are also expressed subsequently in the developing post-implantation embryo and fetus. Embryonic (E) day 7.5 in mice display high expression of GLUT1 and GLUT3 mRNA and protein in extraembryonic tissues rather than the lower amounts in the endoderm [19–21]. By E10-10.5, the expression of GLUT1 is confined to the neural tube, gut, heart, and optic vesicle alone, while GLUT3 is limited to the trophectoderm and embryonic gut [19–21]. GLUT1 and GLUT3 expression is reduced by E14.5, with GLUT3 mRNA being below the sensitivity of detection [19]. Subsequently, expression of GLUT1 and GLUT3 mRNA and protein is evident in the brain, gradually increasing with advancing gestation to E18 and continuing to increase postnatally (PN), attaining peak concentrations at PN14, and remaining constant thereafter into the adult stage [22]. These observations lend fuel to the importance of GLUT3 in the early stages of embryonic development and subsequent late gestation fetal and postnatal neurodevelopment.

GLUTs' expression in the placenta mediates glucose transport from mother to fetus via the human syncytiotrophoblastic microvilli or murine labyrinthine region, both of which primarily bear the GLUT1 isoform. In contrast, GLUT3 is noted in cytotrophoblasts of the human and syncytiotrophoblasts of the labyrinthine region, localized on the maternal facing fetal layers of the murine placenta [23–25]. In addition, we and others have demonstrated the presence of GLUT8 and GLUT10 in the murine placenta, but their expression is much more restricted [26–28]. Given their location and essential function, it is reasonable to connect any changes in the maternal diet or the presence of a metabolic aberration with altered GLUT expression pattern in the placenta, early embryo, and/or the brain of the fetus/offspring. These maternal perturbations set the offspring up for either experiencing fetal growth restriction or ultimately a perturbed neurodevelopmental state underlying altered long-term neurobehavioral outcomes [29,30]. This review focuses first on GLUT3's expression and function in human and animal models, particularly in the brain as it relates to neurodevelopmental disorders. Second, the focus is on maternal dietary effects and genetic modifications of GLUT3 with a propensity towards developing neurodevelopmental disorders.

2. GLUT3

2.1. Glucose Transporters (GLUTs and SGLTs Family)

GLUTs are encoded by the *SLC2* gene family and belong to the facilitative superfamily of membrane-spanning glycoproteins [31]. The human GLUT family consists of 14 members, and they are categorized into three classes according to sequence similarity [31,32]. They are further subdivided into three subfamilies, namely class I (glucose transporters GLUT1-4 and GLUT14), class II (fructose transporter GLUT5, GLUT7, GLUT9, and GLUT11), and class III (GLUT6, 8, 10, 12, and H^+/myo-inositol co-transporter

(HMIT)) [33–35]. The individual isotypes show different characteristics of substrate specificity, kinetic characteristics, and expression profiles through regulation of their gene expression and they enable tissue/cell-specific monosaccharide (glucose and fructose) uptake [32] (Table 1). GLUT1 was the first membrane transporter detected, purified, and cloned. GLUT1 is expressed in many tissues; as shown in Table 1, the most important biological function in the brain is to transport glucose across the BBB and into cells of glial lineage [31,36–38]. GLUT2 is involved in regulation of food intake and the median eminence glucose influx into glucose-sensing cells related to the central nervous system's regulation of glucose homeostasis [39–43]. GLUT3 is a neuronal glucose transporter due to its exclusive expression in neurons but not glia, including oligodendrocytes or microvascular endothelial cells [2,31]. GLUT4 is expressed in specific anatomic regions of the cerebrum in addition to being present peripherally in insulin-responsive tissues such as muscle and adipose cells, contributing towards maintaining whole-body insulin-regulated glucose homeostasis [44–46]. GLUT6 (previously referred to as GLUT9) is also expressed in the brain as well as in white adipose tissue and the spleen [41,42,47,48]. The role of GLUT8 (intracellular) in the brain remains an enigma, but it is perhaps involved in supplying energy to hippocampal neurons [47–51]. GLUT9 is expressed as two differentially spliced variants, GLUT9a and GLUT9b, with each of them being expressed in different tissues and both functioning as a urate transporter [31,52]. GLUT10 is predominantly expressed in the liver and pancreas, although is also observed in the brain, and its gene *SLC2A10* localizes to a chromosomal region previously linked with type 2 diabetes [53,54]. GLUT12 is a glucose transporter widely expressed in the skeletal muscle, adipose tissue, small intestine, and placenta [55].

In addition to the GLUTs, there is another class of glucose transporters, namely the Na^+/glucose co-transporters (SGLTs). These proteins are a family of membrane-bound glucose transporters that are energy-dependent and function as active transporters. SGLTs transport glucose against a glucose concentration gradient but are dependent on co-transport of sodium. One molecule of glucose is transported with one or two sodium ions which are transported down a sodium concentration gradient [41,56]. These proteins are encoded by the *SLC5* gene with 12 members of a human gene family including 6 SGLTs [56]. SGLT1 is mainly expressed in intestinal mucosa mediating transport of glucose and galactose. In the brain, it contributes to glucose uptake and efflux into certain neurons lining the choroid plexus and periventricular region [56,57]. SGLT2 expression is displayed in the early portion of the proximal renal tubule mediating glucose reabsorption. SGLT2 inhibitors are employed as an adjunct in the treatment of type 2 diabetes mellitus [58,59]. Given its low expression in the cerebellum as well, it has the potential of functioning with SGLT1, although the biological role is questionable at the present time [56]. SGLT3 is not a glucose transporter but rather a glucose sensor in cholinergic neurons and found in skeletal muscle [60]. SGLT4 is primarily expressed in the small intestine and skeletal muscle transporting glucose and mannose. SGLT5 is expressed in the kidney transporting glucose and galactose. Both SGLT4 and SGLT5 are not found in the brain. SGLT6, which is known as the Na^+/inositol cotransporter (SMIT) 2, is expressed in the brain hypothalamus and substantia nigra. These locations of expression suggest a role for transporting glucose and inositol in the control of food intake and reward processing by recognizing nutrients [57,61,62]. While the members of this family of Na^+/glucose transporters are biologically important, we will focus mainly on specific members of the GLUT family for the purposes of this review.

Table 1. GLUT and SGLT family.

Classification	Transporters	Km (mM)	Tissue Distribution	Substrate	Function in Brain
GLUT family class I	GLUT1	6.9	Fibroblasts, erythrocytes, brain (endothelial cells, astrocytic processes and oligodendrocytes) >skeletal and cardiac muscle, white adipose tissue, liver	Glucose/Galactose	Transport glucose through BBB and into astrocyte
	GLUT2	11.2	Liver, pancreas, kidney, small intestine, brain (brainstem, thalamus, cortex, hypothalamus, hippocampus) [39,40,43]	Glucose/Galactose /Fructose	Regulation of food and glucose intake
	GLUT3	1.4	Brain (hippocampus, temporal neocortex, gyrus) >testis, placenta, white blood cells, platelets [31]	Glucose/Galactose	Transport glucose to neurons
	GLUT4	4.6	White adipose tissue, skeletal and cardiac muscle cells > brain (basal ganglia, neocortex, hypothalamus, hippocampus)	Glucose	Insulin-dependent regulation of active neuronal circuits
	GLUT14	-	Testis	-	-
GLUT family class II	GLUT5	5	Small intestine >kidney, skeletal muscle, adipose tissue [63,64]	Fructose	-
	GLUT7	0.3	Small intestine, colon [65]	Glucose/Fructose	-
	GLUT9	0.3	GLUT9a: liver, kidney, lung, placenta, leukocytes GLUT9b: kidney, placenta [31,52]	Glucose/Fructose	-
	GLUT11	0.2	Heart, skeletal muscle, pancreas, kidney [66,67]	Glucose/Fructose	-
GLUT family class III	GLUT6		White adipose, spleen, brain (median eminence), peripheral leucocytes	Glucose	Regulation of glucohomeostasis
	GLUT8	2.4	Testis, skeletal muscle, heart, small intestine >brain (amygdala, primary olfactory cortex, dentate gyrus, dorsal hypothalamic area, pituitary stark, posterior pituitary, dentate gyrus, hippocampus)	Glucose	Energy supply for neurons in hippocampus
	GLUT10	0.3	Liver, pancreas > placenta, heart, lung skeletal muscle, kidney, adipose tissue [31]	Glucose/Galactose	-
	GLUT12	4–5	Skeletal muscle, adipose tissue, small intestine [55]	Glucose/Galactose/Fructose	-
	HMIT GLUT13	0.1	Brain (hippocampus, hypothalamus, cerebellum) >white and brown adipose tissues, kidney [68]	Myoinositol	Control of myo-inositol metabolism in brain
SGLT family	SGLT1	0.5	Intestine, Trachea, kidney, heart, testis, prostate, brain (cortical neurons, hippocampal pyramidal cell, Purkinje cells, BBB)	Glucose/Galactose	Removal of glucose from brain interstitium
	SGLT2	5.0	Kidney, brain (cerebellum), liver, thyroid, muscle, heart	Glucose	Not determined
	SGLT3	20	Skeletal muscle, testis, uterus, small intestine, brain (hypothalamus), thyroid	Glucose	Activation of glucosensitive neurons
	SGLT4	2.0	Small intestine, skeletal muscle [56,57]	Glucose/Mannose	-
	SGLT5	-	Kidney [56,57]	Glucose/Galactose	-
	SGLT6	-	Small intestine, brain (hypothalamus and substantia nigra)	Inositol	Recognize nutrients to control food intake and reward processing

2.2. GLUT3—Structure and Kinetics

The process of glucose transport as mediated by the family of GLUT proteins, is non-energy dependent and down a concentration gradient from higher to lower glucose concentrations. This process is referred to as facilitative diffusion, with a rate that is more rapid than simple trans-membrane diffusion [69]. All GLUTs demonstrate $\geq$50% amino acid identity with a similar predicted structure consisting of 12 membrane-spanning α-helical domains with a cytoplasmic amino (N) terminus and a carboxy (C) terminus, with the latter being generally unique to each isoform. The neuronal glucose transporter isoform GLUT3 is encoded by the *SLC2A3* gene and noted within the human chromosome 12p3.3, with a demonstrated higher affinity than other GLUT isoforms [40]. Michaelis Menten's characteristics depict a low Km of 1.4 mM for GLUT3, which is almost one-fifth of that of the other GLUT isoforms [4,33]. Physiological plasma glucose concentrations are normally maintained between 3.0 and 7.8 mM, whereas glucose concentrations in cerebrospinal fluid (CSF) are much lower around 0.5–2.5 mM [70]. The high affinity of GLUT3 for glucose is critically beneficial in fueling energy-demanding neuronal cells, particularly in circumstances surrounding the availability of lower glucose concentrations than physiologically accepted as normal [71].

2.3. GLUT3—Expression/Investigations in Brain and Placenta

GLUT3 mRNAs/proteins are expressed abundantly in mammalian brains as the neuronal glucose transporter [5]. Lower concentrations are expressed in the testis [71,72], spermatozoa, trophectoderm of preimplantation embryo [20,21], placenta [73,74], white blood cells [75], and platelets [71]. Their expression is mostly in the frontal cortex, thalamus, putamen, caudate, hippocampus, and sub-fornical organ located along the antero-dorsal wall of the third ventricle (gray matter-dominant areas), moderately in the cerebellar folia composed of cerebellar white matter, Purkinje neurons and granular neurons (gray matter and white matter mixed areas), and the least in centrum semi-ovale (white matter-dominant area) [10,71,76]. Abundant GLUT3 expression in gray matter, along with much lower levels in white matter, suggests that GLUT3 provides glucose to regions of high metabolic activity [71]. The protein level changes in GLUT3 correspond with synaptogenesis and neuronal maturation in physiologically normal rats and are regulated by the metabolic demand and the regional cerebral glucose utilization rate [1]. In conditions of glucose deficiency, ketones and lactate are used as alternate fuels for energy production. Ketones and lactate traverse the BBB and enter the astrocytes via the monocarboxylate transporter isoform 1 (MCT1) (Km 4.0 mM), while accessing neurons via the MCT2 isoform (Km 0.7 mM) [12] (Figure 1). In addition to the two GLUT isoforms, other isoforms such as GLUT2 [77], GLUT4 [9,78], GLUT6 [42], GLUT8 [78], and GLUT13 [68] are also noted in specific regions or cell types within the brain, albeit in much smaller amounts mediating specific functions.

Homozygous mutations of the GLUT3 gene have only been examined in the context of cell type-specific conditional null mutations in mice [79,80]. This is because of the embryonic demise encountered during the gastrulation phase of development [15]. Such a presentation may hold some validity in humans when early-gestation spontaneous abortion with loss of pregnancy is encountered. Depending on the cell-type selected, namely nestin-, CaMKII- or Emx-1 expressing neural cells, complete absence of GLUT3 has led to varying presentations [79,80]. Employing antisense oligonucleotides specific to the zebra fish GLUT3 gene, which is deployed early in zygotic development, led to significant disruption of brain development with significant growth restriction [81].

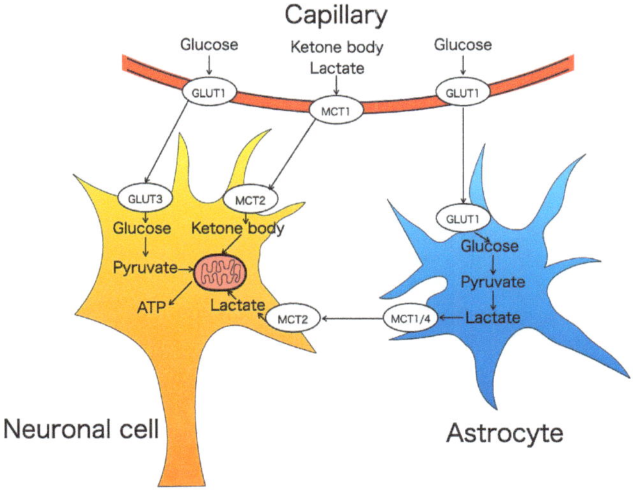

Figure 1. The transport mechanisms underlying transfer of glucose, ketone body, and lactate across the blood–brain barrier from capillary vessels to neurons and astrocytes. GLUT; glucose transporter, MCT; monocarboxylate transporters.

Expression of GLUTs in the placenta is highly regulated throughout pregnancy, which includes GLUT3 and GLUT1 isoforms. GLUT1 and GLUT3 are expressed in both the rodent hemotrichorial and human hemomonochorial placentas. In the human, GLUT1 is expressed by the syncytiotrophoblasts that form the microvilli being highly expressed at the internally located basal membrane during the third trimester of pregnancy [82]; likewise, it is mainly expressed in two layers of syncytiotrophoblasts in the labyrinthine region including the junctional region in rodents [25,74]. In contrast, GLUT3 in humans is mainly observed in cytotrophoblasts that are more enriched during the early gestational period, being 48 $\pm$ 7% in the second trimester and 34 $\pm$ 10% in the third trimester when normalized to 100% of GLUT3 as observed during the first trimester [23]. In the rodent placenta, GLUT3 is expressed in plasma membranes facing the maternal blood supply of the syncytiotrophoblastic layers lining the labyrinthine regions, contributing much more to the total GLUTs concentration [25,74]. This suggests that GLUT3 is important in early gestation of the human pregnancy, due to the presence of actively dividing cytotrophoblasts that impose a higher energy demand than the subsequent fully differentiated syncytiotrophoblasts found more in the second and third trimesters. This early gestation expression of the high-affinity GLUT3 isoform may be necessary for mediating the required glucose transport under an intra-uterine environment of low oxygen and glucose supply prior to the invasion and formation of the intervillous circulation that supplies the early rapidly dividing embryo [24]. In addition to GLUT1 and GLUT3, other isoforms, GLUT4, GLUT8, GLUT9, GLUT10, and GLUT12, are also expressed in the placenta to a limited degree [26–28,82].

2.4. GLUT3 Is Potentially Associated with Neurodevelopmental and Neurodegenerative Disorders

Given the critical role of neuronal metabolism, aberrant GLUT3 expression due to pathological conditions of gene copy number variants (CNVs) or gene mutations, creates the conditions for the emergence of neurodevelopmental disorders. During normal murine development, both GLUT1 and GLUT3 proteins are expressed at low levels in the embryonic and early postnatal brain, only to reach peak concentrations at PN day 10 to 15 [22]. During this phase, hypothyroidism is known to alter expression of these isoforms with a detrimental effect on the postnatal brain [83]. Sp1/Sp3 and phosphorylated CREB were demonstrated to regulate transcription of murine brain GLUT3 gene [84,85].

GLUT3 protein expression increases are paralleled by the corresponding mRNA levels but not associated with the increases in transcriptional rates, whereas GLUT1 protein increase coincides with mRNA levels [22]; however, the processing has been shown to be post-transcriptional [86]. These data suggest that GLUT3 gene is regulated either post-transcriptionally/translationally [22] or there is a lag between transcription and post-transcriptional/translational events. Thus, employing the transgenic GLUT3-luciferase mouse model, we deciphered the developmental timing of transcription to precede the peak levels of brain GLUT3 mRNA and protein [87]. In addition, prior studies have revealed transcriptional control of GLUT3 by various trans-acting nuclear factors [84,85], supporting the idea that transcription occurs before the timing of post-transcription/translation in the case of this gene. Also, other groups have reported that untranslated gene regions carrying mutations have the potential to affect neurodevelopment [88]. These are important to unravel before investigating the impact of either genetic modifications or dietary perturbations in the mother during pregnancy or lactation.

Hypoxic–ischemia (which involves pan-nutritional deficiency including an oxygen-deficient state) early in development or subsequently during juvenile or adult stages enhances brain GLUT3 expression during the early energy-demanding recovery period but is rapidly reduced in the cortex and thalamus, reflecting apoptotic and necrotic injury to the brain during this early response (24 h). The later response (72 h) results in extensive regional area necrosis [89]. Heterozygous GLUT3 null mice with hypoxic–ischemic brain injury is reported to show more severe cellular apoptosis and necrosis than wild-type mice and tend to present with spontaneous clinical seizures [76]. Further, exposure to pentylenetetrazole caused a longer duration of seizures in these genetically modified adult mice [76]. These results suggest that GLUT3 could underlie an adaptive response to hypoxic–ischemia, providing some insights into the development of a therapeutic intervention targeting activation of this isoform in neurons.

In a prior study, pentylenetetrazole- and kainic acid-induced seizures increased both GLUT1 and GLUT3 expression in rat brains [90]. Another group reported that lithium–pilocarpine-induced seizures also increased brain GLUT3 expression, albeit only transiently [91]. Leroy et al. reported on the upregulation of MCT1 and MCT2, suggesting the possibility of ketone utilization as an alternate fuel in the presence of epilepsy [91].

Disruption of glucose metabolism in neuronal cells underlies the pathogenesis and progression of Huntington's disease (HD) [92–94]. In humans, GLUT3 expression was significantly decreased in an advanced stage of HD, while there was no significant difference compared to normal controls in the early stage of the disease despite brain glucose utilization being reduced [95,96]. Li et al. elucidated that Rab11, a Rab family GTP-ase involved in cellular endosomal recycling, influences brain glucose metabolism in 140 CAG repeat knock-in mice [97]. Additionally, they demonstrated that in the presence of increased gene *SLC2A3* CNVs, which led to increasing concentrations of the GLUT3 protein in HD patient's neural cells, the age of onset in acquiring HD clinical features could be delayed [98]. In another neurodegenerative disorder, Alzheimer's disease (AD), reduced GLUT1 and GLUT3 expression has also been reported in the human brain [99]. Liu et al. observed a concordance between brain GLUTs and other established AD markers; GLUT3 decreases in correlation with the decrease in O-GlcNAcylation and the appearance of hyperphosphorylation of the tau protein in the brain [100]. An et al. demonstrated lower brain GLUT3 expression with an associated greater severity of the amyloid plaque and neurofibrillary tangles development, along with increasing severity of the clinical symptoms in AD patients [101]. Importantly, recent studies have emphasized a possible connection between neurodevelopmental and neurodegenerative disorders [102]. For example, in HD, aberrant neurodevelopment sets the stage for future neuronal dysfunction and degeneration [103,104]. Similar findings have been reported for AD [105]. It is thus possible that in both types of disorders, GLUT3 deficiency during brain development plays an important role. Several clinical studies reported that patients presenting with symptoms of attention deficit hyperactivity disorder (ADHD) reveal CNVs of a locus in the *SLC2A3* gene, with the presence of *SLC2A3* gene duplication being associated with altered working memory and cognitive response control, which are features of ADHD [6,106]. Reduced mRNA expression of *SLC2A3* in white blood cells was reported to be negatively associated with a late left-lateralized auditory mismatch [8]. Skeide et al. reported that these SLC2A3 gene variants were associated with a phonological awareness phenotype connected to dyslexia [107]. Heterozygous GLUT3-deficient (GLUT3$^{+/-}$) mice presented with autism spectrum disorder (ASD)-like clinical features and neurobehaviors, namely increased electroencephalographic seizure activity, abnormal spatial learning and working memory, reduced vocalizations, and stereotypies [10]. On the other hand, homozygous GLUT3-deficient mice resulted in embryonic loss at E6.5 due to the critical role of GLUT3 in the trophoectoderm of the early embryo [15,108,109]. However, when conditional null homozygous mutations were created to overcome embryonic demise using the nestin-Cre transgene driving the floxed Slc2A3 gene mutation, no changes were evident until after PN day 10, after which significant growth restriction with microcephaly emerged with demise either before or after weaning from the mother [80]. On the other hand, employing the Emx1-Cre or CaMKII-Cre led to survival into adulthood with successful reproduction. The former demonstrated some features akin to ADHD, whereas the latter expressed lack of fear for spatial exploration or social novelty with some disruption of spatial cognition [79]. These mouse models are essential in teasing out the role of GLUT3 in specific neuron subtypes, thereby affecting different neurobehavioral functions.

3. Maternal and Postnatal Dietary Exposures Affect Offspring's GLUTs

3.1. *High-Fat Diet*

Obesity, with a body mass index (BMI) of 30 or higher, is a global issue, although it is more predominant in Western countries. In the United States, about one-third of reproductive-age women are diagnosed with obesity due to their dietary habits and sedentary lifestyle [110,111]. Many studies have shown that maternal obesity causes long-lasting adverse events in the offspring, such as neurodevelopmental disorders, metabolic derangements, and associated cardiovascular diseases [112–115]. In addition, maternal complications ensue such as gestational hypertension, pre-eclampsia, and gestational diabetes mellitus [116,117]. Recent investigations employing nonhuman primate and rodent models of maternal obesity due to consumption of a high-fat diet demonstrated an increase in inflammatory cytokines, insulin, fatty acids, and triglycerides in the maternal circulation that affect the fetal homeostatic milieu, thereby perturbing the fetal brain melanocortinergic, serotoninergic, and dopaminergic neural networks [30,112,118]. These aberrations acquired in utero are not ameliorated upon postnatal introduction of a regular chow diet, supporting the concept of fetal mal-programming, due to maternal obesity-associated systemic alterations [119]. Upon examination of placental GLUTs, various groups of investigators, including our group, previously demonstrated that wild-type murine placental GLUT1 increases during late gestation when exposed to pre-conceptional and gestational high-fat diet, with no concomitant change in GLUT3 observed [120,121]. While Ganguly et al. observed no change in the immediate postnatal suckling litter body weights [120], Jones et al. reported an increase in body weight gain in response to hyper-caloric high-fat exposure [121]. The difference between the two studies rested on the energy emanating from the dietary carbohydrate composition, being double in the latter compared to the former (52% vs. 27%) [120,121]. Rosario et al. demonstrated an increase in murine placental GLUT1 and GLUT3 concentrations in response to consumption of a high-fat and high-sucrose diet pre-conceptionally and gestationally, resulting in increased postnatal body weights [122]. In contrast to these studies in wild-type mice, a heterozygote null mutation of the Slc2A3 gene with 50% of GLUT3 protein, failed to reduce intra-placental and transplacental glucose transport [123]. Pre-gestation and gestational consumption of a high-fat diet by GLUT3$^{+/-}$ mice increased placental GLUT1 and GLUT3 concentrations (emanating from a single allele), with subsequent postnatal litter body weight increase [120]. Collectively, these studies suggest that while GLUT1 may mediate intra-placental glucose transport, GLUT3 mediates trans-placental glucose transport from mother to fetus, impacting the ultimate weight gain of the offspring.

Supplemental *n*-3 fatty acid in preterm neonatal pigs ameliorates brain immunohistochemical changes by reducing apoptotic cells in the internal granule cell layers [124]. Despite the multiple beneficial effects regarding the intake of *n*-3 fatty acid-rich diets [125–127], one must be aware of the dose-dependent deleterious effects as well, particularly if this exposure is during pregnancy or lactation. We had previously reported that rats on an *n*-3 fatty acid-enriched high-fat diet during lactation, subsequent to maternal *n*-6-enriched high-fat food intake during gestation led to microcephaly with decreased brain GLUT3 concentrations with no difference in GLUT1 [128]. Stachowiak et al. also reported that embryonic day 21 mice exposed to a maternal high-fat diet consisting most probably of *n*-6 fatty acids demonstrated a diminution in migration and maturation of periventricular stem cells within the fetal brain [129]. Thus, despite the reported benefits seen in the metabolic milieu with *n*-3 fatty acids, these studies indicate caution when it comes to neurodevelopment.

3.2. Ketogenic Diet

A ketogenic diet has been established as a therapeutic alternative for anti-epileptic drug (AED)-resistant epilepsy [13,130–132]. Most often, there is either a germline or somatic genetic mutation basis for such epilepsies, warranting surgical resection in the case of focal cortical dysplasias (FCDs). More often, as in the case of the germline Slc2A1 gene mutation (haplodeficiency), infantile-onset epilepsy with persistently low cerebrospinal fluid glucose concentrations, delayed development, microcephaly with intellectual disability, and complex movement difficulties which include gait abnormalities are encountered and referred to as GLUT1 deficiency syndrome [133,134]. In this specific case, while AEDs are ineffective, a ketogenic diet encompassing a high-fat and low-carbohydrate diet, has been effective in controlling seizures. The ketogenic dietary intervention induces a metabolic state of ketosis by increasing the exogenous supply of ketone bodies (β-hydroxybutyrate, acetoacetate, and acetone) and enhancing the endogenous production by fatty acid oxidation. Overall, a 50% or greater reduction in seizure frequency after three or six months of a ketogenic dietary intervention in children has been reported [135–137]. The mechanism of amelioration rests on the provision of a non-glucose alternate source of energy for fueling the metabolism in neurons, restoring impaired mitochondrial function, regulating neurotransmission at pre- and post-synaptic junctions (changing the amount of GABA, glutamate, and adenosine receptors), having anti-inflammatory effects on neurons and reducing the amount of reactive oxygen species, along with having epigenetic effects on DNA and histones [13,131]. The side effects of a ketogenic dietary therapy consist of dehydration, weight loss, and hypertriglyceridemia arising as common early-onset complications, along with osteopenia, renal stones, and cardiomyopathy, setting in as late-onset complications [133,138–140]. Besides epilepsy, the ketogenic diet has been introduced for treatment of other neurological disorders such as Parkinson's disease, multiple sclerosis, AD, and migraine [131]. Autistic behaviors have also been reported to potentially experience amelioration in response to a ketogenic diet [141].

In contrast, isolated GLUT3 deficiency due to a gene mutation has only been reported so far in two children presenting with myelomeningoceles [142]. Thus, not much is known in humans regarding conditions associated with haplodeficiency of GLUT3. Most of the studies thus far have occurred in animal models with genetic modifications. Cheng et al. reported a drastic intervention of a 90% calorie restriction with intake of a ketogenic diet over a period of 7 days which increased rat brain GLUT1 and GLUT3 mRNA expression when compared to the control diet with 90% calorie restriction alone [143]. Classical GLUT3$^{+/-}$ mice presented with a neurodevelopmental disorder akin to ASD as suggested by neurobehaviors, such as increased electroencephalographic seizure activity, abnormal spatial learning and working memory, cognitive inflexibility, stereotypic behaviors of low frequency, abnormal socialization, and reduced vocalizations. Otherwise, homozygous

GLUT3 knock-out mice could have pregnancy loss [10,15]. GLUT3$^{+/-}$ mice revealed an earlier developmental increase in neuronal MCT2 expression at PN 14 through PN60 than that encountered in wild-type mice [10]. Gestational and postnatal ketogenic dietary intervention in the case of these GLUT3$^{+/-}$ mice improved electroencephalographic seizures and abnormal sociability but failed to affect abnormalities in spatial learning, working memory, cognitive inflexibility, and reduced vocalization, suggesting only a partial amelioration of the neurobehavioral presentation by enhanced utilization of ketones as an energy fuel when neurons experience glucopenia [144,145]. Such partial amelioration attests to the successful transfer to fetus of maternal ketones that build up when exposed to a ketogenic diet [145]. Unlike these reports, exposure to a ketogenic diet in normal wild-type mice can prove detrimental to murine neurodevelopment [144]. In addition, Sussman et al. described maternal infertility subsequently when ketoacidosis ensued during the lactation phase. What is most concerning is the ultimate change in the postnatal brain structure encountered in response to prenatal and early postnatal (before weaning) exposure to the ketogenic diet in the normal state. Such an exposure decreased the volume of the cortex, hippocampus, corpus callosum, and lateral ventricle, with relative enlargement of the hypothalamus and medulla at PN11.5 and PN21.5 [146]. These changes persisted into later adult life, where differences in brain morphology were associated with behavioral alterations such as affecting susceptibility to anxiety and depression with elevated hyperactivity, despite reverting to a normal diet post-weaning [147]. Such reports raise the question of whether a ketogenic diet during pregnancy and lactation can program the offspring's neurodevelopment. While extrapolation to the human may be premature, it raises concerns and suggests steering away from a ketogenic diet during pregnancy.

On the other hand, activating *CNVs* in the GLUT3 gene have been reported in individuals with ADHD [6,106], and while no activating GLUT3 mutation murine models exist or have been studied so far, it is imperative to determine this clinical association in a cause-and-effect manner.

3.3. *Energy Restriction*

Inadequate maternal calorie intake causes intrauterine growth restriction (IUGR), which describes a condition of inadequate fetal growth rate that prevents infants from reaching their optimal growth potential [29,148,149]. Etiologies of IUGR may be due to multiple causes with various detrimental outcomes; however, aberrant neurodevelopment is a major risk factor. IUGR infants are known to develop adverse neurodevelopmental outcomes such as neurodevelopmental delay, behavioral problems, motor and cognitive deficiencies, and cerebral palsy [148,150–158]. Genetic mechanisms for neurodevelopmental disabilities with IUGR are suggested [159–162], but remain to be elucidated. Thus, an explosion of animal models to examine the state of IUGR has occurred. Iskusnykh et al. reported that IUGR pigs showed reduced cerebellar weight and the number of granule cells and the JamC/Pard3a molecular pathway mediates compromised initiation of granule cellular radial migration, which contributes to the cerebellar pathology [163].

In the case of placental GLUTs, there is some variability in the results depending on the model and severity of the IUGR state. However, studies have also emanated in the post-parturient human placenta, where increased placental GLUT3 with no change in GLUT1 was observed in the late gestation presentation of a milder form of IUGR [164]. In contrast, Kainulaineu et al. observed no change in human placental GLUTs in a moderately severe form of IUGR [165]. In a large animal model of epitheliochorial placentas such as ewes, when 50% nutrient restriction was imposed during the first half of gestation, increased placental GLUT1 and GLUT3 mRNA expression was noted during mid-gestation [166]. Das et al. reported that late gestational chronic hypoglycemia induced by insulin infusion in sheep, rather than calorie restriction, did not change placental GLUT3 expression but decreased GLUT1 with no difference in transplacental glucose uptake [167]. In small animal models with hemochorial placenta, such as mice with 80% nutrient restriction from early gestation onwards throughout pregnancy, increased placental GLUT1 expression with no change in fetal glucose clearance [168]. In contrast, mid-to-late gestation dietary restriction in mice decreased placental GLUT3, with no change in GLUT1 expression and maternal–fetal glucose transport [169,170]. Comparing mild (~25%) and moderate (~50%) calorie restriction only during mid-to-late gestation led to a differential response, where the mild condition increased and moderate condition decreased placental GLUT3 with a concomitant effect on transplacental glucose transport [123]. Though maternal dexamethasone administration is commonly used to improve mortality and critical morbidity in preterm neonates, it is known to reduce birth weight and multiple dosing regimens of administration in animal models (unlike dosing in human pregnancies) are used to induce IUGR [171–173]. Late-gestation repetitiously dosed dexamethasone-induced IUGR in mice also decreased placental GLUT1 and GLUT3 [174]. Collectively, what is apparent is that the placental GLUTs are reliant on maternal diet, and its effect is dependent on the gestational timing and severity of IUGR. All these factors play a role in the adaptive change in placental GLUTs, which is required for maintaining transplacental glucose transport, towards fueling fetal survival at the expense of fetal growth.

Brain GLUTs are also affected by IUGR. A rat IUGR model consisting of maternal uterine artery ligation causing uteroplacental insufficiency increased fetal brain GLUT1 protein concentrations which persisted until PN21 [175].

Dietary based energy-restricted mice during mid-to-late gestation (~50%) reduced fetal brain GLUT3 protein concentrations by 50% along with a reduction in brain serotonin (5-HT) and serotonin transporter (SERT) concentrations [176]. In addition to changes in brain GLUTs and an imbalanced 5-HT-SERT axis, a reduction in cortical thickness and microcephaly was encountered [177]. In addition, a reduction in nestin (progenitor marker), β-III Tubulin (immature neurons), GFAP (astrocyte marker), and O4 (oligodendrocyte marker) -expressing cells emerged. Maternal dietary restriction has the potential for disturbing neural progenitors' differentiation into cerebral cortical brain cells [177]. Further, the postnatal offspring of the dietary-restricted rats displayed an adaptive increase in brain GLUT1, GLUT3, and brain-derived neurotrophic factor with a concomitant reduction in GLUT4 protein concentrations [9,178] (Table 2). Of importance is the emergence of perturbed neurobehaviors subsequently during adult life such as heightened anxiety and some cognitive impairment [9]. Further, during aging, these rat offspring demonstrated reduced brain IRS-2 and pAkt and increased GFAP and amyloid-p42, akin to that observed in AD. Imposition of postnatal calorie restriction on IUGR, while considered therapeutic in controlling metabolic derangements, is highly detrimental to brain development. While most of the studies described here involve calorie restriction, selective protein restriction and other micronutrient deficiencies have also been shown to affect neurodevelopment adversely [9,178].

In addition to dietary restriction, energy deprivation also occurs under hypoxic–ischemic conditions. We have previously observed that 45 min of hypoxic exposure followed by carotid arterial ligation-induced ischemia led to GLUT3$^{+/-}$ more than wild-type mice incurring brain nuclear pyknosis and cellular necrosis. These GLUT3$^{+/-}$ mice were also observed to display clinical seizures or non-symptomatic EEG seizures alone, while the wild-type mice had no seizures [76]. In vitro studies demonstrated a role for HIF-1α and CREB in inducing GLUT3 expression in response to hypoxia in murine neuroblastoma cells, and in vivo studies in mice corroborated these findings [179]. These reports assign a protective role for neuronal GLUT3 against hypoxic–ischemia, since a reduction in neuronal GLUT3, which worsens brain injury in response to hypoxic–ischemia, is seen as increased cellular apoptosis and necrosis. To determine the relevance to human infants, we undertook a study employing blood cells in hypoxic–ischemic newborn infants subjected to therapeutic hypothermia. Hypoxic–ischemia led to changes in red cell GLUT1 but not in white blood cell GLUT3 [180]. What is important to note is that at this age, while red blood cell GLUT1 concentrations are high, white blood cell GLUT3 concentrations are low [75]. Thus, such studies later in development when white blood cell GLUT3 concentrations are much higher are likely to yield differing results in regard to the role played by both GLUT1 and GLUT3.

Table 2. Effect on GLUTs expression in placenta and brain and neurodevelopment by maternal dietary change.

		Brain GLUTs Expression and Neurodevelopment	Placenta GLUTs Expression
High-fat diet	Maternal	- Reduced GLUT3 expression (rat) [129]. - *n*-3 fatty acids improve vision development (human) [126,127]. - No significant change in the first 2 years of age, but significant positive effects in cognitive tests 3–6 years of age (human) [125–127].	- Increased GLUT1, no change GLUT3(mouse) [120,121]. - High-fat + high-sucrose diet increased GLUT1 and GLUT3 (mouse) [122]. - GLUT3$^{+/-}$ mice increased GLUT1 and GLUT3 [120].
	Postnatal	- Exposure to postnatal *n*-3 fatty acid-enriched high-fat diet after maternal *n*-6 fatty acid-enriched high-fat diet reduced GLUT3, with no change in GLUT1 (mouse) [128].	-
Ketogenic diet	Maternal	- Brain structural change (decreased the volume of cortex, hippocampus, corpus callosum) (mouse) [146]. - Reduced susceptibility to anxiety and depression, elevated hyperactivity (mouse) [147].	- No data regarding GLUTs.
	Maternal and Postnatal	- GLUT3$^{+/-}$ mice decreased ASD-like behaviors and decreased sociability in wild-type mice [144].	-
Energy restriction	Maternal	- Maternal uterine artery ligation in late gestation decreased GLUT1 (rat) [175]. - 50% dietary restriction during mid-to-late gestation decreased fetal brain GLUT3 with reduction in brain 5-HT and SERT concentrations with anxiety and reduced cortical thickness (mouse) [176,177].	Variable results depending on the model and severity of the IUGR state [164–170,174]. - Late-gestation mild-form IUGR showed increased GLUT3, with no change in GLUT1 (human) [164]. - Moderately severe-form IUGR showed no change in GLUT3 and GLUT4 (human) [165]. - 50% nutrient restriction during the first half of gestation increased GLUT1 and GLUT3 during mid-gestation (ewe) [166]. - Chronic hypoglycemia by insulin decreased GLUT1, with no GLUT3 change (sheep) [167]. - 80% nutrient restriction throughout pregnancy increased GLUT1 (mouse) [168]. - Mid-to-late gestation 25% dietary restriction increased GLUT3, and 50% restriction decreased GLUT3 (mouse) [169,170]. - Late gestation dexamethasone-induced IUGR decreased GLUT1 and GLUT3 (mouse) [174].
	Postnatal	- Offspring of 50% dietary-restricted rats displayed an adaptive increase in GLUT1, GLUT3, and BDNF with heightened anxiety and cognitive impairment (rat) [9,178].	-

4. Conclusions

GLUT3 is a high-affinity glucose transporter that plays an important role in the brain and placenta, transporting the primary fuel, namely glucose, to neuronal cells or trans-placentally to the fetus, respectively. Malfunction or deficiency of GLUT3 has the propensity to interfere with sustenance of a pregnancy and ultimately result in intrauterine growth restriction and neurodevelopmental disorders. It also has the capacity to alter the clinical course of adult-onset disorders such as HD and AD. The ketogenic diet has the potential of serving as an alternate fuel sustaining cellular energy metabolism in the presence of a dysfunctional GLUT1 or GLUT3, whether in response to dietary changes or genetic mutations. However, it is imperative to develop newer therapeutic modalities to address these conditions that interfere with the well-being of the mother and developing fetus during pregnancy and the postnatal development of these disorders, with a higher risk of developing aberrant neurobehavioral and subsequent age-related disorders.

Author Contributions: Conceptualization, T.D., B.-C.S. and S.U.D.; writing—original draft preparation, T.D.; writing—review and editing, B.-C.S., C.C. and S.U.D.; visualization, T.D. and B.-C.S.; supervision, S.U.D.; funding acquisition, S.U.D. and C.C. All authors have read and agreed to the published version of the manuscript.

Funding: This research was funded by grants from the National Institute of Health, HD-81206, to S.U.D. and National Institute of Health, NS123883, to S.U.D. and C.C.

Institutional Review Board Statement: The animal study protocol was approved by the Animal Research Committee of the University of California, Los Angeles, protocol# 1999-105 on 29 January 2024. The human study protocol which included obtaining informed parental consent of all parents of subjects was approved by the University of California, Los Angeles, Institutional Review Board protocol# 13–000820 on 13 March 2020.

Conflicts of Interest: The authors declare no conflicts of interest.

References

1. Vannucci, S.J.; Clark, R.R.; Koehler-Stec, E.; Li, K.; Smith, C.B.; Davies, P.; Maher, F.; Simpson, I.A. Glucose transporter expression in brain: Relationship to cerebral glucose utilization. *Dev. Neurosci.* **1998**, *20*, 369–379. [CrossRef] [PubMed]
2. Leino, R.L.; Gerhart, D.Z.; van Bueren, A.M.; McCall, A.L.; Drewes, L.R. Ultrastructural localization of GLUT 1 and GLUT 3 glucose transporters in rat brain. *J. Neurosci. Res.* **1997**, *49*, 617–626. [CrossRef]
3. Maher, F.; Simpson, I.A. The GLUT3 glucose transporter is the predominant isoform in primary cultured neurons: Assessment by biosynthetic and photoaffinity labelling. *Biochem. J.* **1994**, *301 Pt 2*, 379–384. [CrossRef] [PubMed]
4. Simpson, I.A.; Dwyer, D.; Malide, D.; Moley, K.H.; Travis, A.; Vannucci, S.J. The facilitative glucose transporter GLUT3: 20 years of distinction. *Am. J. Physiol. Endocrinol. Metab.* **2008**, *295*, E242–E253. [CrossRef] [PubMed]
5. Nagamatsu, S.; Kornhauser, J.M.; Burant, C.F.; Seino, S.; Mayo, K.E.; Bell, G.I. Glucose transporter expression in brain. cDNA sequence of mouse GLUT3, the brain facilitative glucose transporter isoform, and identification of sites of expression by in situ hybridization. *J. Biol. Chem.* **1992**, *267*, 467–472. [CrossRef] [PubMed]
6. Lesch, K.P.; Selch, S.; Renner, T.J.; Jacob, C.; Nguyen, T.T.; Hahn, T.; Romanos, M.; Walitza, S.; Shoichet, S.; Dempfle, A.; et al. Genome-wide copy number variation analysis in attention-deficit/hyperactivity disorder: Association with neuropeptide Y gene dosage in an extended pedigree. *Mol. Psychiatry* **2011**, *16*, 491–503. [CrossRef] [PubMed]
7. Peng, W.; Tan, C.; Mo, L.; Jiang, J.; Zhou, W.; Du, J.; Zhou, X.; Liu, X.; Chen, L. Glucose transporter 3 in neuronal glucose metabolism: Health and diseases. *Metabolism* **2021**, *123*, 154869. [CrossRef] [PubMed]
8. Roeske, D.; Ludwig, K.U.; Neuhoff, N.; Becker, J.; Bartling, J.; Bruder, J.; Brockschmidt, F.F.; Warnke, A.; Remschmidt, H.; Hoffmann, P.; et al. First genome-wide association scan on neurophysiological endophenotypes points to trans-regulation effects on SLC2A3 in dyslexic children. *Mol. Psychiatry* **2011**, *16*, 97–107. [CrossRef] [PubMed]
9. Tomi, M.; Zhao, Y.; Thamotharan, S.; Shin, B.C.; Devaskar, S.U. Early life nutrient restriction impairs blood-brain metabolic profile and neurobehavior predisposing to Alzheimer's disease with aging. *Brain Res.* **2013**, *1495*, 61–75. [CrossRef]
10. Zhao, Y.; Fung, C.; Shin, D.; Shin, B.C.; Thamotharan, S.; Sankar, R.; Ehninger, D.; Silva, A.; Devaskar, S.U. Neuronal glucose transporter isoform 3 deficient mice demonstrate features of autism spectrum disorders. *Mol. Psychiatry* **2010**, *15*, 286–299. [CrossRef]
11. Wu, A.; Lee, D.; Xiong, W.C. Lactate Metabolism, Signaling, and Function in Brain Development, Synaptic Plasticity, Angiogenesis, and Neurodegenerative Diseases. *Int. J. Mol. Sci.* **2023**, *24*, 13398. [CrossRef] [PubMed]
12. Simpson, I.A.; Carruthers, A.; Vannucci, S.J. Supply and demand in cerebral energy metabolism: The role of nutrient transporters. *J. Cereb. Blood Flow Metab.* **2007**, *27*, 1766–1791. [CrossRef] [PubMed]

13. Rho, J.M.; Boison, D. The metabolic basis of epilepsy. *Nat. Rev. Neurol.* **2022**, *18*, 333–347. [CrossRef] [PubMed]
14. Aghayan, M.; Rao, L.V.; Smith, R.M.; Jarett, L.; Charron, M.J.; Thorens, B.; Heyner, S. Developmental expression and cellular localization of glucose transporter molecules during mouse preimplantation development. *Development* **1992**, *115*, 305–312. [CrossRef] [PubMed]
15. Ganguly, A.; McKnight, R.A.; Raychaudhuri, S.; Shin, B.C.; Ma, Z.; Moley, K.; Devaskar, S.U. Glucose transporter isoform-3 mutations cause early pregnancy loss and fetal growth restriction. *Am. J. Physiol. Endocrinol. Metab.* **2007**, *292*, E1241–E1255. [CrossRef] [PubMed]
16. Heilig, C.W.; Saunders, T.; Brosius, F.C., 3rd; Moley, K.; Heilig, K.; Baggs, R.; Guo, L.; Conner, D. Glucose transporter-1-deficient mice exhibit impaired development and deformities that are similar to diabetic embryopathy. *Proc. Natl. Acad. Sci. USA* **2003**, *100*, 15613–15618. [CrossRef] [PubMed]
17. Ohtsuki, S.; Kikkawa, T.; Hori, S.; Terasaki, T. Modulation and compensation of the mRNA expression of energy related transporters in the brain of glucose transporter 1-deficient mice. *Biol. Pharm. Bull.* **2006**, *29*, 1587–1591. [CrossRef] [PubMed]
18. Adastra, K.L.; Frolova, A.I.; Chi, M.M.; Cusumano, D.; Bade, M.; Carayannopoulos, M.O.; Moley, K.H. Slc2a8 deficiency in mice results in reproductive and growth impairments. *Biol. Reprod.* **2012**, *87*, 49. [CrossRef] [PubMed]
19. Smith, D.E.; Gridley, T. Differential screening of a PCR-generated mouse embryo cDNA library: Glucose transporters are differentially expressed in early postimplantation mouse embryos. *Development* **1992**, *116*, 555–561. [CrossRef]
20. Pantaleon, M.; Kaye, P.L. Glucose transporters in preimplantation development. *Rev. Reprod.* **1998**, *3*, 77–81. [CrossRef]
21. Matsumoto, K.; Akazawa, S.; Ishibashi, M.; Trocino, R.A.; Matsuo, H.; Yamasaki, H.; Yamaguchi, Y.; Nagamatsu, S.; Nagataki, S. Abundant expression of GLUT1 and GLUT3 in rat embryo during the early organogenesis period. *Biochem. Biophys. Res. Commun.* **1995**, *209*, 95–102. [CrossRef] [PubMed]
22. Khan, J.Y.; Rajakumar, R.A.; McKnight, R.A.; Devaskar, U.P.; Devaskar, S.U. Developmental regulation of genes mediating murine brain glucose uptake. *Am. J. Physiol.* **1999**, *276*, R892–R900. [CrossRef] [PubMed]
23. Brown, K.; Heller, D.S.; Zamudio, S.; Illsley, N.P. Glucose transporter 3 (GLUT3) protein expression in human placenta across gestation. *Placenta* **2011**, *32*, 1041–1049. [CrossRef] [PubMed]
24. Kamei, Y.; Tsutsumi, O.; Yamakawa, A.; Oka, Y.; Taketani, Y.; Imaki, J. Maternal epidermal growth factor deficiency causes fetal hypoglycemia and intrauterine growth retardation in mice: Possible involvement of placental glucose transporter GLUT3 expression. *Endocrinology* **1999**, *140*, 4236–4243. [CrossRef] [PubMed]
25. Shin, B.C.; Fujikura, K.; Suzuki, T.; Tanaka, S.; Takata, K. Glucose transporter GLUT3 in the rat placental barrier: A possible machinery for the transplacental transfer of glucose. *Endocrinology* **1997**, *138*, 3997–4004. [CrossRef] [PubMed]
26. Dawson, P.A.; Mychaleckyj, J.C.; Fossey, S.C.; Mihic, S.J.; Craddock, A.L.; Bowden, D.W. Sequence and functional analysis of GLUT10: A glucose transporter in the Type 2 diabetes-linked region of chromosome 20q12-13.1. *Mol. Genet. Metab.* **2001**, *74*, 186–199. [CrossRef] [PubMed]
27. Janzen, C.; Lei, M.Y.Y.; Jeong, I.S.D.; Ganguly, A.; Sullivan, P.; Paharkova, V.; Capodanno, G.; Nakamura, H.; Perry, A.; Shin, B.C.; et al. Humanin (HN) and glucose transporter 8 (GLUT8) in pregnancies complicated by intrauterine growth restriction. *PLoS ONE* **2018**, *13*, e0193583. [CrossRef]
28. Limesand, S.W.; Regnault, T.R.; Hay, W.W., Jr. Characterization of glucose transporter 8 (GLUT8) in the ovine placenta of normal and growth restricted fetuses. *Placenta* **2004**, *25*, 70–77. [CrossRef] [PubMed]
29. Devaskar, S.U.; Chu, A. Intrauterine Growth Restriction: Hungry for an Answer. *Physiology* **2016**, *31*, 131–146. [CrossRef]
30. Sullivan, E.L.; Smith, M.S.; Grove, K.L. Perinatal exposure to high-fat diet programs energy balance, metabolism and behavior in adulthood. *Neuroendocrinology* **2011**, *93*, 1–8. [CrossRef]
31. Mueckler, M.; Thorens, B. The SLC2 (GLUT) family of membrane transporters. *Mol. Aspects Med.* **2013**, *34*, 121–138. [CrossRef] [PubMed]
32. Scheepers, A.; Joost, H.G.; Schurmann, A. The glucose transporter families SGLT and GLUT: Molecular basis of normal and aberrant function. *JPEN J. Parenter. Enteral Nutr.* **2004**, *28*, 364–371. [CrossRef]
33. Manolescu, A.R.; Witkowska, K.; Kinnaird, A.; Cessford, T.; Cheeseman, C. Facilitated hexose transporters: New perspectives on form and function. *Physiology* **2007**, *22*, 234–240. [CrossRef] [PubMed]
34. Joost, H.G.; Thorens, B. The extended GLUT-family of sugar/polyol transport facilitators: Nomenclature, sequence characteristics, and potential function of its novel members (review). *Mol. Membr. Biol.* **2001**, *18*, 247–256. [CrossRef]
35. Holman, G.D. Structure, function and regulation of mammalian glucose transporters of the SLC2 family. *Pflug. Arch.* **2020**, *472*, 1155–1175. [CrossRef] [PubMed]
36. Kasahara, M.; Hinkle, P.C. Reconstitution and purification of the D-glucose transporter from human erythrocytes. *J. Biol. Chem.* **1977**, *252*, 7384–7390. [CrossRef]
37. Mann, G.E.; Yudilevich, D.L.; Sobrevia, L. Regulation of amino acid and glucose transporters in endothelial and smooth muscle cells. *Physiol. Rev.* **2003**, *83*, 183–252. [CrossRef] [PubMed]
38. Mueckler, M.; Caruso, C.; Baldwin, S.A.; Panico, M.; Blench, I.; Morris, H.R.; Allard, W.J.; Lienhard, G.E.; Lodish, H.F. Sequence and structure of a human glucose transporter. *Science* **1985**, *229*, 941–945. [CrossRef]
39. Fukumoto, H.; Seino, S.; Imura, H.; Seino, Y.; Eddy, R.L.; Fukushima, Y.; Byers, M.G.; Shows, T.B.; Bell, G.I. Sequence, tissue distribution, and chromosomal localization of mRNA encoding a human glucose transporter-like protein. *Proc. Natl. Acad. Sci. USA* **1988**, *85*, 5434–5438. [CrossRef]

40. Kayano, T.; Fukumoto, H.; Eddy, R.L.; Fan, Y.S.; Byers, M.G.; Shows, T.B.; Bell, G.I. Evidence for a family of human glucose transporter-like proteins. Sequence and gene localization of a protein expressed in fetal skeletal muscle and other tissues. *J. Biol. Chem.* **1988**, *263*, 15245–15248. [CrossRef]
41. Koepsell, H. Glucose transporters in brain in health and disease. *Pflug. Arch.* **2020**, *472*, 1299–1343. [CrossRef] [PubMed]
42. Martinez, F.; Cifuentes, M.; Tapia, J.C.; Nualart, F. The median eminence as the hypothalamic area involved in rapid transfer of glucose to the brain: Functional and cellular mechanisms. *J. Mol. Med.* **2019**, *97*, 1085–1097. [CrossRef] [PubMed]
43. Thorens, B.; Mueckler, M. Glucose transporters in the 21st Century. *Am. J. Physiol. Endocrinol. Metab.* **2010**, *298*, E141–E145. [CrossRef] [PubMed]
44. Cushman, S.W.; Wardzala, L.J. Potential mechanism of insulin action on glucose transport in the isolated rat adipose cell. Apparent translocation of intracellular transport systems to the plasma membrane. *J. Biol. Chem.* **1980**, *255*, 4758–4762. [CrossRef] [PubMed]
45. Suzuki, K.; Kono, T. Evidence that insulin causes translocation of glucose transport activity to the plasma membrane from an intracellular storage site. *Proc. Natl. Acad. Sci. USA* **1980**, *77*, 2542–2545. [CrossRef] [PubMed]
46. Wallberg-Henriksson, H.; Zierath, J.R. GLUT4: A key player regulating glucose homeostasis? Insights from transgenic and knockout mice (review). *Mol. Membr. Biol.* **2001**, *18*, 205–211. [CrossRef] [PubMed]
47. Doege, H.; Bocianski, A.; Joost, H.G.; Schurmann, A. Activity and genomic organization of human glucose transporter 9 (GLUT9), a novel member of the family of sugar-transport facilitators predominantly expressed in brain and leucocytes. *Biochem. J.* **2000**, *350 Pt 3*, 771–776. [CrossRef] [PubMed]
48. Lisinski, I.; Schurmann, A.; Joost, H.G.; Cushman, S.W.; Al-Hasani, H. Targeting of GLUT6 (formerly GLUT9) and GLUT8 in rat adipose cells. *Biochem. J.* **2001**, *358*, 517–522. [CrossRef] [PubMed]
49. Ibberson, M.; Riederer, B.M.; Uldry, M.; Guhl, B.; Roth, J.; Thorens, B. Immunolocalization of GLUTX1 in the testis and to specific brain areas and vasopressin-containing neurons. *Endocrinology* **2002**, *143*, 276–284. [CrossRef]
50. Scheepers, A.; Doege, H.; Joost, H.G.; Schurmann, A. Mouse GLUT8: Genomic organization and regulation of expression in 3T3-L1 adipocytes by glucose. *Biochem. Biophys. Res. Commun.* **2001**, *288*, 969–974. [CrossRef]
51. Schmidt, S.; Gawlik, V.; Holter, S.M.; Augustin, R.; Scheepers, A.; Behrens, M.; Wurst, W.; Gailus-Durner, V.; Fuchs, H.; Hrabe de Angelis, M.; et al. Deletion of glucose transporter GLUT8 in mice increases locomotor activity. *Behav. Genet.* **2008**, *38*, 396–406. [CrossRef] [PubMed]
52. Augustin, R.; Carayannopoulos, M.O.; Dowd, L.O.; Phay, J.E.; Moley, J.F.; Moley, K.H. Identification and characterization of human glucose transporter-like protein-9 (GLUT9): Alternative splicing alters trafficking. *J. Biol. Chem.* **2004**, *279*, 16229–16236. [CrossRef] [PubMed]
53. McVie-Wylie, A.J.; Lamson, D.R.; Chen, Y.T. Molecular cloning of a novel member of the GLUT family of transporters, SLC2a10 (GLUT10), localized on chromosome 20q13.1: A candidate gene for NIDDM susceptibility. *Genomics* **2001**, *72*, 113–117. [CrossRef] [PubMed]
54. Segade, F.; Allred, D.C.; Bowden, D.W. Functional characterization of the promoter of the human glucose transporter 10 gene. *Biochim. Biophys. Acta* **2005**, *1730*, 147–158. [CrossRef] [PubMed]
55. Rogers, S.; Macheda, M.L.; Docherty, S.E.; Carty, M.D.; Henderson, M.A.; Soeller, W.C.; Gibbs, E.M.; James, D.E.; Best, J.D. Identification of a novel glucose transporter-like protein-GLUT-12. *Am. J. Physiol. Endocrinol. Metab.* **2002**, *282*, E733–E738. [CrossRef] [PubMed]
56. Wright, E.M.; Loo, D.D.; Hirayama, B.A. Biology of human sodium glucose transporters. *Physiol. Rev.* **2011**, *91*, 733–794. [CrossRef]
57. Chen, J.; Williams, S.; Ho, S.; Loraine, H.; Hagan, D.; Whaley, J.M.; Feder, J.N. Quantitative PCR tissue expression profiling of the human SGLT2 gene and related family members. *Diabetes Ther.* **2010**, *1*, 57–92. [CrossRef] [PubMed]
58. Ferrannini, E.; Solini, A. SGLT2 inhibition in diabetes mellitus: Rationale and clinical prospects. *Nat. Rev. Endocrinol.* **2012**, *8*, 495–502. [CrossRef] [PubMed]
59. Wright, E.M. Renal Na(+)-glucose cotransporters. *Am. J. Physiol. Ren. Physiol.* **2001**, *280*, F10–F18. [CrossRef]
60. Diez-Sampedro, A.; Hirayama, B.A.; Osswald, C.; Gorboulev, V.; Baumgarten, K.; Volk, C.; Wright, E.M.; Koepsell, H. A glucose sensor hiding in a family of transporters. *Proc. Natl. Acad. Sci. USA* **2003**, *100*, 11753–11758. [CrossRef]
61. Baader-Pagler, T.; Eckhardt, M.; Himmelsbach, F.; Sauer, A.; Stierstorfer, B.E.; Hamilton, B.S. SGLT6—A pharmacological target for the treatment of obesity? *Adipocyte* **2018**, *7*, 277–284. [CrossRef] [PubMed]
62. Lin, X.; Ma, L.; Fitzgerald, R.L.; Ostlund, R.E., Jr. Human sodium/inositol cotransporter 2 (SMIT2) transports inositols but not glucose in L6 cells. *Arch. Biochem. Biophys.* **2009**, *481*, 197–201. [CrossRef] [PubMed]
63. Burant, C.F.; Takeda, J.; Brot-Laroche, E.; Bell, G.I.; Davidson, N.O. Fructose transporter in human spermatozoa and small intestine is GLUT5. *J. Biol. Chem.* **1992**, *267*, 14523–14526. [CrossRef] [PubMed]
64. Kayano, T.; Burant, C.F.; Fukumoto, H.; Gould, G.W.; Fan, Y.S.; Eddy, R.L.; Byers, M.G.; Shows, T.B.; Seino, S.; Bell, G.I. Human facilitative glucose transporters. Isolation, functional characterization, and gene localization of cDNAs encoding an isoform (GLUT5) expressed in small intestine, kidney, muscle, and adipose tissue and an unusual glucose transporter pseudogene-like sequence (GLUT6). *J. Biol. Chem.* **1990**, *265*, 13276–13282. [PubMed]
65. Cheeseman, C. GLUT7: A new intestinal facilitated hexose transporter. *Am. J. Physiol. Endocrinol. Metab.* **2008**, *295*, E238–E241. [CrossRef] [PubMed]

66. Wu, X.; Li, W.; Sharma, V.; Godzik, A.; Freeze, H.H. Cloning and characterization of glucose transporter 11, a novel sugar transporter that is alternatively spliced in various tissues. *Mol. Genet. Metab.* **2002**, *76*, 37–45. [CrossRef] [PubMed]
67. Doege, H.; Bocianski, A.; Scheepers, A.; Axer, H.; Eckel, J.; Joost, H.G.; Schurmann, A. Characterization of human glucose transporter (GLUT) 11 (encoded by SLC2A11), a novel sugar-transport facilitator specifically expressed in heart and skeletal muscle. *Biochem. J.* **2001**, *359*, 443–449. [CrossRef]
68. Uldry, M.; Ibberson, M.; Horisberger, J.D.; Chatton, J.Y.; Riederer, B.M.; Thorens, B. Identification of a mammalian H(+)-myo-inositol symporter expressed predominantly in the brain. *EMBO J.* **2001**, *20*, 4467–4477. [CrossRef] [PubMed]
69. Carruthers, A.; DeZutter, J.; Ganguly, A.; Devaskar, S.U. Will the original glucose transporter isoform please stand up! *Am. J. Physiol. Endocrinol. Metab.* **2009**, *297*, E836–E848. [CrossRef]
70. Watts, A.G.; Donovan, C.M. Sweet talk in the brain: Glucosensing, neural networks, and hypoglycemic counterregulation. *Front. Neuroendocrinol.* **2010**, *31*, 32–43. [CrossRef]
71. Haber, R.S.; Weinstein, S.P.; O'Boyle, E.; Morgello, S. Tissue distribution of the human GLUT3 glucose transporter. *Endocrinology* **1993**, *132*, 2538–2543. [CrossRef] [PubMed]
72. Burant, C.F.; Davidson, N.O. GLUT3 glucose transporter isoform in rat testis: Localization, effect of diabetes mellitus, and comparison to human testis. *Am. J. Physiol.* **1994**, *267*, R1488–R1495. [CrossRef] [PubMed]
73. Devaskar, S.U.; Devaskar, U.P.; Schroeder, R.E.; deMello, D.; Fiedorek, F.T., Jr.; Mueckler, M. Expression of genes involved in placental glucose uptake and transport in the nonobese diabetic mouse pregnancy. *Am. J. Obstet. Gynecol.* **1994**, *171*, 1316–1323. [CrossRef] [PubMed]
74. Zhou, J.; Bondy, C.A. Placental glucose transporter gene expression and metabolism in the rat. *J. Clin. Investig.* **1993**, *91*, 845–852. [CrossRef]
75. Mantych, G.J.; James, D.E.; Chung, H.D.; Devaskar, S.U. Cellular localization and characterization of Glut 3 glucose transporter isoform in human brain. *Endocrinology* **1992**, *131*, 1270–1278. [CrossRef] [PubMed]
76. Fung, C.; Evans, E.; Shin, D.; Shin, B.C.; Zhao, Y.; Sankar, R.; Chaudhuri, G.; Devaskar, S.U. Hypoxic-ischemic brain injury exacerbates neuronal apoptosis and precipitates spontaneous seizures in glucose transporter isoform 3 heterozygous null mice. *J. Neurosci. Res.* **2010**, *88*, 3386–3398. [CrossRef] [PubMed]
77. Choeiri, C.; Staines, W.; Messier, C. Immunohistochemical localization and quantification of glucose transporters in the mouse brain. *Neuroscience* **2002**, *111*, 19–34. [CrossRef] [PubMed]
78. Sankar, R.; Thamotharan, S.; Shin, D.; Moley, K.H.; Devaskar, S.U. Insulin-responsive glucose transporters-GLUT8 and GLUT4 are expressed in the developing mammalian brain. *Brain Res. Mol. Brain Res.* **2002**, *107*, 157–165. [CrossRef] [PubMed]
79. Shin, B.C.; Cepeda, C.; Eghbali, M.; Byun, S.Y.; Levine, M.S.; Devaskar, S.U. Adult glut3 homozygous null mice survive to demonstrate neural excitability and altered neurobehavioral responses reminiscent of neurodevelopmental disorders. *Exp. Neurol.* **2021**, *338*, 113603. [CrossRef]
80. Shin, B.C.; Cepeda, C.; Estrada-Sanchez, A.M.; Levine, M.S.; Hodaei, L.; Dai, Y.; Jung, J.; Ganguly, A.; Clark, P.; Devaskar, S.U. Neural Deletion of Glucose Transporter Isoform 3 Creates Distinct Postnatal and Adult Neurobehavioral Phenotypes. *J. Neurosci.* **2018**, *38*, 9579–9599. [CrossRef]
81. Carayannopoulos, M.O.; Xiong, F.; Jensen, P.; Rios-Galdamez, Y.; Huang, H.; Lin, S.; Devaskar, S.U. GLUT3 gene expression is critical for embryonic growth, brain development and survival. *Mol. Genet. Metab.* **2014**, *111*, 477–483. [CrossRef] [PubMed]
82. Stanirowski, P.J.; Lipa, M.; Bomba-Opoń, D.; Wielgoś, M. Expression of placental glucose transporter proteins in pregnancies complicated by fetal growth disorders. *Adv. Protein Chem. Struct. Biol.* **2021**, *123*, 95–131. [CrossRef]
83. Khan, J.Y.; Rajakumar, R.A.; Devaskar, U.P.; Weissfeld, L.A.; Devaskar, S.U. Effect of primary congenital hypothyroidism upon expression of genes mediating murine brain glucose uptake. *Pediatr. Res.* **1999**, *45*, 718–725. [CrossRef]
84. Rajakumar, A.; Thamotharan, S.; Raychaudhuri, N.; Menon, R.K.; Devaskar, S.U. Trans-activators regulating neuronal glucose transporter isoform-3 gene expression in mammalian neurons. *J. Biol. Chem.* **2004**, *279*, 26768–26779. [CrossRef] [PubMed]
85. Rajakumar, R.A.; Thamotharan, S.; Menon, R.K.; Devaskar, S.U. Sp1 and Sp3 regulate transcriptional activity of the facilitative glucose transporter isoform-3 gene in mammalian neuroblasts and trophoblasts. *J. Biol. Chem.* **1998**, *273*, 27474–27483. [CrossRef]
86. Boado, R.J. Post-transcription modulation of the blood-brain barrier GLUT1 glucose transporter by brain-derived factors. *J. Neural Transm. Suppl.* **2000**, *59*, 255–261. [CrossRef]
87. Thamotharan, S.; Stout, D.; Shin, B.C.; Devaskar, S.U. Temporal and spatial distribution of murine placental and brain GLUT3-luciferase transgene as a readout of in vivo transcription. *Am. J. Physiol. Endocrinol. Metab.* **2013**, *304*, E254–E266. [CrossRef] [PubMed]
88. Plassmeyer, S.P.; Florian, C.P.; Kasper, M.J.; Chase, R.; Mueller, S.; Liu, Y.; White, K.M.; Jungers, C.F.; Djuranovic, S.P.; Djuranovic, S.; et al. A Massively Parallel Screen of 5′UTR Mutations Identifies Variants Impacting Translation and Protein Production in Neurodevelopmental Disorder Genes. *medRxiv* **2023**. [CrossRef]
89. Vannucci, S.J.; Reinhart, R.; Maher, F.; Bondy, C.A.; Lee, W.H.; Vannucci, R.C.; Simpson, I.A. Alterations in GLUT1 and GLUT3 glucose transporter gene expression following unilateral hypoxia-ischemia in the immature rat brain. *Brain Res. Dev. Brain Res.* **1998**, *107*, 255–264. [CrossRef]
90. Gronlund, K.M.; Gerhart, D.Z.; Leino, R.L.; McCall, A.L.; Drewes, L.R. Chronic seizures increase glucose transporter abundance in rat brain. *J. Neuropathol. Exp. Neurol.* **1996**, *55*, 832–840. [CrossRef]

91. Leroy, C.; Pierre, K.; Simpson, I.A.; Pellerin, L.; Vannucci, S.J.; Nehlig, A. Temporal changes in mRNA expression of the brain nutrient transporters in the lithium-pilocarpine model of epilepsy in the immature and adult rat. *Neurobiol. Dis.* **2011**, *43*, 588–597. [CrossRef]
92. McClory, H.; Williams, D.; Sapp, E.; Gatune, L.W.; Wang, P.; DiFiglia, M.; Li, X. Glucose transporter 3 is a rab11-dependent trafficking cargo and its transport to the cell surface is reduced in neurons of CAG140 Huntington's disease mice. *Acta Neuropathol. Commun.* **2014**, *2*, 179. [CrossRef]
93. Iuliano, M.; Seeley, C.; Sapp, E.; Jones, E.L.; Martin, C.; Li, X.; DiFiglia, M.; Kegel-Gleason, K.B. Disposition of Proteins and Lipids in Synaptic Membrane Compartments Is Altered in Q175/Q7 Huntington's Disease Mouse Striatum. *Front. Synaptic Neurosci.* **2021**, *13*, 618391. [CrossRef]
94. Acuna, A.I.; Esparza, M.; Kramm, C.; Beltran, F.A.; Parra, A.V.; Cepeda, C.; Toro, C.A.; Vidal, R.L.; Hetz, C.; Concha, I.I.; et al. A failure in energy metabolism and antioxidant uptake precede symptoms of Huntington's disease in mice. *Nat. Commun.* **2013**, *4*, 2917. [CrossRef]
95. Ciarmiello, A.; Cannella, M.; Lastoria, S.; Simonelli, M.; Frati, L.; Rubinsztein, D.C.; Squitieri, F. Brain white-matter volume loss and glucose hypometabolism precede the clinical symptoms of Huntington's disease. *J. Nucl. Med.* **2006**, *47*, 215–222.
96. Gamberino, W.C.; Brennan, W.A., Jr. Glucose transporter isoform expression in Huntington's disease brain. *J. Neurochem.* **1994**, *63*, 1392–1397. [CrossRef]
97. Li, X.; Valencia, A.; McClory, H.; Sapp, E.; Kegel, K.B.; Difiglia, M. Deficient Rab11 activity underlies glucose hypometabolism in primary neurons of Huntington's disease mice. *Biochem. Biophys. Res. Commun.* **2012**, *421*, 727–730. [CrossRef]
98. Vittori, A.; Breda, C.; Repici, M.; Orth, M.; Roos, R.A.; Outeiro, T.F.; Giorgini, F.; Hollox, E.J.; Network, R.i.o.t.E.H.s.D. Copy-number variation of the neuronal glucose transporter gene SLC2A3 and age of onset in Huntington's disease. *Hum. Mol. Genet.* **2014**, *23*, 3129–3137. [CrossRef]
99. Simpson, I.A.; Chundu, K.R.; Davies-Hill, T.; Honer, W.G.; Davies, P. Decreased concentrations of GLUT1 and GLUT3 glucose transporters in the brains of patients with Alzheimer's disease. *Ann. Neurol.* **1994**, *35*, 546–551. [CrossRef]
100. Liu, Y.; Liu, F.; Iqbal, K.; Grundke-Iqbal, I.; Gong, C.X. Decreased glucose transporters correlate to abnormal hyperphosphorylation of tau in Alzheimer disease. *FEBS Lett.* **2008**, *582*, 359–364. [CrossRef]
101. An, Y.; Varma, V.R.; Varma, S.; Casanova, R.; Dammer, E.; Pletnikova, O.; Chia, C.W.; Egan, J.M.; Ferrucci, L.; Troncoso, J.; et al. Evidence for brain glucose dysregulation in Alzheimer's disease. *Alzheimers Dement.* **2018**, *14*, 318–329. [CrossRef]
102. Shabani, K.; Hassan, B.A. The brain on time: Links between development and neurodegeneration. *Development* **2023**, *150*, dev200397. [CrossRef]
103. Cepeda, C.; Oikonomou, K.D.; Cummings, D.; Barry, J.; Yazon, V.W.; Chen, D.T.; Asai, J.; Williams, C.K.; Vinters, H.V. Developmental origins of cortical hyperexcitability in Huntington's disease: Review and new observations. *J. Neurosci. Res.* **2019**, *97*, 1624–1635. [CrossRef]
104. Ratie, L.; Humbert, S. A developmental component to Huntington's disease. *Rev. Neurol.* **2024**, *180*, 357–362. [CrossRef]
105. Arendt, T.; Stieler, J.; Ueberham, U. Is sporadic Alzheimer's disease a developmental disorder? *J. Neurochem.* **2017**, *143*, 396–408. [CrossRef]
106. Merker, S.; Reif, A.; Ziegler, G.C.; Weber, H.; Mayer, U.; Ehlis, A.C.; Conzelmann, A.; Johansson, S.; Muller-Reible, C.; Nanda, I.; et al. SLC2A3 single-nucleotide polymorphism and duplication influence cognitive processing and population-specific risk for attention-deficit/hyperactivity disorder. *J. Child Psychol. Psychiatry* **2017**, *58*, 798–809. [CrossRef]
107. Skeide, M.A.; Kirsten, H.; Kraft, I.; Schaadt, G.; Muller, B.; Neef, N.; Brauer, J.; Wilcke, A.; Emmrich, F.; Boltze, J.; et al. Genetic dyslexia risk variant is related to neural connectivity patterns underlying phonological awareness in children. *Neuroimage* **2015**, *118*, 414–421. [CrossRef]
108. Schmidt, S.; Richter, M.; Montag, D.; Sartorius, T.; Gawlik, V.; Hennige, A.M.; Scherneck, S.; Himmelbauer, H.; Lutz, S.Z.; Augustin, R.; et al. Neuronal functions, feeding behavior, and energy balance in *Slc2a3*$^{+/-}$ mice. *Am. J. Physiol. Endocrinol. Metab.* **2008**, *295*, E1084–E1094. [CrossRef]
109. Stuart, C.A.; Ross, I.R.; Howell, M.E.; McCurry, M.P.; Wood, T.G.; Ceci, J.D.; Kennel, S.J.; Wall, J. Brain glucose transporter (Glut3) haploinsufficiency does not impair mouse brain glucose uptake. *Brain Res.* **2011**, *1384*, 15–22. [CrossRef]
110. Chu, S.Y.; Bachman, D.J.; Callaghan, W.M.; Whitlock, E.P.; Dietz, P.M.; Berg, C.J.; O'Keeffe-Rosetti, M.; Bruce, F.C.; Hornbrook, M.C. Association between obesity during pregnancy and increased use of health care. *N. Engl. J. Med.* **2008**, *358*, 1444–1453. [CrossRef]
111. Yu, Y.; Ma, Q.; Groth, S.W. Prepregnancy dieting and obstetrical and neonatal outcomes: Findings from a national surveillance project in the United States. *Midwifery* **2024**, *132*, 103972. [CrossRef]
112. Bilbo, S.D.; Tsang, V. Enduring consequences of maternal obesity for brain inflammation and behavior of offspring. *FASEB J.* **2010**, *24*, 2104–2115. [CrossRef]
113. Boney, C.M.; Verma, A.; Tucker, R.; Vohr, B.R. Metabolic syndrome in childhood: Association with birth weight, maternal obesity, and gestational diabetes mellitus. *Pediatrics* **2005**, *115*, e290–e296. [CrossRef]
114. Pinney, S.E.; Simmons, R.A. Metabolic programming, epigenetics, and gestational diabetes mellitus. *Curr. Diabetes Rep.* **2012**, *12*, 67–74. [CrossRef]
115. Urbonaite, G.; Knyzeliene, A.; Bunn, F.S.; Smalskys, A.; Neniskyte, U. The impact of maternal high-fat diet on offspring neurodevelopment. *Front. Neurosci.* **2022**, *16*, 909762. [CrossRef]

116. Sathyapalan, T.; Mellor, D.; Atkin, S.L. Obesity and gestational diabetes. *Semin. Fetal Neonatal Med.* **2010**, *15*, 89–93. [CrossRef]
117. Sweeting, A.; Wong, J.; Murphy, H.R.; Ross, G.P. A Clinical Update on Gestational Diabetes Mellitus. *Endocr. Rev.* **2022**, *43*, 763–793. [CrossRef]
118. Grayson, B.E.; Levasseur, P.R.; Williams, S.M.; Smith, M.S.; Marks, D.L.; Grove, K.L. Changes in melanocortin expression and inflammatory pathways in fetal offspring of nonhuman primates fed a high-fat diet. *Endocrinology* **2010**, *151*, 1622–1632. [CrossRef]
119. Srinivasan, M.; Katewa, S.D.; Palaniyappan, A.; Pandya, J.D.; Patel, M.S. Maternal high-fat diet consumption results in fetal malprogramming predisposing to the onset of metabolic syndrome-like phenotype in adulthood. *Am. J. Physiol. Endocrinol. Metab.* **2006**, *291*, E792–E799. [CrossRef]
120. Ganguly, A.; Devaskar, S.U. High-fat diet affects pregestational adiposity and glucose tolerance perturbing gestational placental macronutrient transporters culminating in an obese offspring in wild-type and glucose transporter isoform 3 heterozygous null mice. *J. Nutr. Biochem.* **2018**, *62*, 192–201. [CrossRef]
121. Jones, H.N.; Woollett, L.A.; Barbour, N.; Prasad, P.D.; Powell, T.L.; Jansson, T. High-fat diet before and during pregnancy causes marked up-regulation of placental nutrient transport and fetal overgrowth in C57/BL6 mice. *FASEB J.* **2009**, *23*, 271–278. [CrossRef]
122. Rosario, F.J.; Kanai, Y.; Powell, T.L.; Jansson, T. Increased placental nutrient transport in a novel mouse model of maternal obesity with fetal overgrowth. *Obesity* **2015**, *23*, 1663–1670. [CrossRef] [PubMed]
123. Ganguly, A.; Touma, M.; Thamotharan, S.; De Vivo, D.C.; Devaskar, S.U. Maternal Calorie Restriction Causing Uteroplacental Insufficiency Differentially Affects Mammalian Placental Glucose and Leucine Transport Molecular Mechanisms. *Endocrinology* **2016**, *157*, 4041–4054. [CrossRef] [PubMed]
124. Chizhikov, D.; Buddington, R.K.; Iskusnykh, I.Y. Effects of Phosphatidylserine Source of Docosahexaenoic Acid on Cerebellar Development in Preterm Pigs. *Brain Sci.* **2020**, *10*, 475. [CrossRef]
125. Colombo, J.; Carlson, S.E.; Cheatham, C.L.; Shaddy, D.J.; Kerling, E.H.; Thodosoff, J.M.; Gustafson, K.M.; Brez, C. Long-term effects of LCPUFA supplementation on childhood cognitive outcomes. *Am. J. Clin. Nutr.* **2013**, *98*, 403–412. [CrossRef]
126. Neuringer, M.; Connor, W.E. n-3 fatty acids in the brain and retina: Evidence for their essentiality. *Nutr. Rev.* **1986**, *44*, 285–294. [CrossRef]
127. Uauy, R.; Birch, E.; Birch, D.; Peirano, P. Visual and brain function measurements in studies of n-3 fatty acid requirements of infants. *J. Pediatr.* **1992**, *120*, S168–S180. [CrossRef]
128. Shin, B.C.; Ghosh, S.; Dai, Y.; Byun, S.Y.; Calkins, K.L.; Devaskar, S.U. Early life high-fat diet exposure maintains glucose tolerance and insulin sensitivity with a fatty liver and small brain size in the adult offspring. *Nutr. Res.* **2019**, *69*, 67–81. [CrossRef] [PubMed]
129. Stachowiak, E.K.; Srinivasan, M.; Stachowiak, M.K.; Patel, M.S. Maternal obesity induced by a high fat diet causes altered cellular development in fetal brains suggestive of a predisposition of offspring to neurological disorders in later life. *Metab. Brain Dis.* **2013**, *28*, 721–725. [CrossRef]
130. Boison, D. New insights into the mechanisms of the ketogenic diet. *Curr. Opin. Neurol.* **2017**, *30*, 187–192. [CrossRef]
131. Dynka, D.; Kowalcze, K.; Paziewska, A. The Role of Ketogenic Diet in the Treatment of Neurological Diseases. *Nutrients* **2022**, *14*, 5003. [CrossRef] [PubMed]
132. Wheless, J.W. History of the ketogenic diet. *Epilepsia* **2008**, *49* (Suppl. S8), 3–5. [CrossRef] [PubMed]
133. Klepper, J.; Akman, C.; Armeno, M.; Auvin, S.; Cervenka, M.; Cross, H.J.; De Giorgis, V.; Della Marina, A.; Engelstad, K.; Heussinger, N.; et al. Glut1 Deficiency Syndrome (Glut1DS): State of the art in 2020 and recommendations of the international Glut1DS study group. *Epilepsia Open* **2020**, *5*, 354–365. [CrossRef] [PubMed]
134. Seidner, G.; Alvarez, M.G.; Yeh, J.I.; O'Driscoll, K.R.; Klepper, J.; Stump, T.S.; Wang, D.; Spinner, N.B.; Birnbaum, M.J.; De Vivo, D.C. GLUT-1 deficiency syndrome caused by haploinsufficiency of the blood-brain barrier hexose carrier. *Nat. Genet.* **1998**, *18*, 188–191. [CrossRef] [PubMed]
135. Kim, S.H.; Shaw, A.; Blackford, R.; Lowman, W.; Laux, L.C.; Millichap, J.J.; Nordli, D.R., Jr. The ketogenic diet in children 3 years of age or younger: A 10-year single-center experience. *Sci. Rep.* **2019**, *9*, 8736. [CrossRef] [PubMed]
136. Lyons, L.; Schoeler, N.E.; Langan, D.; Cross, J.H. Use of ketogenic diet therapy in infants with epilepsy: A systematic review and meta-analysis. *Epilepsia* **2020**, *61*, 1261–1281. [CrossRef] [PubMed]
137. Martin-McGill, K.J.; Bresnahan, R.; Levy, R.G.; Cooper, P.N. Ketogenic diets for drug-resistant epilepsy. *Cochrane Database Syst. Rev.* **2020**, *6*, CD001903. [CrossRef] [PubMed]
138. Bertoli, S.; Trentani, C.; Ferraris, C.; De Giorgis, V.; Veggiotti, P.; Tagliabue, A. Long-term effects of a ketogenic diet on body composition and bone mineralization in GLUT-1 deficiency syndrome: A case series. *Nutrition* **2014**, *30*, 726–728. [CrossRef] [PubMed]
139. Kang, H.C.; Chung, D.E.; Kim, D.W.; Kim, H.D. Early- and late-onset complications of the ketogenic diet for intractable epilepsy. *Epilepsia* **2004**, *45*, 1116–1123. [CrossRef]
140. Paoli, A.; Rubini, A.; Volek, J.S.; Grimaldi, K.A. Beyond weight loss: A review of the therapeutic uses of very-low-carbohydrate (ketogenic) diets. *Eur. J. Clin. Nutr.* **2013**, *67*, 789–796. [CrossRef]

141. Evangeliou, A.; Vlachonikolis, I.; Mihailidou, H.; Spilioti, M.; Skarpalezou, A.; Makaronas, N.; Prokopiou, A.; Christodoulou, P.; Liapi-Adamidou, G.; Helidonis, E.; et al. Application of a ketogenic diet in children with autistic behavior: Pilot study. *J. Child. Neurol.* **2003**, *18*, 113–118. [CrossRef]
142. Connealy, B.D.; Northrup, H.; Au, K.S. Genetic variations in the GLUT3 gene associated with myelomeningocele. *Am. J. Obstet. Gynecol.* **2014**, *211*, 305.e1–305.e8. [CrossRef]
143. Cheng, C.M.; Kelley, B.; Wang, J.; Strauss, D.; Eagles, D.A.; Bondy, C.A. A ketogenic diet increases brain insulin-like growth factor receptor and glucose transporter gene expression. *Endocrinology* **2003**, *144*, 2676–2682. [CrossRef]
144. Dai, Y.; Zhao, Y.; Tomi, M.; Shin, B.C.; Thamotharan, S.; Mazarati, A.; Sankar, R.; Wang, E.A.; Cepeda, C.; Levine, M.S.; et al. Sex-Specific Life Course Changes in the Neuro-Metabolic Phenotype of Glut3 Null Heterozygous Mice: Ketogenic Diet Ameliorates Electroencephalographic Seizures and Improves Sociability. *Endocrinology* **2017**, *158*, 936–949. [CrossRef]
145. Herrera, E.; Gomez-Coronado, D.; Lasuncion, M.A. Lipid metabolism in pregnancy. *Biol. Neonate* **1987**, *51*, 70–77. [CrossRef]
146. Sussman, D.; Ellegood, J.; Henkelman, M. A gestational ketogenic diet alters maternal metabolic status as well as offspring physiological growth and brain structure in the neonatal mouse. *BMC Pregnancy Childbirth* **2013**, *13*, 198. [CrossRef]
147. Sussman, D.; Germann, J.; Henkelman, M. Gestational ketogenic diet programs brain structure and susceptibility to depression & anxiety in the adult mouse offspring. *Brain Behav.* **2015**, *5*, e00300. [CrossRef]
148. Brodsky, D.; Christou, H. Current concepts in intrauterine growth restriction. *J. Intensive Care Med.* **2004**, *19*, 307–319. [CrossRef]
149. Mandruzzato, G.; Antsaklis, A.; Botet, F.; Chervenak, F.A.; Figueras, F.; Grunebaum, A.; Puerto, B.; Skupski, D.; Stanojevic, M. Intrauterine restriction (IUGR). *J. Perinat. Med.* **2008**, *36*, 277–281. [CrossRef]
150. Barker, D.J.; Godfrey, K.M.; Fall, C.; Osmond, C.; Winter, P.D.; Shaheen, S.O. Relation of birth weight and childhood respiratory infection to adult lung function and death from chronic obstructive airways disease. *BMJ* **1991**, *303*, 671–675. [CrossRef]
151. Baschat, A.A. Neurodevelopment following fetal growth restriction and its relationship with antepartum parameters of placental dysfunction. *Ultrasound Obstet. Gynecol.* **2011**, *37*, 501–514. [CrossRef] [PubMed]
152. Jacobsson, B.; Ahlin, K.; Francis, A.; Hagberg, G.; Hagberg, H.; Gardosi, J. Cerebral palsy and restricted growth status at birth: Population-based case-control study. *BJOG* **2008**, *115*, 1250–1255. [CrossRef] [PubMed]
153. Jarvis, S.; Glinianaia, S.V.; Torrioli, M.G.; Platt, M.J.; Miceli, M.; Jouk, P.S.; Johnson, A.; Hutton, J.; Hemming, K.; Hagberg, G.; et al. Cerebral palsy and intrauterine growth in single births: European collaborative study. *Lancet* **2003**, *362*, 1106–1111. [CrossRef] [PubMed]
154. McCowan, L.; Horgan, R.P. Risk factors for small for gestational age infants. *Best Pract. Res. Clin. Obstet. Gynaecol.* **2009**, *23*, 779–793. [CrossRef] [PubMed]
155. Miller, S.L.; Huppi, P.S.; Mallard, C. The consequences of fetal growth restriction on brain structure and neurodevelopmental outcome. *J. Physiol.* **2016**, *594*, 807–823. [CrossRef] [PubMed]
156. Pryor, J.; Silva, P.A.; Brooke, M. Growth, development and behaviour in adolescents born small-for-gestational-age. *J. Paediatr. Child Health* **1995**, *31*, 403–407. [CrossRef] [PubMed]
157. Vollmer, B.; Edmonds, C.J. School Age Neurological and Cognitive Outcomes of Fetal Growth Retardation or Small for Gestational Age Birth Weight. *Front. Endocrinol.* **2019**, *10*, 186. [CrossRef] [PubMed]
158. Wang, Y.; Fu, W.; Liu, J. Neurodevelopment in children with intrauterine growth restriction: Adverse effects and interventions. *J. Matern. Fetal Neonatal Med.* **2016**, *29*, 660–668. [CrossRef] [PubMed]
159. Sharma, D.; Sharma, P.; Shastri, S. Genetic, metabolic and endocrine aspect of intrauterine growth restriction: An update. *J. Matern. Fetal Neonatal Med.* **2017**, *30*, 2263–2275. [CrossRef]
160. Gazzolo, D.; Marinoni, E.; Di Iorio, R.; Lituania, M.; Marras, M.; Bruschettini, M.; Bruschettini, P.; Frulio, R.; Michetti, F.; Petraglia, F.; et al. High maternal blood S100B concentrations in pregnancies complicated by intrauterine growth restriction and intraventricular hemorrhage. *Clin. Chem.* **2006**, *52*, 819–826. [CrossRef]
161. Gazzolo, D.; Marinoni, E.; di Iorio, R.; Lituania, M.; Bruschettini, P.L.; Michetti, F. Circulating S100beta protein is increased in intrauterine growth-retarded fetuses. *Pediatr. Res.* **2002**, *51*, 215–219. [CrossRef] [PubMed]
162. Florio, P.; Marinoni, E.; Di Iorio, R.; Bashir, M.; Ciotti, S.; Sacchi, R.; Bruschettini, M.; Lituania, M.; Serra, G.; Michetti, F.; et al. Urinary S100B protein concentrations are increased in intrauterine growth-retarded newborns. *Pediatrics* **2006**, *118*, e747–e754. [CrossRef] [PubMed]
163. Iskusnykh, I.Y.; Fattakhov, N.; Buddington, R.K.; Chizhikov, V.V. Intrauterine growth restriction compromises cerebellar development by affecting radial migration of granule cells via the JamC/Pard3a molecular pathway. *Exp. Neurol.* **2021**, *336*, 113537. [CrossRef] [PubMed]
164. Janzen, C.; Lei, M.Y.; Cho, J.; Sullivan, P.; Shin, B.C.; Devaskar, S.U. Placental glucose transporter 3 (GLUT3) is up-regulated in human pregnancies complicated by late-onset intrauterine growth restriction. *Placenta* **2013**, *34*, 1072–1078. [CrossRef] [PubMed]
165. Kainulainen, H.; Jarvinen, T.; Heinonen, P.K. Placental glucose transporters in fetal intrauterine growth retardation and macrosomia. *Gynecol. Obstet. Investig.* **1997**, *44*, 89–92. [CrossRef] [PubMed]
166. Ma, Y.; Zhu, M.J.; Uthlaut, A.B.; Nijland, M.J.; Nathanielsz, P.W.; Hess, B.W.; Ford, S.P. Upregulation of growth signaling and nutrient transporters in cotyledons of early to mid-gestational nutrient restricted ewes. *Placenta* **2011**, *32*, 255–263. [CrossRef] [PubMed]
167. Das, U.G.; He, J.; Ehrhardt, R.A.; Hay, W.W., Jr.; Devaskar, S.U. Time-dependent physiological regulation of ovine placental GLUT-3 glucose transporter protein. *Am. J. Physiol. Regul. Integr. Comp. Physiol.* **2000**, *279*, R2252–R2261. [CrossRef] [PubMed]

168. Coan, P.M.; Vaughan, O.R.; Sekita, Y.; Finn, S.L.; Burton, G.J.; Constancia, M.; Fowden, A.L. Adaptations in placental phenotype support fetal growth during undernutrition of pregnant mice. *J. Physiol.* **2010**, *588*, 527–538. [CrossRef] [PubMed]
169. Ganguly, A.; Collis, L.; Devaskar, S.U. Placental glucose and amino acid transport in calorie-restricted wild-type and Glut3 null heterozygous mice. *Endocrinology* **2012**, *153*, 3995–4007. [CrossRef]
170. Lesage, J.; Hahn, D.; Leonhardt, M.; Blondeau, B.; Breant, B.; Dupouy, J.P. Maternal undernutrition during late gestation-induced intrauterine growth restriction in the rat is associated with impaired placental GLUT3 expression, but does not correlate with endogenous corticosterone levels. *J. Endocrinol.* **2002**, *174*, 37–43. [CrossRef]
171. Reinisch, J.M.; Simon, N.G.; Karow, W.G.; Gandelman, R. Prenatal exposure to prednisone in humans and animals retards intrauterine growth. *Science* **1978**, *202*, 436–438. [CrossRef] [PubMed]
172. Motta, K.; Gomes, P.R.L.; Sulis, P.M.; Bordin, S.; Rafacho, A. Dexamethasone Administration During Late Gestation Has No Major Impact on Lipid Metabolism, but Reduces Newborn Survival Rate in Wistar Rats. *Front. Physiol.* **2018**, *9*, 783. [CrossRef] [PubMed]
173. Crowther, C.A.; Ashwood, P.; Andersen, C.C.; Middleton, P.F.; Tran, T.; Doyle, L.W.; Robinson, J.S.; Harding, J.E.; Group, A.S. Maternal intramuscular dexamethasone versus betamethasone before preterm birth (ASTEROID): A multicentre, double-blind, randomised controlled trial. *Lancet Child Adolesc. Health* **2019**, *3*, 769–780. [CrossRef] [PubMed]
174. Alawadhi, M.; Mouihate, A.; Kilarkaje, N.; Al-Bader, M. Progesterone partially recovers placental glucose transporters in dexamethasone-induced intrauterine growth restriction. *Reprod. Biomed. Online* **2022**, *44*, 595–607. [CrossRef] [PubMed]
175. Sadiq, H.F.; Das, U.G.; Tracy, T.F.; Devaskar, S.U. Intra-uterine growth restriction differentially regulates perinatal brain and skeletal muscle glucose transporters. *Brain Res.* **1999**, *823*, 96–103. [CrossRef]
176. Ye, X.; Shin, B.C.; Baldauf, C.; Ganguly, A.; Ghosh, S.; Devaskar, S.U. Developing Brain Glucose Transporters, Serotonin, Serotonin Transporter, and Oxytocin Receptor Expression in Response to Early-Life Hypocaloric and Hypercaloric Dietary, and Air Pollutant Exposures. *Dev. Neurosci.* **2021**, *43*, 27–42. [CrossRef] [PubMed]
177. Baldauf, C.; Sondhi, M.; Shin, B.C.; Ko, Y.E.; Ye, X.; Lee, K.W.; Devaskar, S.U. Murine maternal dietary restriction affects neural Humanin expression and cellular profile. *J. Neurosci. Res.* **2020**, *98*, 902–920. [CrossRef]
178. Garg, M.; Thamotharan, M.; Dai, Y.; Lagishetty, V.; Matveyenko, A.V.; Lee, W.N.; Devaskar, S.U. Glucose intolerance and lipid metabolic adaptations in response to intrauterine and postnatal calorie restriction in male adult rats. *Endocrinology* **2013**, *154*, 102–113. [CrossRef]
179. Thamotharan, S.; Raychaudhuri, N.; Tomi, M.; Shin, B.C.; Devaskar, S.U. Hypoxic adaptation engages the CBP/CREST-induced coactivator complex of Creb-HIF-1alpha in transactivating murine neuroblastic glucose transporter. *Am. J. Physiol. Endocrinol. Metab.* **2013**, *304*, E583–E598. [CrossRef]
180. Maggiotto, L.V.; Sondhi, M.; Shin, B.C.; Garg, M.; Devaskar, S.U. Circulating blood cellular glucose transporters—Surrogate biomarkers for neonatal hypoxic-ischemic encephalopathy assessed by novel scoring systems. *Mol. Genet. Metab.* **2019**, *127*, 166–173. [CrossRef]

nutrients

MDPI

Review

Neuronutrition and Its Impact on Post-Stroke Neurorehabilitation: Modulating Plasticity Through Diet

Irene Ciancarelli [1,2], Giovanni Morone [1,3,*], Marco Iosa [4,5], Antonio Cerasa [6,7], Rocco Salvatore Calabrò [8] and Maria Giuliana Tozzi Ciancarelli [1]

1 Department of Life, Health and Environmental Sciences, University of L'Aquila, 67100 L'Aquila, Italy; irene.ciancarelli@univaq.it (I.C.); mariagiuliana.tozzi@guest.univaq.it (M.G.T.C.)
2 ASL 1 Abruzzo (Avezzano-Sulmona-L'Aquila), 67100 L'Aquila, Italy
3 San Raffaele Institute of Sulmona, 67039 Sulmona, Italy
4 Department of Psychology, Sapienza University of Rome, 00185 Rome, Italy; marco.iosa@uniroma1.it
5 IRCCS Fondazione Santa Lucia, 00179 Rome, Italy
6 Institute of BioImaging and Complex Biological Systems (IBSBC-CNR), Via T. Campanella, 88100 Catanzaro, Italy; antonio.cerasa@cnr.it
7 S. Anna Institute, 88900 Crotone, Italy
8 IRCCS Centro Neurolesi Bonino Pulejo, 98124 Messina, Italy; roccos.calabro@irccsme.it
* Correspondence: giovanni.morone@univaq.it

Abstract: The recovery of neurological deficits after ischemic stroke largely depends on the brain's ability to reorganize its undamaged neuronal circuits and neuronal plasticity phenomena. The consolidated evidence highlights the involvement of the patient's impaired nutritional conditions in post-stroke recovery and unsatisfying rehabilitative outcomes. Standardized nutritional protocols usually applied in hospitalized patients in a rehabilitation setting aim mainly to improve the general health conditions of patients, do not consider the high inter-individual variability in neurorehabilitation outcomes, and are not sufficiently modifiable to provide neuroprotective and restorative dietary patterns that could promote neuronal plasticity and functional recovery during neurorehabilitation. Neuronutrition, an emergent scientific field of neuroscience, represents a valid model of a personalized nutritional approach, assuring, for each patient, nutrients having antioxidant and anti-inflammatory properties, ensuring a balanced microbiota composition, and providing adequate neurotrophic support, essential for improving neuronal plasticity, brain functional recovery, and rehabilitative outcomes. In the present narrative review, we provide an overview of the current knowledge on neuronutrition as an adjuvant strategy of a personalized nutritional approach potentially effective in improving post-stroke neuroplasticity and neurorehabilitation by counteracting or at least limiting post-stroke oxidative/nitrosative stress, neuroinflammation, and gut–brain axis disturbance.

Keywords: stroke; rehabilitation; neuronutrition; oxidative stress; inflammation; gut microbiota; gut–brain axis

Citation: Ciancarelli, I.; Morone, G.; Iosa, M.; Cerasa, A.; Calabrò, R.S.; Tozzi Ciancarelli, M.G. Neuronutrition and Its Impact on Post-Stroke Neurorehabilitation: Modulating Plasticity Through Diet. *Nutrients* **2024**, *16*, 3705. https://doi.org/10.3390/nu16213705

Academic Editor: Arved Weimann

Received: 30 September 2024
Revised: 21 October 2024
Accepted: 25 October 2024
Published: 30 October 2024

1. Introduction

The recovery of neurological deficits after ischemic stroke, maximal in the subacute phase and much less effective in the chronic phase, largely depends on neuronal plasticity phenomena that trigger the brain's capacity to reorganize its undamaged circuits through new connections, particularly increased in the cerebral tissue surrounding the necrotic area [1,2]. Parallel processes of the remodelling of neurovascular units start to allow connections among neurons and blood vessels, essential for providing nutritional substances to the brain [3–5]. Neurorehabilitation facilitates post-stroke brain reorganization and modulates neuronal excitability in damaged networks by developing neurobiologically guided therapies that exploit behavioural and neural signals to stimulate neuroplasticity [4–7]. Functional recovery after stroke and the effectiveness of rehabilitation treatment are strongly characterized by a high inter-individual variability dependent, at least in part, on neural signals driving plasticity that is modulated by genetic polymorphisms and epigenetic modifications of DNA that can "switch on" or "switch off" the gene-mediated response to internal or external bodily factors [8–10]. Moreover, different biological and clinical variables, pre-existing or resulting from ischemic brain damage, interfere with each other, thus influencing the rehabilitation response of each patient and the progress of the functional recovery [7,10,11]. Among the verifiable post-stroke complications, some of them could be avoided as reported and recommended by numerous stroke guidelines [7,12,13]. A poor nutritional status/malnutrition is one of the most frequent and common problems among stroke patients upon admission to hospital in a rehabilitation setting. The sequelae of the stroke such as dysphagia, hemiparesis, reduced mobility, sarcopenia, cognitive impairment/depression, and/or pre-existing stroke comorbidities, indeed, contribute to the deterioration of nutritional conditions also in patients not malnourished before the stroke's occurrence, and impair the neurorehabilitation effectiveness [14–16]. Optimizing nutritional management and monitoring the nutritional status in all phases of stroke are, therefore, out of the question and among the urgent purposes in stroke care. Clinical evidence shows that the nutritional condition on admission predicts the rehabilitation outcomes. For patients with an adequate nutritional status at admission, there is insufficient evidence to support nutritional interventions [17], while they are strongly recommended for patients with malnutrition and for those at risk [17,18]. The link between the effectiveness of nutrition interventions for patients with an impaired nutritional status and rehabilitation effectiveness is also underlined by studies showing improved conventional outcome measures (the NIH Stroke Scale, the Barthel Index, the modified Rankin Scale, and the Functional Independence Measure), used to examine the neurological results and functional independence of patients after nutritional treatment [19–23]. Therefore, nutrition, due to its pleiotropic properties and in compliance with the neuroprotective and restorative needs required by the brain recovery process, is confirmed as a crucial exigency for post-stroke rehabilitative outcomes. Standardized nutritional protocols usually applied in hospitalized patients and in rehabilitation settings aim to improve mostly general health conditions of patients, namely, those with a poor nutritional status or with evident malnutrition, to reduce common clinical comorbidities, and avoid a delay in starting neurorehabilitation treatment and its decreased effectiveness. Nutritional interventions, in fact, often translates only into an increase in caloric and nutritional intake, various types of food supplementation, and a supplementation of minerals and vitamins, with particular emphasis on protein intake essential for correcting the protein–energy imbalance and counteracting muscle atrophy and sarcopenia [24–27]. In addition, homologated nutrition interventions, generally used for hospitalized patients, do not consider the high inter-individual variability in rehabilitation outcomes and are not changeable enough to provide dietary patterns that, owing to their specific neuroprotective properties, may favour neuroplasticity and, therefore, functional recovery during neurorehabilitation [17]. Oxidative stress and inflammation are strongly involved in the mechanisms underlying ischemic injury and repair processes following brain damage as well in the alterations in the nutritional status of stroke patients [5]. Based on this evidence, reinforced antioxidant and anti-inflammatory defence has been proposed as a strategy to facilitate brain recovery and improve the nutritional status. Accordingly, the experimental findings endorse the potential of this approach. Evidence from non-human studies suggests that docosahexaenoic acid (DHA) enhances the expression of brain-derived neurotrophic factor (BDNF) and provides a positive influence against tissue damage induced by brain injury [28]. Positive effects on neuroplasticity, neurogenesis, and cerebral blood flow were attributed to flavonoids, a family of compounds present in several edible plants with antioxidant and anti-inflammatory properties [29–31]. However, the translation of these experimental results into clinical practice still requires the definition of several aspects, and it is not conclusive [29]. There is now a great deal of interest in considering the conceptual framework of neuronutrition, an emerging scientific field of nutritional systems biology that places at the centre of its objectives the need for a personalized intervention and the consequent tailored dietetic program [5,32,33]. Technologies collectively called "-omics" enable the simultaneous measurement of an impressive number of biomolecules that can be potential markers for both the inter-individual capacity with which each patient responds to rehabilitation treatment, and the mechanisms with which dietary patterns are able to activate cellular signaling pathways involved in neuroplasticity [34,35]. Furthermore, the opportunity to empower patients to take an active role in their neurorehabilitative program, according to the principles of 5P medicine (predictive, preventive, participatory, personalized, and precision medicine) [36], could facilitate the adherence to consume a personalized diet based on the daily intake of nutrients promoting functional recovery and neurorehabilitation outcomes (Table 1). In this narrative review, we report the available evidence on the potential properties of some neuronutrients to influence positively the recovery processes and rehabilitative outcomes by interfering with post-stroke oxidative/nitrosative stress, neuroinflammation, and gut–brain axis disturbance.

Table 1. Dietary sources of nutrients with potential influence on the mechanisms involved on post-stroke recovery and rehabilitation effectiveness.

Food Sources	Bioactive Substances	Specific Effects	References
Legumes, fruits, vegetables, fish, extra virgin olive oil, fish and nut oils, and leafy vegetables	Omega-3 fatty acids: EPA, DHA, and DPA	Improved neurotransmission, neuronal membrane fluidity, cell signalling, neuronal plasticity, BDNF, and microbiota composition (taxonomic groups producing SCFA); improved rehabilitation outcomes	[5,28,29,31,35,37–41]
Vegetables, green tea, coffee, wine, extra virgin olive oil, and well-balanced diet (the Mediterranean diet, MD)	Polyphenols	Antioxidant and anti-inflammatory properties; neuroprotection; scavenging free radicals, chelating metals, dampening pro-oxidative enzymes	[27,32,35,37–39,42,43]
Fruits, legumes, animal red meats, poultry, beef or sheep liver, seafood, eggs, herbs, spices, high dietary fiber intake, nuts, seeds, and whole grain products	Minerals (Zn, Mg, Se, and Cu)	Co-factors of antioxidant enzyme, long-term regulation of systemic inflammation, and metabolic homeostasis	[24–27,43–49]
Well-balanced diet, vegetables, fruits, dairy products, egg yolk, and offal and liver of pigs, sheep, and cattle.	Vitamins (A, C, E, D, B group, and K2)	Antioxidants and anti-inflammatory; anti-apoptosis; and neurorestorative (post-stroke recovery, rehabilitation effectiveness)	[27,44,47,50,51]
Diet with high fat, moderate protein content, and low carbohydrates (ketogenic diet)	Ketone bodies (acetone, and β hydroxybutyrate acetoacetate)	Prevention of mitochondrial dysfunction, decreased oxidative and inflammatory damage, and GABA release	[52–55]
Fruits, legumes, and vegetables	dietary fiber (carbohydrate polymers, and non-digestible carbohydrates)	Gut microbiome composition, intestinal peristalsis, acid–base balance, and decreased proinflammatory cytokines	[5,27,47]

2. General Overview on Functional Recovery Mechanism after Stroke

After cerebral ischemic injury, neural plasticity and brain tissue reorganization intervene in damaged and non-damaged areas of the brain. Cellular and molecular mechanisms with multiple underlying pathways, highly interconnected among themselves, are involved at restoring, replacing, and compensating brain-damaged structures and lost functions, albeit within certain limits, thus allowing neurorehabilitation training to use neural circuits modelled on new functional connections and the pruning of non-functional ones [11]. More understanding of the biological basis of this complex process is essential in order to develop new therapeutic approaches and rehabilitative strategies pivotal to improving functional recovery. As is known, the interruption of blood flow and the consequent deprivation of O_2 and nutrients to the ischemic area lead to metabolic changes of the surrounding neurons, altered mitochondrial activity, the disruption of the blood–brain barrier, oedema, inflammation, and a strong imbalance of the vulnerable equilibrium between the generation of free radicals and the antioxidant defence [56–58]. The persistence after ischemic onset of the excessive generation and release of reactive oxygen species (ROS) and reactive nitrogen species (RNS), together with a long-lasting depletion of endogenous antioxidant defences, triggers cellular cytotoxic pathways responsible for neuronal necrosis and apoptosis, and remodelling cell–cell signalling, such as neurogenesis and angiogenesis [59]. The activation of transcription factors and proinflammatory gene expression results in an increased secretion of inflammatory cytokines [5,42]. Inflammation exacerbates the ischemic injury in the early phase and influences post-stroke recovery in the late phase, persisting for days and gradually fading away within weeks after the stroke's onset. Microglia undergo activation and assume the role of one of the most important cellular components of post-stroke inflammation. Moreover, brain-resident cell-mediated inflammation represents the main source of oxidative stress after a stroke's onset [5,42]. Oxidative stress and inflammation after stroke onset could represent, therefore, an interesting target to develop nutritional procedures as an adjuvant strategy to support post-stroke recovery and neuronal plasticity. Many bioactive molecules found in foods offer a potential positive influence on cerebral recovery as antioxidant and anti-inflammatory agents [35,60,61], even though their molecular structure, solubility, food matrix, and gut microbiota metabolism limit their bioavailability and absorption. Interestingly, efficacious technologies, now tested, may improve the above-mentioned limiting factors [62].

In concert with cerebral tissue repair and neuronal plasticity, vascular remodeling patterns occur. Angiogenesis is a protective tissue mechanism that promotes neural regeneration and functional recovery after stroke. Neurons and astrocytes express angiogenic factors to promote microvascular growth, and newly formed microvessels influence brain tissue repair via the release of growth factors such as BDNF [63–68]. In this scenario, the brain's capacity for restoring lost functions and recovery proceeds spontaneously in the early period after stroke and then with compensatory neuronal plasticity based on the reorganization of neural circuits, the creation of new functional communications in the remaining neuronal circuits, and the enhancement of neuronal activity in pre-existing damaged networks [1,5]. Notably, the effectiveness of neuron plasticity depends on many factors including the patient's clinical history, age, and education. Interestingly, evidence supports that there is a sort of brain cognitive reserve in skilled individuals that may have an impact on the recovery process [67]. Neurorehabilitation, as already reported, facilitates post-stroke brain reorganization and exerts a positive influence over ongoing neuronal plasticity. Of note, individual variability in response to rehabilitation treatment depends on different factors among which the patient's nutritional status and clinical history are determinants. A rehabilomic approach, based on the analysis of candidate biomarkers expressing the mechanisms of functional recovery, may provide a valid integration of the patient's clinical data to offer personalized nutritional interventions needed to optimize individual neurorehabilitation outcomes [69].

3. Neuronutrition as an Adjuvant Strategy in Post-Stroke Neurorehabilitation

Eating disabilities are frequent clinical complications that affect the nutritional status of patients after stroke, namely, aged individuals, and result in the development of unsatisfactory adherence to neurorehabilitation treatment because of stroke-associated sarcopenia with the consequent exacerbated loss of physical strength and fatigue, as well depressive behavioural aspects [70]. Moreover, the frequent aging- and stroke-induced impairment of taste and smell decreasing the physiologic pleasure of palatable foods further results in a decreased daily dietary intake [71]. Behind dysphagia, which is one of the most important complications following a stroke, the penalizing dependence on help for eating, together with disempowerment, boredom, frustration, and, in more serious cases, cognitive impairment, has, in fact, a detrimental impact on the proper quantity and composition of everyday food intake. The consequent nutritional deficiencies, specific or global, are crucial for the patient's nutritional condition and negatively influence neurorehabilitation effectiveness [22–24]. The benefits of proper dietary patterns underline how the synergic interactions between diet components and the adequate intake of macronutrients, micronutrients, and bioactive substances contained in them are a fundamental requirement for maintaining one's health status that, however, cannot be separated from a healthy lifestyle, especially regular physical activity [72,73]. Furthermore, the long-term consumption of balanced diets could prevent or attenuate the deterioration of cognitive functions and, possibly, the onset and progression of neurodegenerative diseases frequent, namely, in aging individuals [33]. The mechanisms associated with the benefits of proper dietary patterns are multiple, and include antioxidant and anti-inflammatory activity, the modulation of gut microbiota and gut functions, and increased neurotrophic support, as well as decreased neuronal damage [5]. Neuronutrition represents a valid model of a personalized nutritional approach toward optimizing neurological health, preventing neurological diseases, and favoring brain recovery in the event of damage, as occurs for neurodegenerative diseases and stroke [33,74]. Improving eating behavior through the correction of the patient's diet altered by stroke and adopting dietary patterns with selected and appropriate foods with antioxidant and anti-inflammatory activity are essential in order to enhance post-stroke brain structural and functional recovery so as create clinical conditions favorable to rehabilitation outcomes. Oxidative/nitrosative stress, inflammation, gut–brain axis disturbance, and neurotransmitter imbalance are the more significant targets of neuronutrition [33,75–77]. According to the neuronutrition conceptual purpose, dietary patterns based on foods having bioactive components interfering with the main mechanisms induced by stroke onset could positively influence brain repair, and improve plasticity and functional recovery, thus favouring rehabilitative effectiveness.

4. Neuronutrition and Crosstalk Between Oxidative/Nitrosative Stress and Inflammation

Determining nutritional needs to support recovery and metabolic demands for post-stroke patients undergoing neurorehabilitation is difficult due to multifactorial conditions, including the altered patient feeding behaviour, altered levels of autonomic dysfunction, and hypercatabolic state, which interfere with brain recovery and all bodily repair processes [33,77–80]. Studies performed mainly on neurodegenerative diseases have emphasized the promising influence of a variety of foods, individual nutrients, and dietary habits on stemming or, at least, limiting oxidative/nitrosative stress and inflammation, as well as on strengthening antioxidant defences [74–78]. The hypothesis that nutrients or dietary patterns influencing the crosstalk between oxidative stress and inflammation could provide a neuroprotective influence on post-stroke recovery mechanisms and improve rehabilitative responsiveness remains of great interest. The relative findings are few, in fact, and there is no evidence, as far as we know, of the involvement of specific dietary patterns or single nutrients, present normally in foods, on rehabilitation outcomes because of their antioxidant and anti-inflammatory properties [27,57,81,82].

4.1. *Oxidative/Nitrosative Stress and Inflammation*

As is widely known, physiologic amounts of ROS and RNS are generated by all cells to act as signaling molecules, while the release of large amounts triggers or amplifies inflammation via an upregulation of different genes that code for proinflammatory cytokines and adhesion molecules working in the immune defense mechanism [83,84]. The consequent crosstalk between oxidative/nitrosative stress and inflammation is dynamically modulated by oxidative metabolites that activate inflammatory-signaling pathways, and by inflammatory cytokines that keep the oxidative stress "on" [5]. The development of brain-resident cell-mediated inflammation promotes the expansion of the ischemic lesion, blood–brain barrier dysfunction, and systemic inflammatory response that negatively affect the brain repair process [42,57–59]. A variety of enzymes and non-enzymatic molecules widely distributed in the intra- and extra-cellular compart constitutes the powerful antioxidant body's system. Antioxidants, both endogenous and derived from diet, may mitigate the oxidative/nitrosative stress by removing potential oxidants or transforming them into less reactive compounds and tone down the cytokine storm and inflammation [77,78,84].

Superoxide dismutase (SOD), catalase, glutathione (GSH), GSH peroxidase (GPx), thioreductase, and uric acid are the main endogenous antioxidants. Of note, albumin, whose oxidized form is considered as a marker of oxidative stress, is actively involved in the redox status via its multiple-binding sites and free-radical-trapping properties that, overall, potentiate the bodily antioxidant status. The most relevant are connected to its ability to bind and transport in the systemic circulation bilirubin, polyunsaturated fatty acids, many dietary flavonoids, and polyvalent metal ions [85]. Main dietary sources of antioxidants include vitamins A, C, and E, as well as polyphenolic compounds and minerals. Folate and the B vitamins, crucial in the metabolism of methionine, exert a positive influence on antioxidant GSH, central to a variety of processes [44]. An excessive ROS amount induces the activation of the nuclear factor erythroid 2-related factor (Nrf2), a transcription factor recognizing the antioxidant response element that, in turn, increases the expression and activity of superoxide dismutase, glutathione peroxidases, and catalase, and reduces lipid peroxidation in brain tissue. Interestingly, the phytoalexin resveratrol exhibits a neuroprotective influence by inhibiting inflammation via the activation of the Nrf2 pathway [86,87]. Exogenous antioxidants such as polyphenols, polyunsaturated fatty acids (PUFAs), and vitamins A and C, as well as vitamin D could express neurorestorative effects essential for post-stroke recovery and rehabilitation effectiveness [27,42,43]. Therefore, antioxidant- and anti-inflammatory-rich foods could stop or modulate the stroke-associated oxidative and inflammatory chain reactions and provide a neuroprotective influence essential for enhancing the recovery process.

4.2. Role of Minerals in the Oxidative/Nitrosative Stress and Inflammation

The research findings showed the importance of the mineral intake in oxidative stress and inflammation, and mineral homeostasis might be a sensitive indicator of oxidative stress and inflammation in stroke patients [43,45–49]. Many studies underlined the essential role of some minerals such as zinc, magnesium, copper, and selenium, and their potential for antioxidant activity, not through the direct scavenging of free radicals, but instead through their requirement as regulatory co-factors in different antioxidant enzyme functions. The source of these elements is only foods of animal and vegetable origin, and the detrimental impact of eating disabilities on the everyday food intake of patients could account for their frequent deficiency. High levels of zinc (Zn) are present in the brain where it assumes multiples roles. Zinc deficiency results in weight loss and poor food efficiency [43,46]. The restoration of body weight, extremely important in assuring the effectiveness of rehabilitative interventions, should include adequate zinc in the diet [45]. Together with copper (Cu), Zn is a component of Cu/Zn superoxide dismutase that is responsible for scavenging superoxide anions and preventing nitric oxide decomposition at the vascular endothelium level [5]. Moreover, Zn absorption is reduced by a vitamin A deficiency [46]. Selenium (Se) is a dietary trace element that, in the form of selenoproteins, possesses remarkable antioxidant properties, immune functions, and metabolic homeostasis [47]. Glutathione peroxidase is a selenocysteine-dependent enzyme important for scavenging hydrogen peroxide and is strictly dependent on Cu/Zn and Cu/Se molar ratios and the serum availability of these elements [44]. The source of organic Se is mushrooms and foods, both of animal (animal red meats, poultry, beef or sheep liver, seafood, eggs, and dairy products) and plant origin. A deficiency of Se, as for other foods, can easily occur in stroke patients who are less likely to consume a variety of beneficial foods, have poorer eating habits, and have an impoverished dietary quality [47]. Magnesium (Mg) maintains cell membrane stability, participates as a cofactor of several enzymes involved in energy metabolism, controls the calcium influx to the neurons as a NMDA receptor blocker, and works as an antioxidant mitigating the effects of oxidative stress [48]. Fruits and vegetables, as well as nuts, seeds, and whole grain products, are the main natural sources of magnesium. However, its absorption is only 30–40% of what is consumed [48]. Inadequate levels of magnesium, zinc, copper, iron, and selenium impair immune competence and the long-term regulation of systemic inflammation [49]. Overall, the improper eating habits that often occur because of the patients' insufficient food intake contribute to the long-lasting cytotoxic effects of stroke-induced oxidative stress and impair the regulation of inflammation.

4.3. *Effects of Antioxidant and Anti-Inflammatory Diets: The Mediterranean Diet and Ketogenic Diet*

As already mentioned, reducing some of the post-stroke malnutrition-associated consequences is essential so as not to hinder rehabilitation programs. Restoring nutritional deficiencies and re-accustoming the patient to correct eating behavior are an integral part of stroke management. The apparent benefits of the Mediterranean diet (MD) are ascribed to the variety of foods, including aromatic herbs and spices (phytochemicals, vitamins, poly-unsaturated fatty acids, dietary fibers, trace elements, etc.), which, and not individually, work as powerful modulators of oxidative stress and inflammation and endothelial function [27,47]. It is widely known that the consumption of legumes, fruits, vegetables, fish, extra virgin olive oil, fish and nut oils, and leafy vegetables for their content of omega-3 (n-3) fatty acids docosahexaenoic acid (DHA) and eicosapentaenoic acid (EPA), polyphenols, vitamins, and minerals could improve neurotransmission and modulate neuronal membrane fluidity, essential for supporting cell signaling and neuronal plasticity [32,35,37–39]. Furthermore, adherence to the MD is associated with a high microbiota diversity, with a positive balance between commensal and pathogenic bacteria, and a proper production of neurotransmitters and SCFAs, necessary to ensure the correct functioning of the intestinal barrier [40]. Of interest, re-accustoming the patient to the palatable foods that characterize the core constituent of this eco-sustainable dietary model could contribute to lessening the impairment of taste and smell frequently observed in post-stroke patients.

The hypothesis that the ketogenic diet can supply necessary calories to all body functions shifting the physiologic energetic source from carbohydrate to fat has recently suggested its use, beyond epilepsy and weight loss, as a treatment of neurologic diseases in which the neuron mitochondria are dysfunctional and the impairment of energy metabolism, increased oxidative stress, and inflammation occur, as is the case with stroke [52,53]. Ketone bodies (KBs) comprise acetone, acetoacetate, and β-hydroxybutyrate, and are produced mostly in the liver and in glial cells, namely, astrocytes [53]. Many experimental studies underlined the pleiotropic properties of KBs in animal models and their positive influence in improving or preventing mitochondrial dysfunction as well as in mitigating oxidative and inflammatory damage [88]. There is evidence that KBs can inhibit increased neuronal excitability by modifying pre-synaptic concentrations and the release of the inhibitory γ-aminobutyric acid neurotransmitter (GABA) [54]. A ketogenic diet may also provide neuroprotective effects by improving the mitochondrial function that results in increased mitochondrial energy reserves, with anti-inflammatory effects, together with a Nrf2-induced decrease of ROS generation [88,89]. Accordingly, with the above reported evidence, a ketogenic diet could be an alternative strategy with which to improve rehabilitative outcomes by targeting the crosstalk between oxidative stress and inflammation, particularly burdensome in obese and type II diabetic patients [55].

5. Neuronutrition and Stroke-Induced Gut–Brain Axis Disturbance

A schematic representation of the impact of neuronutrition on stroke-induced gut–brain axis disturbance is reported in the Figure 1.

In stroke, the brain–gut axis is altered, and morphological and functional consequences in both directions occur. Stroke-induced oxidative stress and inflammation are involved in the gut dysbiosis and in malnutrition, compromising brain functional repair and rehabilitation effectiveness. Neuronutrition can revert the dysbiosis, positively influence the gut–brain axis signalling, and improve post-stroke recovery by reducing the neuroinflammation oxidative stress, and restoring the microbiota composition improves rehabilitative outcomes.

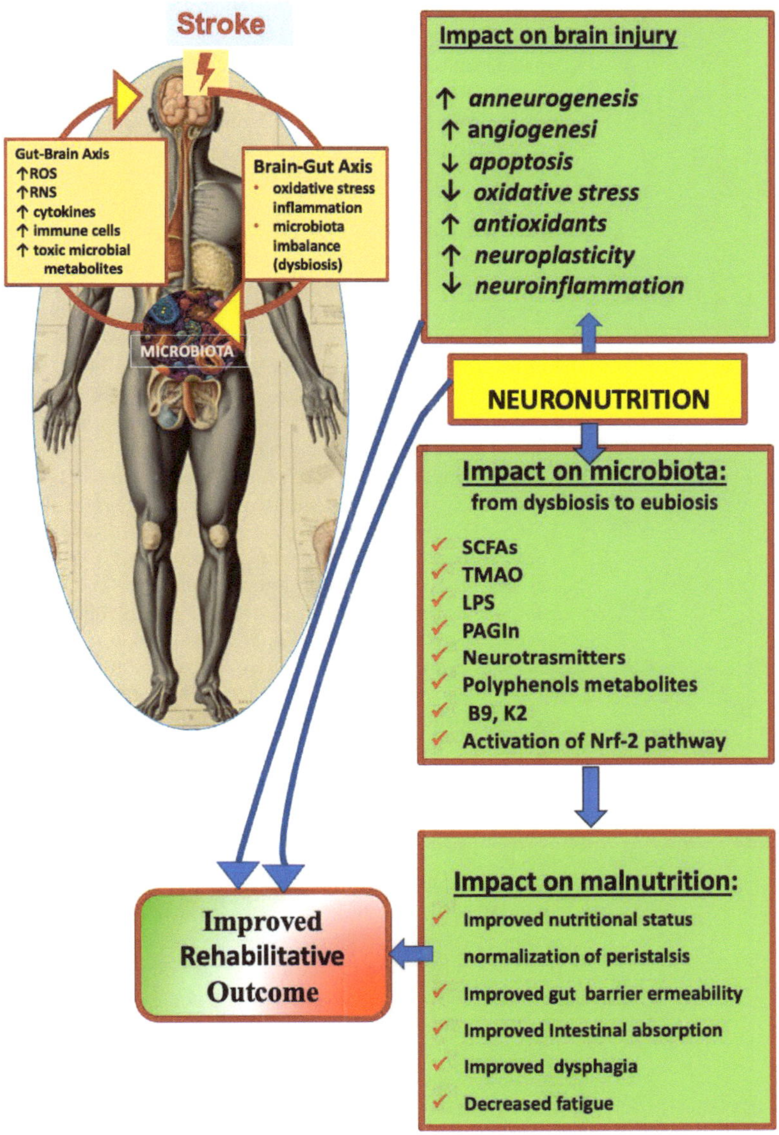

Figure 1. Schematic representation of the impact of neuronutrition on stroke-induced gut–brain axis disturbance.

ROS, reactive oxygen species; RNS, reactive nitrogen species; Nrf-2: nuclear factor erythroid 2-related factor; SCFAs: short-chain fatty acids; BAs: bile acids; TMAO: trimethylamine. *N*-oxide; LPSs: lipopolysaccharides; PAGln: phenylacetylglutamine. ↓ decreasese; ↑ increase.

5.1. The Gut–Brain Axis, the Gut Microbiota, and Eubiosis

Articulate bidirectional mechanisms, known as brain-to-gut and gut-to-brain signaling pathways, allow an efficient connection between the brain and the gut and vice versa. In the top-down mechanism, the brain strongly controls the functions of the entire gastrointestinal tract (from peristaltic movements, to the permeability of the intestinal barrier, to the release of neurotransmitters and stress hormones, to the activation of resident immune cells, to the gut microbiome) by means of a multiple signaling system (the vagus nerve, sympathetic prevertebral ganglia, endocrine, immune, humoral links, and gut microbiota) [90]. The gut-to-brain signaling mechanism, also known as the microbiota–gut–brain axis, on the other hand, is, overall, a dynamic system of humoral and nervous afferents to the brain to elicit adequate responses to a vast number of humoral signals coming from the environment. It involves different neural pathways involving vagal and/or spinal afferent fibers, the endocrine system, the hypothalamic–pituitary–adrenal axis, the immune system, and the microbiota and microbiome-derived metabolites [91]. The modulating factor that fulfills a predominant role in gut–brain communication is the gut microbiota, an intestinal ecosystem of a population of fungi, archaea, virus, bacteria, and parasites that, together with a diverse array of microbiome-derived metabolites, interacts with all structures of the intestine to maintain gut homeostasis [91]. The human gut microbiome (1 kg in a healthy and adult subject) is a complex system that resides primarily in the lower gut and lives in a symbiotic relationship with the human host. It consists of approximately more than trillions of microorganisms in a stable ratio themselves. The Firmicutes (F) (e.g., Lactobacillus, Clostridium, and Enterococcus) and Bacteroidetes (B) (e.g., Bacteroides) phyla represent the majority of these intestinal taxonomic categories [92–94]. Changes in the abundance of some bacterial taxa were observed in many diseases associated with inflammation [95]. The features of the entire gastrointestinal tract (pH, mucus layer, intestinal redox potential, age of the subject, etc.) and a sensible feedback mechanism cooperating within the microbial community assure a balanced gut microbiota composition, eubiosis, and regulate microbiota growth and stability [93]. Diet and host characteristics including the nutritional status, age, and genetics interfere with the composition of the intestinal microbiota and modify their signaling activity [94,95]. The gut microbiota produces a variety of compounds such as short-chain fatty acids (SCFAs), bile acids (BAs), trimethylamine N-oxide (TMAO), lipopolysaccharides (LPSs), and phenylacetylglutamine (PAGln) [92]. Of note, evidence underlined that the gut microbiota has the capability to produce a range of neurotransmitters as γ-aminobutyric acid, noradrenaline, and dopamine, and that neurotransmitter modulation represents the ways by which the microbiota communicates along the gut–brain axis [94–96]. Moreover, efficacious antioxidants, such as bioactive polyphenol-derived metabolites and vitamins such B9 and K2, are also produced by specific microbiota components [50,51]. Interestingly, Lactobacillus spp., a component of the gut microbiota and major group of lactic acid bacteria, play an important antioxidant role by activating the Nrf-2 pathway in response to an excessive ROS/NRS availability in the gut tract, resulting from both the ability of some commensal and pathogenic bacteria to alter their basal generation of mitochondrial ROS, and from the oxidative damage associated with neuroinflammation that characterizes neurodegenerative diseases and ischemic stroke [97,98]. There are multiple and significant factors, independent of pathological conditions, that contribute to shaping the microbiota composition. Dietary eating patterns and the gut microbiota composition are closely connected to each other. Interestingly, a short-term dietary change can alter gut microbial populations within 24 h, although the main enterotypes remain largely unmodified [41,99,100]. Dietary eating patterns (e.g., a high intake of saturated fat and simple sugars) are determinant factors, which are, above all, modifiable, that may modify the biodiversity and representation of taxa with a prevalence of Bacteroidetes, and decreased levels of Firmicutes in humans, as well as preclinical models [101]. On the other hand, the regular consumption of omega-3 fatty acids, found in fatty fish or leafy vegetables, led to increased circulating acids docosahexaenoic acid (DHA) and eicosapentaenoic acid (EPA) that may revert the microbiota composition by stimulating taxonomic groups producing SCFA, thus influencing the gut–brain axis [41]. Macronutrient and fiber contents are important in determining the microbiota composition and its effect on health outcomes and behavior. In addition to the composition of nutrients, the time of food intake and eating patterns have been shown to affect the gut microbiota. The mechanisms through which the microbiota exerts its beneficial or detrimental influences are yet to be better defined, but the elaboration of signaling molecules and the recognition of bacterial epitopes by both intestinal epithelial and mucosal immune cells could be involved [93]. Compelling evidence shows that the gut microbiota influences the nutritional and metabolic homeostasis modulating appetite and food intake, thus preserving a proper nutritional status [5].

5.2. Stroke-Induced Modifications of the Gut–Brain Axis and Dysbiosis

Deregulated, the microbiota–gut–brain axis depends on many factors leading to a series of structural and functional consequences, among which, essentially, are the decreased expression of tight junction proteins with a consequent increased intestinal barrier permeability (leaky gut syndrome), increased secretion of pro-inflammatory cytokines, and modified blood–brain barrier permeability with the consequent excessive translocation of immune cells and toxic microbial metabolites into the brain, [91,93,102]. Qualitative and quantitative changes of the microbiota species, each of them with a different catabolism capacity, determine the dysbiosis that is involved in several inflammatory diseases such as obesity, type 2 diabetes, several cardiovascular diseases, neurodegenerative diseases, and ischemic stroke [101–104]. Evidence suggests that stroke-associated oxidative stress and inflammation can be involved in the destruction of the balanced and physiologic composition of the gut microbiota and can trigger the harmful condition of gut microbiota dysbiosis [5,76,105]. Experimental studies from animal models of stroke showed a significant alteration in the bacterial composition characterized by an excessive growth and amount of the Bacteroidetes phylum and Prevotella genus, together with a significant decrease in the Firmicutes phylum, as well as the Faecalibacterium, Oscillospira, and Lactobacillus genera [106–109]. Clinical evidence supports the experimental studies and shows that the gut microbiota in patients with stroke was significantly changed in quantitative and qualitative composition [110–112]. Dysbiosis in stroke patients consists in an increase of opportunistic pathogens (Streptococcus and Bacteroide) and a decreased number of SCFA-producing bacteria with a consequent decreased plasma concentration of butyrate, essential for the integrity of the intestinal barrier, in the inhibition of the pro-inflammatory cytokine production, and involved in neurogenesis and angiogenesis mechanisms. Of interest, significant associations have been found between the alterations in distinctive gut microbiota and the severity of the neurologic impairment and global functional prognosis [109,110]. Central is also the role of dysbiosis for modifications of appetite and satiety-regulating systems precipitating or worsening malnutrition due to an altered function of the gut–microbiota–brain axis [5,103,104]. Malnutrition and stroke-related symptoms, such as fatigue syndrome, and sarcopaenia, as well as cardio–respiratory–muscle deconditioning are recognized as useful predictors of limited mobility and negatively affect neuronal plasticity and functional recovery, constituting, thus, a real barrier to stroke rehabilitation, namely, physical exercise training [103].

5.3. The Gut Microbiota as a Potential Target for Post-Stroke Functional Recovery

Many studies report evidence that the gut microbiota and their metabolites might be considered as an interesting target for post-stroke functional recovery because of their influence on multiple mechanisms via the gut–microbiota–brain axis. Although the relationship between the gut microbiota and post-stroke brain remodeling is yet to be defined, restoring post-stroke dysbiosis is the initial approach for promoting neuroplasticity, stroke recovery, and rehabilitation effectiveness [76,113–115]. Findings in animal stroke models show that the normalization of stroke-induced dysbiosis (e.g., a reduction in the levels of Bacteroidetes and an increase in the Proteobacteria and Firmicutes population or SCFA-producing bacteria) mitigates neurological deficits, and improves post-stroke recovery by decreasing inflammation oxidative stress and restoring the SCFA-producing bacteria amount that regulate the levels of BDNF, a well-known neurotrophic factor involved as a keystone molecule in neuroplasticity, learning, and memory [116–119]. It is known that the recovery of motor function after stroke is mediated by neuroplasticity [120]. Studies on developing rehabilitation strategies aimed at facilitating and maximizing functional outcomes post-stroke showed an emergent role of BDNF as a key facilitator of neuroplasticity involved in motor learning and rehabilitation after stroke [121]. Experimental findings showed that probiotic or prebiotic supplementation improves the microbiota composition that, in turn, increases BDNF levels in various brain regions [2,122]. Their role as inflammatory modulators has been well-evidenced in experimental studies [123]. Evidence demonstrated that the immune modulation performed by probiotics might be due to the release in the gut of the anti-inflammatory cytokine [120]. Therefore, the regular intake of probiotics, especially in malnourished stroke patients, might be useful for maintaining the homeostasis of the gut microbiota, and then the proper working of the gut–brain axis, by preventing the destruction of tight junction proteins and inhibiting pathogenic bacterial overgrowth and the consequent infections. Among the natural compounds enhancing neuroplasticity, polyphenols, a wide family of molecules present in many food sources (vegetables, red fruits, green tea, coffee, and wine), show neuroprotective properties such as strong antioxidants and anti-inflammatory molecules [27,60]. However, the beneficial effectiveness of these compounds for the brain repair mechanisms after a stroke is strictly dependent on the amount consumed and their effective availability, via the systemic circulation, on the neurovascular units adjacent to the ischemic lesion. Further investigation and controlled clinical studies are necessary in order to validate their therapeutic efficacy.

6. Conclusions

Stroke-related long-term sequelae and their high social and economic burden require effective and affordable measures, improving brain functional recovery and the effectiveness of rehabilitative treatment. The recognition of the role of neuronutrition as an adjuvant strategy for integrating the brain recovery processes emerges from experimental research findings that have demonstrated how the properties of some nutrients and dietary patterns can contribute to influencing the post-stroke recovery processes by interfering with oxidative stress, inflammation, and gut–brain axis disturbance. Limited information is still available on how experimental results might translate to the recovery of patients after stroke. Rigorous studies in prospective clinical trials are therefore required in order to verify whether the experimental nutritional interventions on animal models or in vitro research can find clinical applications. Of note, the complexity of human nutritional intervention makes it difficult to attribute a role/function to isolated dietary components by extrapolating them from the context of the multiple interactions occurring between the different components of a single food and, even more, of the entire dietary pattern. The improvements in the technology and implementation of omics sciences in terms of nutrition and rehabilitation allow us to apply personalized nutrition-based care and a personalized approach to rehabilitation. Indeed, the simultaneous measurement of an enormous number of biomolecules that can "capture" many potential biological factors that contribute to the high inter-individual variability of the stroke recovery course and rehabilitation outcome will be an effective methodologic setting for better results. Advances in our understanding of the mechanisms underlying the impact of nutrition on the brain and the microbiota–gut–brain axis will facilitate the real development of neuronutritional interventions and their clinical application to optimizing post-stroke functional recovery.

Author Contributions: Conceptualization, M.G.T.C. and I.C.; methodology, G.M.; software, M.I.; validation, M.G.T.C., I.C., G.M. and M.I.; investigation, M.G.T.C.; data curation, G.M.; writing—original draft preparation, M.G.T.C.; writing—review and editing, M.G.T.C., I.C. and G.M.; supervision, M.G.T.C., I.C., G.M., A.C. and R.S.C. All authors have read and agreed to the published version of the manuscript.

Funding: This research received no external funding.

Conflicts of Interest: The authors declare no conflicts of interest.

References

1. Cheatwood, J.L.; Emerick, A.J.; Kartje, G.L. Neuronal plasticity and functional recovery after ischemic stroke. *Top. Stroke Rehabil.* **2008**, *15*, 42–50. [CrossRef] [PubMed]
2. Joy, M.T.; Carmichael, S.T. Encouraging an excitable brain state: Mechanisms of brain repair in stroke. *Nat. Rev. Neurosci.* **2021**, *22*, 38–53. [CrossRef] [PubMed]
3. Dąbrowski, J.; Czajka, A.; Zielińska-Turek, J.; Jaroszyński, J.; Furtak-Niczyporuk, M.; Mela, A.; Poniatowski, Ł.A.; Drop, B.; Dorobek, M.; Barcikowska-Kotowicz, M.; et al. Brain Functional Reserve in the Context of Neuroplasticity after Stroke. *Neural Plast.* **2019**, *2019*, 9708905. [CrossRef] [PubMed]
4. Warraich, Z.; Kleim, J.A. Neural plasticity: The biological substrate for neurorehabilitation. *PM&R J. Inj. Funct. Rehabil.* **2010**, *2* (Suppl. 2), S208–S219. [CrossRef]
5. Ciancarelli, I.; Morone, G.; Iosa, M.; Cerasa, A.; Calabrò, R.S.; Iolascon, G.; Gimigliano, F.; Tonin, P.; Tozzi Ciancarelli, M.G. Influence of Oxidative Stress and Inflammation on Nutritional Status and Neural Plasticity: New Perspectives on Post-Stroke Neurorehabilitative Outcome. *Nutrients* **2022**, *15*, 108. [CrossRef]
6. Malik, A.N.; Tariq, H.; Afridi, A.; Rathore, F.A. Technological advancements in stroke rehabilitation. *J. Pak. Med. Assoc.* **2022**, *72*, 1672–1674. [CrossRef] [PubMed]
7. Platz, T. Evidence-based guidelines and clinical pathways in stroke rehabilitation—An international perspective. *Front. Neurol.* **2019**, *10*, 200. [CrossRef]
8. Prabhakaran, S.; Zarahn, E.; Riley, C.; Speizer, A.; Chong, J.Y.; Lazar, R.M.; Marshall, R.S.; Krakauer, J.W. Inter-individual variability in the capacity for motor recovery after ischemic stroke. *Neurorehabil. Neural Repair.* **2008**, *22*, 64–71. [CrossRef]
9. Carnwath, T.P.; Demel, S.L.; Prestigiacomo, C.J. Genetics of ischemic stroke functional outcome. *J. Neurol.* **2024**, *271*, 2345–2369. [CrossRef]
10. Feys, H.; De Weerdt, W.; Nuyens, G.; van de Winckel, A.; Selz, B.; Kiekens, C. Predicting motor recovery of the upper limb after stroke rehabilitation: Value of a clinical examination. *Physiother. Res. Int.* **2000**, *5*, 1–18. [CrossRef]
11. Boyd, L.A.; Hayward, K.S.; Ward, N.S.; Stinear, C.M.; Rosso, C.; Fisher, R.J.; Carter, A.R.; Le, A.P.; Copland, D.A.; Carey, L.M.; et al. Biomarkers of Stroke Recovery: Consensus-Based Core Recommendations from the Stroke Recovery and Rehabilitation Roundtable. *Int. J. Stroke* **2017**, *12*, 480–493. [CrossRef]
12. Winstein, C.J.; Stein, J.; Arena, R.; Bates, B.; Cherney, L.R.; Cramer, S.C.; Deruyter, F.; Eng, J.J.; Fisher, B.; Harvey, R.L.; et al. Guidelines for adult stroke rehabilitation and recovery: A guideline for healthcare professionals from the American Heart Association/American Stroke Association. *Stroke* **2016**, *47*, e98–e169. [CrossRef] [PubMed]
13. Rehman, M.U.; Wali, A.F.; Ahmad, A.; Shakeel, S.; Rasool, S.; Ali, R.; Rashid, S.M.; Madkhali, H.; Ganaie, M.A.; Khan, R. Neuroprotective Strategies for Neurological Disorders by Natural Products: An update. *Curr. Neuropharmacol.* **2019**, *17*, 247–267. [CrossRef] [PubMed]
14. Hao, R.; Qi, X.; Xia, X.; Wang, L.; Li, X. Malnutrition on admission increases the in-hospital mortality and length of stay in elder adults with acute ischemic stroke. *J. Clin. Lab. Anal.* **2021**, *36*, e24132. [CrossRef] [PubMed]
15. Sabbouh, T.; Torbey, M.T. Malnutrition in Stroke Patients: Risk Factors, Assessment, and Management. *Neurocrit. Care* **2017**, *29*, 374–384. [CrossRef]
16. Yoo, S.-H.; Kim, J.S.; Kwon, S.U.; Yun, S.-C.; Koh, J.-Y.; Kang, D.-W. Undernutrition as a Predictor of Poor Clinical Outcomes in Acute Ischemic Stroke Patients. *Arch. Neurol.* **2008**, *65*, 39–43. [CrossRef]
17. Ko, S.H.; Shin, Y.I. Nutritional Supplementation in Stroke Rehabilitation: A Narrative Review. *Brain Neurorehabil.* **2022**, *15*, e3. [CrossRef]
18. Dennis, M.; Lewis, S.; Cranswick, G.; Forbes, J.; FOOD Trial Collaboration. FOOD: A multicenter randomized animals trial evaluating feeding policies in patients admitted to hospital with a recent stroke. *Health Technol. Assess.* **2006**, *10*, iii–iv; ix–x; 1–120. [CrossRef] [PubMed]
19. Scrutinio, D.; Lanzillo, B.; Guida, P.; Passantino, A.; Spaccavento, S.; Battista, P. Association Between Malnutrition and Outcomes in Patients with Severe Ischemic Stroke Undergoing Rehabilitation. *Arch. Phys. Med. Rehabil.* **2020**, *101*, 852–860. [CrossRef]
20. Liu, J.; Dong, J.; Guo, J. The effects of nutrition supplement on rehabilitation for patients with stroke: Analysis based on 16 randomized controlled trials. *Medicine* **2022**, *101*, e29651. [CrossRef]
21. Huppertz, V.; Guida, S.; Holdoway, A.; Strilciuc, S.; Baijens, L.; Schols, J.M.G.A.; van Helvoort, A.; Lansink, M.; Muresanu, D.F. Impaired Nutritional Condition After Stroke from the Hyperacute to the Chronic Phase: A Systematic Review and Meta-Analysis. *Front. Neurol.* **2022**, *12*, 780080. [CrossRef] [PubMed]
22. Rabadi, M.H.; Coar, P.L.; Lukin, M.; Lesser, M.; Blass, J.P. Intensive nutritional supplements can improve outcomes in stroke rehabilitation. *Neurology* **2008**, *71*, 1856–1861. [CrossRef] [PubMed]
23. Kishimoto, H.; Yozu, A.; Khono, Y.; Oose, H. Nutritional improvement is associated with better functional outcome in stroke rehabilitation: A cross-sectional study using controlling in nutritional status. *J. Rehabil. Med.* **2020**, *52*, jrm00028. [CrossRef] [PubMed]
24. Lieber, A.C.; Hong, E.; Putrino, D.; Nistal, D.A.; Pan, J.S.; Kellner, C.P. Nutrition, Energy Expenditure, Dysphagia, and Self-Efficacy in Stroke Rehabilitation: A Review of the Literature. *Brain Sci.* **2018**, *8*, 218. [CrossRef] [PubMed]

25. Yoshimura, Y.; Bise, T.; Shimazu, S.; Tanoue, M.; Tomioka, Y.; Araki, M.; Nishino, T.; Kuzuhara, A.; Takatsuki, F. Effects of a leucine-enriched amino acid supplement on muscle mass; muscle strength; and physical function in post-stroke patients with sarcopenia: A randomized controlled trial. *Nutrition* **2018**, *58*, 1–6. [CrossRef]
26. Aquilani, R.; Scocchi, M.; Iadarola, P.; Franciscone, P.; Verri, M.; Boschi, F.; Pasini, E.; Viglio, S. Protein supplementation may enhance the spontaneous recovery of neurological alterations in patients with ischaemic stroke. *Clin. Rehabil.* **2008**, *22*, 1042–1050. [CrossRef]
27. Zielinska-Nowak, E.; Cichon, N.; Saluk-Bijak, J.; Bijak, M.; Miller, E. Nutritional Supplements and Neuroprotective Diets and Their Potential Clinical Significance in Post-Stroke Rehabilitation. *Nutrients* **2021**, *13*, 2704. [CrossRef]
28. Sun, G.Y.; Simonyi, A.; Fritsche, K.L.; Chuang, D.Y.; Hannink, M.; Gu, Z.; Greenlief, C.M.; Yao, J.K.; Lee, J.C.; Beversdorf, D.Q. Docosahexaenoic acid (DHA): An essential nutrient and a nutraceutical for brain health and diseases. *Prostaglandins Leukot. Essent. Fat. Acids* **2018**, *136*, 3–13. [CrossRef] [PubMed] [PubMed Central]
29. Briones-Valdivieso, C.; Briones, F.; Orellana-Urzúa, S.; Chichiarelli, S.; Saso, L.; Rodrigo, R. Novel Multi-Antioxidant Approach for Ischemic Stroke Therapy Targeting the Role of Oxidative Stress. *Biomedicines* **2024**, *12*, 501. [CrossRef] [PubMed] [PubMed Central]
30. Grabska-Kobyłecka, I.; Szpakowski, P.; Król, A.; Książek-Winiarek, D.; Kobyłecki, A.; Głąbiński, A.; Nowak, D. Polyphenols and Their Impact on the Prevention of Neurodegenerative Diseases and Development. *Nutrients* **2023**, *15*, 3454. [CrossRef]
31. Gomes, F.; Emery, P.W.; Weekes, C.E. Risk of malnutrition is an independent predictor of mortality, length of hospital stay, and hospitalization costs in stroke patients. *J. Stroke Cerebrovasc. Dis.* **2016**, *25*, 799–806. [CrossRef] [PubMed]
32. Simmons, L.A.; Dinan, M.A.; Robinson, T.J.; Snyderman, R. Personalized medicine is more than genomic medicine: Confusion over terminology impedes progress towards personalized healthcare. *Pers. Med.* **2012**, *9*, 85–91. [CrossRef] [PubMed]
33. Badaeva, A.V.; Danilov, A.B.; Clayton, P.; Moskalev, A.A.; Karasev, A.V.; Tarasevich, A.F.; Vorobyeva, Y.D.; Novikov, V.N. Perspectives on Neuronutrition in Prevention and Treatment of Neurological Disorders. *Nutrients* **2023**, *15*, 2505. [CrossRef] [PubMed]
34. Adams, S.H.; Anthony, J.C.; Carvajal, R.; Chae, L.; Khoo, C.S.H.; Latulippe, M.E.; Matusheski, N.V.; McClung, H.L.; Rozga, M.; Schmid, C.H.; et al. Perspective: Guiding Principles for the Implementation of Personalized Nutrition Approaches That Benefit Health and Function. *Adv. Nutr.* **2020**, *11*, 25–34. [CrossRef] [PubMed] [PubMed Central]
35. Chen, H.; He, Y.; Chen, S.; Qi, S.; Shen, J. Therapeutic targets of oxidative/nitrosative stress and neuroinflammation in ischemic stroke: Applications for natural product efficacy with omics and systemic biology. *Pharmacol. Res.* **2020**, *158*, 104877. [CrossRef]
36. Pires, I.M.; Denysyuk, H.V.; Villasana, M.V.; Sá, J.; Lameski, P.; Chorbev, I.; Zdravevski, E.; Trajkovik, V.; Morgado, J.F.; Garcia, N.M. Mobile 5P-Medicine Approach for Cardiovascular Patients. *Sensors* **2021**, *21*, 6986. [CrossRef] [PubMed] [PubMed Central]
37. Tozzi Ciancarelli, M.G.; Di Massimo, C.; De Amicis, D.; Ciancarelli, I. Mediterranean Diet and Health Promotion: Evidence and Current Concerns. *Med. Res. Arch.* **2017**, *5*, 1–16. Available online: https://esmed.org/MRA/mra/article/view/1385 (accessed on 1 October 2024). [CrossRef]
38. Gantenbein, K.; Kanaka-Gantenbein, C. Mediterranean Diet as an Antioxidant: The Impact on Metabolic Health and Overall Wellbeing. *Nutrients* **2021**, *13*, 1951. [CrossRef]
39. Nani, A.; Murtaza, B.; Sayed Khan, A.; Khan, N.A.; Hichami, A. Antioxidant and Anti-Inflammatory Potential of Polyphenols Contained in Mediterranean Diet in Obesity: Molecular Mechanisms. *Molecules* **2021**, *26*, 985. [CrossRef]
40. Seethaler, B.; Nguyen, N.K.; Basrai, M.; Kiechle, M.; Walter, J.; Delzenne, N.M.; Bischoff, S.C. Short-chain fatty acids are key mediators of the favorable effects of the Mediterranean diet on intestinal barrier integrity: Data from the randomized controlled LIBRE trial. *Am. J. Clin. Nutr.* **2022**, *116*, 928–942. [CrossRef] [PubMed]
41. Hills, R.D., Jr.; Pontefract, B.A.; Mishcon, H.R.; Black, C.A.; Sutton, S.C.; Theberge, C.R. Gut Microbiome: Profound Implications for Diet and Disease. *Nutrients* **2019**, *11*, 1613. [CrossRef] [PubMed] [PubMed Central]
42. Sanchez-Moreno, C.; Dashe, J.F.; Scott, T.; Thaler, D.; Folstein, M.F.; Martin, A. Decreased Levels of Plasma Vitamin C and Increased Concentrations of Inflammatory and Oxidative Stress Markers After Stroke. *Stroke* **2004**, *35*, 163–168. [CrossRef] [PubMed]
43. Potocnik, F.C.; van Rensburg, S.J.; Hon, D.; Emsley, R.A.; Moodie, I.M.; Erasmus, R.T. Oral zinc augmentation with vitamins A and D increases plasma zinc concentration: Implications for burden of disease. *Metab. Brain Dis.* **2006**, *21*, 139–147. [CrossRef] [PubMed]
44. Miro'nczuk, A.; Kapica-Topczewska, K.; Socha, K.; Soroczy'nska, J.; Jamiołkowski, J.; Kułakowska, A.; Kochanowicz, J. Selenium, Copper, Zinc Concentrations and Cu/Zn, Cu/Se Molar Ratios in the Serum of Patients with Acute Ischemic Stroke in Northeastern Poland-A New Insight into Stroke Pathophysiology. *Nutrients* **2021**, *13*, 2139. [CrossRef] [PubMed]
45. Baltaci, A.K.; Mogulkoc, R. Leptin and zinc relation: In regulation of food intake and immunity. *Indian J. Endocrinol. Metab.* **2012**, *16*, S611–S616. [CrossRef]
46. Hess, S.Y.; McLain, A.C.; Lescinsky, H.; Brown, K.H.; Afshin, A.; Atkin, R.; Osendarp, S.J. Basis for changes in the disease burden estimates related to vitamin A and zinc deficiencies in the 2017 and 2019 Global Burden of Disease Studies. *Public Health Nutr.* **2021**, *25*, 2225–2231. [CrossRef]
47. Bjørklund, G.; Shanaida, M.; Lysiuk, R.; Antonyak, H.; Klishch, I.; Shanaida, V.; Peana, M. Selenium: An Antioxidant with a Critical Role in Anti-Aging. *Molecules* **2022**, *27*, 6613. [CrossRef]
48. Veronese, N.; Barbagallo, M. Magnesium and Micro-Elements in Older Persons. *Nutrients* **2021**, *13*, 847. [CrossRef]

49. Stefanache, A.; Lungu, I.-I.; Butnariu, I.-A.; Calin, G.; Gutu, C.; Marcu, C.; Grierosu, C.; Goroftei, E.R.B.; Duceac, L.-D.; Dabija, M.G.; et al. Understanding How Minerals Contribute to Optimal Immune Function. *J. Immunol. Res.* **2023**, *2023*, 3355733. [CrossRef]
50. Gholami, H.; Chmiel, J.A.; Burton, J.P.; Maleki Vareki, S. The Role of Microbiota-Derived Vitamins in Immune Homeostasis and Enhancing Cancer Immunotherapy. *Cancers* **2023**, *15*, 1300. [CrossRef] [PubMed] [PubMed Central]
51. Wang, D.; Ho, L.; Faith, J.; Ono, K.; Janle, E.M.; Lachcik, P.J.; Cooper, B.R.; Jannasch, A.H.; R D'Arcy, B.; Williams, B.A.; et al. Role of intestinal microbiota in the generation of polyphenol derived phenolic acid mediated attenuation of Alzheimer's disease b-amyloid oligomerization. *Mol. Nutr. Food Res.* **2015**, *59*, 1025–1040. [CrossRef] [PubMed]
52. Haces, M.L.; Hernández-Fonseca, K.; Medina-Campos, O.N.; Montiel, T.; Pedraza-Chaverri, J.; Massieu, L. Antioxidant capacity contributes to protection of ketone bodies against oxidative damage induced during hypoglycemic conditions. *Exp. Neurol.* **2008**, *211*, 85–96. [CrossRef] [PubMed]
53. Jang, J.; Kim, S.R.; Lee, J.E.; Lee, S.; Son, H.J.; Choe, W.; Yoon, K.-S.; Kim, S.S.; Yeo, E.-J.; Kang, I. Molecular Mechanisms of Neuroprotection by Ketone Bodies and Ketogenic Diet in Cerebral Ischemia and Neurodegenerative Diseases. *Int. J. Mol. Sci.* **2024**, *25*, 124. [CrossRef] [PubMed]
54. Dahlin, M.; Elfving, Å.; Ungerstedt, U.; Åmark, P. The ketogenic diet influences the levels of excitatory and inhibitory amino acids in the CSF in children with refractory epilepsy. *Epilepsy Res.* **2005**, *64*, 115–125. [CrossRef] [PubMed]
55. Szili-Torok, T.; de Borst, M.H.; Garcia, E.; Gansevoort, R.T.; Dullaart, R.P.F.; Connelly, M.A.; Bakker, S.J.L.; Tietge, U.J.F. Fasting Ketone Bodies and Incident Type 2 Diabetes in the General Population. *Diabetes* **2023**, *72*, 1187–1192. [CrossRef] [PubMed] [PubMed Central]
56. Ko, S.B.; Yoon, B.W. Mechanisms of functional recovery after stroke. *Front. Neurol. Neurosci.* **2013**, *32*, 1–8. [CrossRef] [PubMed]
57. Siotto, M.; Germanotta, M.; Santoro, M.; Canali, R.; Pascali, S.; Insalaco, S.; Cipollini, V.; Papadopoulou, D.; Antonacci, E.; Aprile, I. Oxidative Stress Status in Post Stroke Patients: Sex Differences. *Healthcare* **2022**, *10*, 869. [CrossRef]
58. Lakhan, S.E.; Kirchgessner, A.; Hofer, M. Inflammatory mechanisms in ischemic stroke: Therapeutic approaches. *J. Transl. Med.* **2009**, *7*, 97. [CrossRef]
59. Ciancarelli, I.; Di Massimo, C.; De Amicis, D.; Carolei, A.; Ciancarelli, M.G.T. Evidence of redox unbalance in post-acute ischemic stroke patients. *Curr. Neurovasc. Res.* **2012**, *9*, 85–90. [CrossRef]
60. Cichon, N.; Saluk-Bijak, J.; Gorniak, L.; Przyslo, L.; Bijak, M. Flavonoids as a Natural Enhancer of Neuroplasticity—An Overview of the Mechanism of Neurorestorative Action. *Antioxidants* **2020**, *9*, 1035. [CrossRef]
61. Li, H.; Wang, J.; Wang, P.; Rao, Y.; Chen, L. Resveratrol Reverses the Synaptic Plasticity Deficits in a Chronic Cerebral Hypoperfusion Rat Model. *J. Stroke Cerebrovasc. Dis.* **2016**, *25*, 122–128. [CrossRef] [PubMed]
62. Li, L.; Zeng, Y.; Chen, M.; Liu, G. Application of Nanomicelles in Enhancing Bioavailability and Biological Efficacy of Bioactive Nutrients. *Polymers* **2022**, *14*, 3278. [CrossRef] [PubMed] [PubMed Central]
63. Hermann, D.M.; Zechariah, A. Implications of vascular endothelial growth factor for postischemic neurovascular remodeling. *J. Cereb. Blood Flow Metab.* **2009**, *29*, 1620–1643. [CrossRef] [PubMed]
64. Guo, H.; Zhou, H.; Lu, J.; Qu, Y.; Yu, D.; Tong, Y. Vascular endothelial growth factor: An attractive target in the treatment of hypoxic/ischemic brain injury. *Neural Regen. Res.* **2016**, *11*, 174–179. [CrossRef] [PubMed] [PubMed Central]
65. Moon, S.; Chang, M.-S.; Koh, S.-H.; Choi, Y.K. Repair Mechanisms of the Neurovascular Unit after Ischemic Stroke with a Focus on VEGF. *Int. J. Mol. Sci.* **2021**, *22*, 8543. [CrossRef]
66. Hermann, D.M.; Chopp, M. Promoting brain remodelling and plasticity for stroke recovery: Therapeutic promise and potential pitfalls of clinical translation. *Lancet Neurol.* **2012**, *11*, 369–380. [CrossRef] [PubMed] [PubMed Central]
67. Dodich, A.; Carli, G.; Cerami, C.; Iannaccone, S.; Magnani, G.; Perani, D. Social and cognitive control skills in long-life occupation activities modulate the brain reserve in the behavioural variant of frontotemporal dementia. *Cortex* **2018**, *99*, 311–318. [CrossRef] [PubMed]
68. Hara, Y. Brain plasticity and rehabilitation in stroke patients. *J. Nippon. Med. Sch.* **2015**, *82*, 4–13. [CrossRef] [PubMed]
69. Cao, W.; Zhang, X.; Qiu, H. Rehabilomics: A state-of-the-art review of framework; application; and future considerations. *Front. Neurol.* **2023**, *14*, 1103349. [CrossRef]
70. Hazelton, C.; McGill, K.; Campbell, P.; Todhunter-Brown, A.; Thomson, K.; Nicolson, D.J.; Cheyne, J.D.; Chung, C.; Dorris, L.; Gillespie, D.C.; et al. Perceptual Disorders After Stroke: A Scoping Review of Interventions. *Stroke* **2022**, *53*, 1772–1787. [CrossRef]
71. Dutta, T.M.; Josiah, A.F.; Cronin, C.A.; Wittenberg, G.F.; Cole, J.W. Altered taste and stroke: A case report and literature review. *Top. Stroke Rehabil.* **2013**, *20*, 78–86. [CrossRef] [PubMed]
72. Norman, K.; Haß, U.; Pirlich, M. Malnutrition in Older Adults—Recent Advances and Remaining Challenges. *Nutrients* **2021**, *13*, 2764. [CrossRef] [PubMed]
73. Melzer, T.M.; Manosso, L.M.; Yau, S.Y.; Gil-Mohapel, J.; Brocardo, P.S. In Pursuit of Healthy Aging: Effects of Nutrition on Brain Function. *Int. J. Mol. Sci.* **2021**, *22*, 5026. [CrossRef] [PubMed]
74. Devi, A.; Narayanan, R. A Review on Neuronutrition. *Asian J. Dairy Food Res.* **2019**, *38*, 128–133. [CrossRef]
75. Holton, K. F Micronutrients May Be a Unique Weapon Against the Neurotoxic Triad of Excitotoxicity, Oxidative Stress and Neuroinflammation: A Perspective. *Front. Neurosci.* **2021**, *15*, 726457. [CrossRef]

76. Chidambaram, S.B.; Rathipriya, A.G.; Mahalakshmi, A.M.; Sharma, S.; Hediyal, T.A.; Ray, B.; Sunanda, T.; Rungratanawanich, W.; Kashyap, R.S.; Qoronfleh, M.W.; et al. The Influence of Gut Dysbiosis in the Pathogenesis and Management of Ischemic Stroke. *Cells* **2022**, *11*, 1239. [CrossRef]
77. Poblete, R.A.; Yaceczko, S.; Aliakbar, R.; Saini, P.; Hazany, S.; Breit, H.; Louie, S.G.; Lyden, P.D.; Partikian, A. Optimization of Nutrition after Brain Injury: Mechanistic and Therapeutic Considerations. *Biomedicines* **2023**, *11*, 2551. [CrossRef]
78. Garbagnati, F.; Cairella, G.; De Martino, A.; Multari, M.; Scognamiglio, U.; Venturiero, V.; Paolucci, S. Is Antioxidant and n–3 Supplementation Able to Improve Functional Status in Poststroke Patients? Results from the Nutristroke Trial. *Cerebrovasc. Dis.* **2009**, *27*, 375–383. [CrossRef]
79. Cha, K.H.; Kang, N.Y.; Huh, S.; Ko, S.H.; Shin, Y.I.; Min, J.H. The Effects of Autonomic Dysfunction on Functional Outcomes in Patients with Acute Stroke. *Brain Sci.* **2023**, *13*, 1694. [CrossRef]
80. Tavarez, T.; Roehl, K.; Koffman, L. Nutrition in the Neurocritical Care Unit: A New Frontier. *Curr. Treat. Options Neurol.* **2021**, *23*, 16–18. [CrossRef]
81. Sakai, K.; Kinoshita, S.; Tsuboi, M.; Fukui, R.; Momosaki, R.; Wakabayashi, H. Effects of Nutrition Therapy in Older Stroke Patients Undergoing Rehabilitation: A Systematic Review and Meta-Analysis. *J. Nutr. Health Aging* **2019**, *23*, 21–26. [CrossRef] [PubMed]
82. Wang, J.; Chang, E.; Jiang, Y. Effects of vitamin C stimulation on rehabilitation of dysphagia after stroke: A randomized trial. *Eur. J. Phys. Rehabil. Med.* **2022**, *58*, 558–564. [CrossRef] [PubMed]
83. Conner, E.M.; Grisham, M.B. Inflammation, free radicals, and antioxidants. *Nutrition* **1996**, *12*, 274–277. [CrossRef] [PubMed]
84. Goszcz, K.; Deakin, S.J.; Duthie, G.G.; Stewart, D.; Leslie, S.J.; Megson, I.L. Antioxidants in cardiovascular therapy: Panacea or false hope? *Front. Cardiovasc. Med.* **2015**, *2*, 29. [CrossRef]
85. Belinskaia, D.A.; Voronina, P.A.; Shmurak, V.I.; Jenkins, R.O.; Goncharov, N.V. Serum Albumin in Health and Disease: Esterase, Antioxidant, Transporting and Signaling Properties. *Int. J. Mol. Sci.* **2021**, *22*, 10318. [CrossRef]
86. Shah, Z.; Li, R.-C.; Thimmulappa, R.; Kensler, T.; Yamamoto, M.; Biswal, S.; Doré, S. Role of reactive oxygen species in modulation of Nrf2 following ischemic reperfusion injury. *Neuroscience* **2007**, *147*, 53–59. [CrossRef]
87. Yang, J.; Huang, J.; Shen, C.; Cheng, W.; Yu, P.; Wang, L.; Tang, F.; Guo, S.; Yang, Q.; Zhang, J. Resveratrol Treatment in Different Time-Attenuated Neuronal Apoptosis After Oxygen and Glucose Deprivation/Reoxygenation via Enhancing the Activation of Nrf-2 Signaling Pathway In Vitro. *Cell Transpl.* **2018**, *27*, 1789–1797. [CrossRef]
88. Lu, Y.; Yang, Y.Y.; Zhou, M.W.; Liu, N.; Xing, H.Y.; Liu, X.X.; Li, F. Ketogenic diet attenuates oxidative stress and inflammation after spinal cord injury by activating Nrf2 and suppressing the NF-κB signaling pathways. *Neurosci. Lett.* **2018**, *683*, 13–18. [CrossRef]
89. Milder, J.B.; Liang, L.P.; Patel, M. Acute oxidative stress and systemic Nrf2 activation by the ketogenic diet. *Neurobiol. Dis.* **2010**, *40*, 238–244. [CrossRef]
90. Arya, A.K.; Hu, B. Brain–gut axis after stroke. *Brain Circ.* **2018**, *4*, 165–173.
91. Osadchiy, V.; Martin, C.R.; Mayer, E.A. The Gut-Brain Axis and the Microbiome: Mechanisms and Clinical Implications. *Clin. Gastroenterol. Hepatol.* **2019**, *17*, 322–332. [CrossRef] [PubMed] [PubMed Central]
92. Thursby, E.; Juge, N. Introduction to the human gut microbiota. *Biochem. J.* **2017**, *474*, 1823–1836. [CrossRef] [PubMed] [PubMed Central]
93. Sekirov, I.; Russell, S.L.; Antunes, L.C.; Finlay, B.B. Gut microbiota in health and disease. *Physiol. Rev.* **2010**, *90*, 859–904. [CrossRef] [PubMed]
94. Strandwitz, P. Neurotransmitter modulation by the gut microbiota. *Brain Res.* **2018**, *1693 Pt B*, 128–133. [CrossRef] [PubMed] [PubMed Central]
95. Dicks, L.M.T. Gut Bacteria and Neurotransmitters. *Microorganisms* **2022**, *10*, 1838. [CrossRef]
96. Asano, Y.; Hiramoto, T.; Nishino, R.; Aiba, Y.; Kimura, T.; Yoshihara, K.; Koga, Y.; Sudo, N. Critical role of gut microbiota in the production of biologically active, free catecholamines in the gut lumen of mice. *Am. J. Physiol. Gastrointest. Liver Physiol.* **2012**, *303*, G1288–G1295. [CrossRef]
97. Chu, Z.; Zhu, L.; Zhou, Y.; Yang, F.; Hu, Z.; Luo, Y.; Li, W.; Luo, F. Targeting Nrf2 by bioactive peptides alleviate inflammation: Expanding the role of gut microbiota and metabolites. *Crit. Rev. Food Sci. Nutr.* **2024**, *17*, 1–20. [CrossRef] [PubMed]
98. Kong, Y.; Olejar, K.J.; On, S.L.W.; Chelikani, V. The potential of *Lactobacillus* spp. for modulating oxidative stress in the gastrointestinal tract. *Antioxidants* **2020**, *9*, 610. [CrossRef]
99. Turnbaugh, P.J.; Ridaura, V.K.; Faith, J.J.; Rey, F.E.; Knight, R.; Gordon, J.I. The effect of diet on the human gut microbiome: A metagenomic analysis in humanized gnotobiotic mice. *Sci. Transl. Med.* **2009**, *1*, 6ra14. [CrossRef]
100. David, L.A.; Maurice, C.F.; Carmody, R.N.; Gootenberg, D.B.; Button, J.E.; Wolfe, B.E.; Ling, A.V.; Devlin, A.S.; Varma, Y.; Fischbach, M.A.; et al. Diet rapidly and reproducibly alters the human gut microbiome. *Nature* **2014**, *505*, 559–563. [CrossRef]
101. Hou, K.; Wu, Z.X.; Chen, X.Y.; Wang, J.Q.; Zhang, D.; Xiao, C.; Zhu, D.; Koya, J.B.; Wei, L.; Li, J.; et al. Microbiota in health and diseases. *Signal Transduct. Target. Ther.* **2022**, *7*, 135. [CrossRef] [PubMed] [PubMed Central]
102. Cryan, J.F.; O'Riordan, K.J.; Cowan, C.S.M.; Sandhu, K.V.; Bastiaanssen, T.F.S.; Boehme, M.; Codagnone, M.G.; Cussotto, S.; Fulling, C.; Golubeva, A.V.; et al. The microbiota-gut-brain axis. *Physiol. Rev.* **2019**, *99*, 1877–2013. [CrossRef] [PubMed]
103. Bauer, P.V.; Hamr, S.C.; Duca, F.A. Regulation of energy balance by a gut–brain axis and involvement of the gut microbiota. *Cell. Mol. Life Sci.* **2016**, *73*, 737–755. [CrossRef] [PubMed]

104. Romaní-Pérez, M.; Bullich-Vilarrubias, C.; López-Almela, I.; Liébana-García, R.; Olivares, M.; Sanz, Y. The Microbiota and the Gut–Brain Axis in Controlling Food Intake and Energy Homeostasis. *Int. J. Mol. Sci.* **2021**, *22*, 5830. [CrossRef]
105. Dumitrescu, L.; Popescu-Olaru, I.; Cozma, L.; Tulba, D.; Hinescu, M.E.; Ceafalan, L.C.; Gherghiceanu, M.; Popescu, B.O. Oxidative Stress and the Microbiota-Gut-Brain Axis. Oxidative Med. *Cell. Longev.* **2018**, *2018*, 2406594. [CrossRef]
106. Houlden, A.; Goldrick, M.; Brough, D.; Vizi, E.S.; Lénárt, N.; Martinecz, B.; Roberts, I.S.; Denes, A. Brain injury induces specific changes in the caecal microbiota of mice via altered autonomic activity and mucoprotein production. *Brain Behav. Immun.* **2016**, *57*, 10–20. [CrossRef]
107. Singh, V.; Roth, S.; Llovera, G.; Sadler, R.; Garzetti, D.; Stecher, B.; Dichgans, M.; Liesz, A. Microbiota Dysbiosis Controls the Neuroinflammatory Response after Stroke. *J. Neurosci.* **2016**, *36*, 7428–7440. [CrossRef] [PubMed] [PubMed Central]
108. Pluta, R.; Januszewski, S.; Czuczwar, S.J. The Role of Gut Microbiota in an Ischemic Stroke. *Int. J. Mol. Sci.* **2021**, *22*, 915. [CrossRef]
109. Dang, Y.; Zhang, X.; Zheng, Y.; Yu, B.; Pan, D.; Jiang, X.; Yan, C.; Yu, Q.; Lu, X. Distinctive Gut Microbiota Alteration Is Associated with Poststroke Functional Recovery: Results from a Prospective Cohort Study. *Neural Plast.* **2021**, *2021*, 1469339. [CrossRef] [PubMed] [PubMed Central]
110. Zeng, X.; Gao, X.; Peng, Y.; Wu, Q.; Zhu, J.; Tan, C.; Xia, G.; You, C.; Xu, R.; Pan, S.; et al. Higher risk of stroke is correlated with increased opportunistic pathogen load and reduced levels of butyrate-producing bacteria in the gut. *Front. Cell. Infect. Microbiol.* **2019**, *9*, 4. [CrossRef]
111. Chang, Y.; Woo, H.G.; Jeong, J.H.; Kim, G.H.; Park, K.D.; Song, T.J. Microbiota dysbiosis and functional outcome in acute ischemic stroke patients. *Sci. Rep.* **2021**, *11*, 10977. [CrossRef] [PubMed]
112. Bao, W.; Sun, Y.; Wang, J.; Wei, S.; Mao, L.; Zheng, J.; Liu, P.; Yang, X.; Chen, Z. Relationship Between the Gut Microbiota and Neurological Deficits in Patients with Cerebral Ischemic Stroke. *Neurorehabil. Neural Repair.* **2024**, *38*, 527–538. [CrossRef] [PubMed]
113. Murciano-Brea, J.; Garcia-Montes, M.; Geuna, S.; Herrera-Rincon, C. Gut Microbiota and Neuroplasticity. *Cells* **2021**, *10*, 2084. [CrossRef] [PubMed] [PubMed Central]
114. Sarubbo, F.; Cavallucci, V.; Pani, G. The Influence of Gut Microbiota on Neurogenesis: Evidence and Hopes. *Cells* **2022**, *11*, 382. [CrossRef] [PubMed]
115. Hammond, T.C.; Powell, E.; Green, S.J.; Chlipala, G.; Frank, J.; Yackzan, A.T.; Yanckello, L.M.; Chang, Y.-H.; Xing, X.; Heil, S.; et al. Functional recovery outcomes following acute stroke is associated with abundance of gut microbiota related to inflammation, butyrate and secondary bile acid. *Front. Rehabilit. Sci.* **2022**, *3*, 1017180. [CrossRef]
116. Kowiański, P.; Lietzau, G.; Czuba, E.; Wa'skow, M.; Steliga, A.; Mory ´s, J. BDNF: A key factor with multipotent impact on brain signaling and synaptic plasticity. *Cell. Mol. Neurobiol.* **2018**, *38*, 579–593. [CrossRef]
117. Bekinschtein, P.; Cammarota, M.; Katche, C.; Slipczuk, L.; Rossato, J.I.; Goldin, A.; Izquierdo, I.; Medina, J.H. BDNF is essential to promote persistence of long-term memory storage. *Proc. Natl. Acad. Sci. USA* **2008**, *105*, 2711–2716. [CrossRef]
118. Shandilya, S.; Kumar, S.; Kumar Jha, N.; Kumar Kesari, K.; Ruokolainen, J. Interplay of gut microbiota and oxidative stress: Perspective on neurodegeneration and neuroprotection. *J. Adv. Res.* **2021**, *38*, 223–244. [CrossRef] [PubMed] [PubMed Central]
119. Zhou, Z.; Xu, N.; Matei, N.; McBride, D.W.; Ding, Y.; Liang, H.; Tang, J.; Zhang, J.H. Sodium Butyrate Attenuated Neuronal Apoptosis via GPR41/Gbetagamma/PI3K/Akt Pathway After MCAO in Rats. *J. Cereb. Blood Flow. Metab.* **2021**, *41*, 267–281. [CrossRef]
120. Mang, C.S.; Campbell, K.L.; Ross, C.J.; Boyd, L.A. Promoting neuroplasticity for motor rehabilitation after stroke: Considering the effects of aerobic exercise and genetic variation on brain-derived neurotrophic factor. *Phys. Ther.* **2013**, *93*, 1707–1716. [CrossRef] [PubMed] [PubMed Central]
121. Alcantara, C.C.; García-Salazar, L.F.; Silva-Couto, M.A.; Santos, G.L.; Reisman, D.S.; Russo, T.L. Post-stroke BDNF Concentration Changes Following Physical Exercise: A Systematic Review. *Front. Neurol.* **2018**, *9*, 637. [CrossRef] [PubMed]
122. Savignac, H.M.; Corona, G.; Mills, H.; Chen, L.; Spencer, J.P.E.; Tzortzis, G.; Burnet, P.W.J. Prebiotic feeding elevates central brain derived neurotrophic factor, N-Methyl-d-Aspartate receptor subunits and d-Serine. *Neurochem. Int.* **2013**, *63*, 756–764. [CrossRef] [PubMed]
123. Ziegler, T.; Tsiountsioura, M.; Meixner-Goetz, L.; Cvirn, G.; Lamprecht, M. Polyphenols' Impact on Selected Biomarkers of Brain Aging in Healthy Middle-Aged and Elderly Subjects: A Review of Clinical Trials. *Nutrients* **2023**, *15*, 3770. [CrossRef] [PubMed] [PubMed Central]

nutrients

MDPI

Review

A Narrative Review on the Neurocognitive Profiles in Eating Disorders and Higher Weight Individuals: Insights for Targeted Interventions

Isabel Krug [1,*], An Binh Dang [1], Evonne Lu [2], Wenn Lynn Ooi [1], Jade Portingale [1] and Stephanie Miles [3,4,5]

[1] Melbourne School of Psychological Sciences, The University of Melbourne, Melbourne, VIC 3010, Australia; dangb1@student.unimelb.edu.au (A.B.D.); wennlynn.ooi@gmail.com (W.L.O.); jportingale@student.unimelb.edu.au (J.P.)
[2] Monash Faculty of Medicine, Nursing and Health Sciences, Monash University, Melbourne, VIC 3800, Australia; eluu0007@student.monash.edu
[3] Orygen, Parkville, VIC 3052, Australia; stephanie.miles@orygen.org.au
[4] Centre for Youth Mental Health, The University of Melbourne, Melbourne, VIC 3010, Australia
[5] Department of Psychological Sciences, Swinburne University of Technology, Hawthorn, VIC 3122, Australia
* Correspondence: isabel.krug@unimelb.edu.au; Tel.: +61-390358551; Fax: +61-393264774

Abstract: Background/Objectives: Recent research has increasingly explored the cognitive processes underlying eating disorders (EDs), including anorexia nervosa (AN), bulimia nervosa (BN), binge eating disorder (BED), other specified feeding or eating disorders (OSFEDs), and individuals with higher weight (HW). This critical narrative review focuses on neurocognitive findings derived from mainly experimental tasks to provide a detailed understanding of cognitive functioning across these groups. Where experimental data are lacking, we draw on self-report measures and neuroimaging findings to offer supplementary insights. **Method:** A search of major databases that prioritized meta-analyses and recent publications (last 10 years) was conducted. Using comprehensive search terms related to EDs, HW, and neurocognition, eligible studies focused on human neurocognitive outcomes (e.g., cognitive flexibility, attentional bias, etc.) published in English were selected. **Results:** We found that some neurocognitive characteristics, such as cognitive rigidity, impulsivity, emotion processing difficulties, and dysregulated reward processing, appear transdiagnostic, spanning multiple ED subtypes and HW populations. We also revealed neurocognitive features specific to ED subtypes and HW. For instance, individuals with AN demonstrate an enhanced focus on detail, and BN and BED are characterized by a pronounced attentional bias toward food-related stimuli. In individuals with HW, cognitive processes underpin behaviours associated with overeating and weight gain. **Conclusions:** These findings highlight the critical importance of understanding both the unique and shared neurocognitive patterns across ED subtypes and HW populations. By identifying transdiagnostic factors, such as cognitive rigidity and reward processing, alongside ED subtype/HW-specific vulnerabilities, researchers and clinicians can develop more nuanced, evidence-based interventions that address the core mechanisms driving disordered eating behaviours.

Keywords: anorexia nervosa; bulimia nervosa; binge eating disorder; otherwise specified feeding or eating disorders; higher weight; neurocognitive profile; executive functioning

Citation: Krug, I.; Dang, A.B.; Lu, E.; Ooi, W.L.; Portingale, J.; Miles, S. A Narrative Review on the Neurocognitive Profiles in Eating Disorders and Higher Weight Individuals: Insights for Targeted Interventions. *Nutrients* **2024**, *16*, 4418. https://doi.org/10.3390/nu16244418

Academic Editor: Hubertus Himmerich

Received: 13 November 2024
Revised: 17 December 2024
Accepted: 18 December 2024
Published: 23 December 2024

1. Introduction

Neurocognitive characteristics have been increasingly recognized as significant factors in the development and maintenance of eating disorders (EDs). Deficits in executive functioning and neurocognitive symptoms such as impulsivity [1], cognitive inflexibility [2], and poor emotion regulation [3] have been associated with several EDs. However, it remains unknown if these neurocognitive difficulties are intrinsic to EDs and part of the illness or are secondary consequences of malnutrition and changes in weight.

While EDs, including anorexia nervosa (AN), bulimia nervosa (BN), binge eating disorder (BED), and other specified feeding or eating disorders (OSFEDs), involve distinct behavioural patterns, they all share common underlying disturbances related to eating, body image, and weight [4,5]. Further, when examining EDs, considering people with a higher weight (HW) can provide additional insights—not as an ED, but as a condition situated at one end of the weight spectrum.

In this review, the term HW will refer to individuals whose body weight or body mass index (BMI) exceeds what health guidelines consider the "normal" range. Specifically, the term HW includes individuals with BMIs classified as overweight (BMI 25–29.9) or obese (BMI $\geq$ 30) according to the criteria set forth by the World Health Organization [6]. While HW is not classified as an ED, it is often associated with maladaptive eating behaviours that overlap with the characteristics of EDs, particularly BED and BN. For instance, one previous study found that lifetime obesity was as high as 87% in a treatment-seeking BED sample [7]. HW individuals also often exhibit neurocognitive and emotional dysfunctions like those seen in ED populations, including impaired cognitive flexibility [8], reward processing [9], heightened impulsivity [10], and emotion processing difficulties [11].

AN and HW represent extremes of weight dysregulation, and integrating HW into a broader examination of neurocognitive functioning is both relevant and necessary for understanding the full scope of weight-related problems. While various studies assessing HW have referred to their sample as "suffering from obesity", we use the terminology of HW throughout the review. This term is preferred in scientific and clinical contexts to reduce stigma and bias, promoting a more neutral, person-centred approach that respects body diversity and lessens the emphasis on weight as a sole health measure [12].

Furthermore, it is important to acknowledge potential biases in how HW is categorized in research. BMI, while widely used, does not account for body composition, distribution of fat, or metabolic health, potentially oversimplifying a complex construct [12,13]. Cultural and medical biases in the HW terminology, such as framing HW primarily as a pathological state, can also shape the focus of research and influence the interpretation of findings [13,14]. These biases may perpetuate stigmatizing narratives, overlook protective or neutral factors, and obscure the heterogeneity of HW populations. A critical examination of these issues is essential to accurately interpret findings and ensure that the inclusion of HW populations in ED research advances understanding without reinforcing stereotypes or over-simplifications.

This review will examine neurocognitive domains in different weight categories, including underweight (AN), "normal" weight (BN, OSFED), and HW (BED, HW) by primarily focusing on data from experimental tasks. Where experimental data are limited or unavailable, self-report data will also be considered. By examining neurocognitive profiles across EDs and HW, this review seeks to disentangle whether the observed cognitive patterns are a consequence of extreme weight states (underweight in AN or overweight/HW) or reflect core features of the disorders/conditions themselves. Understanding these distinctions is crucial for identifying the underlying mechanisms driving these conditions and for developing interventions that target the specific neurocognitive processes contributing to their onset and maintenance.

Avoidant/restrictive food intake disorder (ARFID) was not included in this review because it differs from traditional EDs like AN, BN, BED, OSFED, and HW in terms of their clinical presentation. ARFID is characterized by food avoidance based on sensory characteristics rather than body image concerns or binge–purge behaviours [4,5]. Therefore, its exclusion allows for a more focused examination of the neurocognitive characteristics of ED subtypes and HW populations who present with a more similar clinical presentation.

2. Method

Narrative reviews do not follow the same structured approach as systematic reviews using reporting tools such as the Preferred Reporting Items for Systematic Reviews and Meta-Analyses (PRISMA) guidelines [15]. Instead, they allow for a more flexible and qualitative synthesis of the existing literature without strict inclusion/exclusion criteria, with the aim of focusing on interpreting and synthesizing findings in a more narrative manner.

This narrative review was conducted in three steps: search execution, abstract and full-text review, and write-up and discussion of the main findings. We conducted a comprehensive literature search using major scientific databases, including PubMed, PsycINFO, Web of Science, and Google Scholar. Using these databases, a systematic search strategy was employed to identify relevant studies. The search covered mainly publications from the last 10 years to ensure the inclusion of the most current research, but older articles were also considered if they were key to the literature. The final search, completed in November 2024, included international articles, online reports, and electronic books. Where possible, meta-analyses or other reviews were prioritized to summarize the literature, with specific articles selected to provide illustrative examples or to address gaps where reviews were unavailable. Keywords including "eating disorders", "higher weight", "obesity", "anorexia nervosa", "bulimia nervosa", "binge eating disorder", "OSFED", "atypical anorexia nervosa", "purging disorder", "night eating syndrome", "subthreshold bulimia/binge eating disorder" to capture EDs/HW were combined with the following neurocognitive search terms: "cognitive flexibility/inflexibility", "central coherence", "attentional bias", "reward processing", "inhibitory control", "impulsivity", "reward processing", and "emotion regulation/processing". Studies included in this review met the following criteria:

1. Human studies, with a cross-sectional, longitudinal, or experimental design.
2. Research focused on neurocognitive/imaging outcomes related to EDs or HW.
3. Articles published in English.

Studies were excluded if they did not specify neurocognitive/imaging outcomes, were animal studies, lacked primary data, or were not published in English. The initial selection involved screening titles and abstracts to exclude studies that did not meet the criteria. Full-text articles of relevant studies were reviewed for detailed analysis. Reference lists from selected studies were also reviewed for additional sources.

3. Anorexia Nervosa

According to the DSM-5, AN is an ED characterized by a persistent restriction of energy intake, an intense fear of gaining weight or becoming fat, and a distorted body image. AN results in a significantly low body weight for the individual's age, sex, and developmental trajectory. It has two primary subtypes: the restrictive subtype (AN-R), and the binge–purging subtype (AN-BP), which is characterized by cycles of binge eating followed by purging behaviours to prevent weight gain [4,5]. AN is associated with numerous severe complications, including electrolyte imbalances, reduced bone density, cognitive impairments, and psychiatric comorbidities, notably anxiety, depression, and obsessive–compulsive traits [16,17].

Beyond the disorder's characteristic cognitive and behavioural distortions concerning food and body image, AN is also linked to neurocognitive deficits in areas such as cognitive flexibility, decision-making, and central coherence [18]. These impairments may be intrinsic to AN or could result from malnutrition and low BMI [19]. While the role of starvation in AN remains unclear, certain neurocognitive functions appear preserved, with general intelligence typically within normal ranges [20]. This preservation supports treatment engagement and recovery, underscoring the importance of addressing specific deficits while leveraging premorbid cognitive strengths.

3.1. Cognitive Flexibility

Cognitive flexibility refers to the ability to adapt to changing task demands or environmental shifts by adjusting behaviours and/or thoughts [2]. One prominent construct within cognitive flexibility is set shifting, or the capacity to switch between different mental sets or rules. In AN, cognitive inflexibility has been proposed as a mechanism that may perpetuate symptoms and contribute to treatment resistance [2]. Poor cognitive flexibility is reflected in behaviours such as compulsive weight control, restricted eating, ritualized food consumption, resistance to adopting new habits [1], and difficulties in social interactions [21]. While some studies indicate that individuals with AN exhibit poorer cognitive flexibility compared to healthy controls (HCs) [22–24], other research has reported no significant differences between these groups in cognitive flexibility tasks [25–27].

A systematic review by Miles et al. (2020) [2] highlights these mixed findings, showing that adolescents with AN perform comparably to HCs on cognitive flexibility tasks, whereas adults with AN often demonstrate poorer performance on perceptual-based cognitive flexibility tasks, yet no significant group difference was supported for verbal cognitive flexibility tasks. Miles et al. (2020) [2] noted that the 69 studies included in their review used over 30 different measures of cognitive flexibility, creating inconsistencies that hinder synthesis and may contribute to conflicting findings. The review further notes variability in findings for weight-restored and fully recovered AN samples, suggesting that while some aspects of cognitive flexibility may improve, certain deficits may persist even after recovery or weight restoration [2].

Other research has explored the relationship between cognitive flexibility and BMI in AN as BMI is suggested as a severity indicator for AN per both the DSM-5 [4,5] and ICD-11 [28]. A recent systematic review found no association between cognitive flexibility and BMI [20], and this finding was supported by subsequent studies [29,30]. These findings suggest that cognitive inflexibility in AN may not be merely a consequence of low weight or starvation but may instead represent a core feature of the disorder.

Understanding cognitive inflexibility as a central aspect of AN points to promising clinical interventions. Targeting this rigidity through cognitive training such as Cognitive Remediation Therapy (CRT) [31], increasing awareness of inflexible thought patterns, and designing behavioural exercises to improve set-shifting abilities may help address key maintenance factors and support long-term recovery.

3.2. Central Coherence

Central coherence denotes to the ability to grasp complex stimuli or information, often described as "big picture" thinking, and weak central coherence is typified by an excessive focus on small details. A systematic review and meta-analysis conducted by Keegan et al. (2021) [32] concluded that participants with AN exhibited significantly poorer central coherence compared to HCs. Regarding the relationship between central coherence and BMI, studies have produced varied results [20]. For example, López et al. (2008) [33] found in a sample of women with AN that there was a negative association between BMI and errors on the Homograph Reading Task, a measure of central coherence, yet there were no other significant correlations between BMI and the outcomes of other central coherence tasks included in the study. Conversely, Herbrich et al. (2018) [34] observed a negative correlation between BMI and performance on the Group Embedded Figures Test in participants with AN-BP, but not in the AN-R group.

While most findings suggest deficits in central coherence among those with AN, the findings remain somewhat inconsistent. This variability is partly due to the heterogeneity of studies and methodological differences that need to be considered. Various tests have been used to measure central coherence, raising questions about the comparability of results [2]. Different cognitive tests vary in complexity and often target multiple cognitive functions. For instance, the Homograph Reading Task focuses on linguistic and contextual coherence, whereas the Group Embedded Figures Test assesses perceptual and visual-spatial aspects, each providing distinct insights into different components of central coherence.

In summary, although more research is needed to clarify the relationship between BMI and central coherence in AN, the current evidence points to central coherence deficits among those with AN. A deeper understanding of neuropsychological functioning in AN, particularly its link to neural mechanisms and symptoms, could inform more effective treatments.

3.3. Attentional Bias

Attentional bias, the tendency to prioritize processing certain stimuli over others, has been extensively studied in AN. Research investigating attentional processes in AN employs diverse methods, including variations in measurement procedures, types of stimuli (e.g., words or images), threat content, and outcome measures. Despite this methodological diversity, findings consistently show heightened attentional bias toward body shape, weight, and food-related stimuli in individuals with AN compared to HCs [12,35]. Specifically, the Stroop Task and Dot-Probe Task, in combination with eye-tracking paradigms, are commonly used to assess this bias. Eye-tracking research demonstrates that individuals with AN initially display an attentional bias towards food cues that is similar to HCs, but rather than sustaining this attention, individuals with AN quickly switch to attentional avoidance [36]. Werthmann et al. (2019) [36] further found that avoidance was stronger for high-calorie food cues, especially in adults with longer AN illness durations compared to adolescents. This avoidance behaviour tends to become more entrenched as the illness progresses, potentially maintaining the fear of food or restrictive eating behaviours [37].

In terms of BMI, while some work has found no association between BMI and attentional bias [38], other research has revealed that those with a low BMI are more likely to pay attention to high-calorie foods [36]. Future studies should further investigate the relationship between BMI and attentional bias toward food and body shape to better inform treatment approaches for AN, such as the potential benefits of attention training.

3.4. Impulsivity

Impulsivity is a multi-faceted concept used to describe a tendency to act quickly without conscious judgement, focus, or planning and without considering the potential consequences, particularly in emotionally charged situations [39]. However, researchers in EDs have yet to agree on a standard operationalization of impulsivity [40]. Impulsivity is frequently linked to EDs presenting with binge–purge symptomatology, including the AN-BP subtype [1,41].

Studies indicate that individuals with AN-BP display higher impulsivity and greater novelty-seeking behaviours than HCs and those with the AN-R subtype [41,42]. Additionally, those with AN-BP are more likely to engage in impulsive, high-risk activities, such as substance use [42] and shoplifting [43] than HCs and those with AN-R. Impulsivity may contribute to cycles of disordered eating, like bingeing and purging, by making it difficult to resist urges, potentially worsening symptoms [1]. This subtype difference implies that AN-BP interventions may benefit from targeting impulsivity and related behaviours like substance use and binge–purge cycles in addition to other AN training methods such as managing rigidity and overcontrol.

3.5. Emotional Processing Difficulties

Emotional processing difficulties, such as challenges in recognizing and being aware of different emotions, have been linked to AN [25]. Research indicates that individuals with AN often struggle with identifying and managing emotions, which may lead to maladaptive behaviours, such as restrictive eating, as a coping strategy [44,45]. Emotion recognition—the ability to identify and interpret others' emotional expressions—is essential for social functioning and mental health, and emerging evidence suggests that individuals with AN exhibit significant deficits in this area compared to HCs [46,47]. Several systematic reviews have emphasized impaired emotion recognition and altered responses to social-affective stimuli in individuals with EDs, including those with AN [48,49].

Research consistently indicates that individuals with AN also experience significant challenges in emotion regulation, manifesting as difficulties in identifying, expressing, and managing emotions—factors that contribute to the persistence of restrictive eating behaviours and heightened symptom severity [50]. Women with AN have been found to report significantly greater emotion regulation difficulties than HCs [47,50,51]. A central element of these emotional difficulties is alexithymia, defined by an impaired ability to recognize and describe one's emotions, which is notably prevalent in AN and intensifies emotion regulation difficulties by limiting emotional awareness [52,53]. Emotion regulation challenges, coupled with alexithymia, often lead to maladaptive coping strategies such as emotional suppression and avoidance, which further reinforce disordered eating patterns and complicate treatment [53]. Consequently, addressing emotion regulation deficits, particularly by enhancing emotional awareness and fostering adaptive coping strategies, is critical for effective AN treatment.

The relationship between emotion processing (recognition and regulation) deficits and BMI in AN is inconsistent, possibly due to studies being conducted in various phases of the illness [25]. For instance, while one study found a positive correlation between BMI and emotion processing difficulties in AN such that lower BMI was associated with fewer emotion regulation difficulties [51], others have not found a significant relationship between BMI and emotion regulation [46]. A recent 15-year longitudinal study found that as individuals with AN recovered and their BMI increased, there was no significant linear effect on their emotional processing [25]. This finding is consistent with earlier studies that showed no significant association between BMI and impaired emotional functioning, whether in the acute or recovered phases of AN [45,46,54]. From such findings, Castro et al. (2021) [25] suggested that emotional dysfunction in AN may not solely be a result of malnutrition, highlighting the transdiagnostic role of emotion processing in the development and maintenance of psychiatric disorders like AN.

Finally, it is also worth outlining that poor emotion regulation strategies can strain the therapeutic relationship, as individuals with AN may struggle to express overwhelming emotions, potentially making therapy less effective or even invalidating [55]. Consequently, therapy should focus on helping clients recognize, label, and tolerate emotions while building effective coping strategies.

4. Bulimia Nervosa

BN is characterized by recurrent episodes of binge eating, where a person consumes an unusually large amount of food within a short period (e.g., 2 h period) and is accompanied by a sense of loss of control [4,5]. To prevent weight gain, individuals with BN typically engage in compensatory behaviours, such as self-induced vomiting, excessive exercise, or misuse of laxatives. Binge eating episodes and purging behaviours need to occur at least once a week for three months for a diagnosis of BN [4,5]. It has been suggested that the bingeing and purging behaviours reflect deficiencies in inhibitory control [56], a core executive function that overrides impulses through conscious decision-making. The exploration of neurocognition in BN has also highlighted impaired decision-making compared to those with AN [57] and HCs [58–60].

4.1. Cognitive Flexibility

Cognitive flexibility research in BN has shown mixed results. Early research suggested poor cognitive flexibility in people diagnosed with BN compared to HCs [61–64]. In contrast, another study found no significant differences in cognitive flexibility between participants with BN and HCs [65]. It also remains unknown if/how cognitive flexibility may be associated with BMI in BN. Given the limited amount of research that has investigated cognitive flexibility in BN specifically, the potential role of cognitive flexibility in treatment outcomes remains unclear.

4.2. Reward Processing

Reward processing refers to the neural and psychological mechanisms that evaluate, respond to, and guide behaviour based on rewarding stimuli or outcomes [66]. Such processing may be understood using a dual-pathway model [67], wherein decisions are influenced by two processes—an automatic, unconscious process primarily associated with reward sensitivity to food and a reflective, conscious process involving executive functioning that can counteract automatic processing.

In BN, a weakened reflective system is overridden by hyper-responsive automatic reward processing towards food stimuli, which manifests as an "addiction" to highly palatable foods [68]. Such heightened reward sensitivities among individuals with BN are consistently reported in the literature using self-report measures [69]. Studies have also used neurocognitive tasks such as the Game of Dice task [59] and the Iowa Gambling Task [57,58,60] to demonstrate that individuals with BN consistently prefer high-reward options despite the high risk compared to HCs. Some of these studies also showed that performance on the Iowa Gambling Task was negatively correlated with self-reported BN symptomatology [58,60]. Collectively, the evidence suggests that an impaired ability to weigh immediate rewards versus long-term consequences may fuel destructive binge–purge habits in BN.

Another concept that may help inform the abnormalities in BN reward processing is delay discounting. It refers to a phenomenon wherein the value of a reward depreciates with a temporal delay in its delivery [70]. To our knowledge, only four papers to date have studied delay discounting in BN populations [71–74]. A meta-analysis of the three earliest papers showed an elevated discounting of monetary rewards (i.e., greater preference for sooner and smaller amounts of money) in participants with BN compared to controls, reflecting an impulsive preference for immediate rewards over delayed gratification [75]. However, the meta-analysis comprised a small, pooled sample size of 84 BN participants, and the results concerning monetary rewards may not translate to condition-specific triggers (i.e., food).

A more recent study [74] extended experimental stimuli to food rewards and observed decreased delay discounting to both monetary and food rewards in women with BN compared to HCs. That is, women with BN showed a preference for larger/later over smaller/sooner amounts of food and money relative to HCs. Although this finding contradicts previous findings from the earlier meta-analysis [75], decreased delay discounting may explain prolonged periods of food intake restriction in BN, a behaviour that necessitates a high degree of cognitive control.

4.3. Impulsivity

Impulsivity is implicated in BN, but findings from behavioural tasks are mixed. For example, using the Go/No-Go task, which is proposed to measure action inhibition and restraint, Rosval et al. (2006) [76] found that BN individuals did not differ significantly in overall performance compared to HCs and individuals diagnosed with AN, while Van den Eynde et al. (2012) [77] found that BN individuals showed no significant difference in commission errors when compared to HCs only. Another task, the Stroop Test, which evaluates interference/inhibitory control, was used in two studies, one of which found that BN individuals performed comparably to HCs [77] while the other study found that BN individuals performed significantly poorer than HCs [78]. Overall, the evolving body of evidence has prompted a critical re-evaluation of BN as simply a disorder of impulsivity (for more details, see the systematic review by Howard et al. (2020) [1]).

In recognition of the multi-faceted nature of impulsivity and the general nature of the aforementioned behavioural tasks, some studies have used symptom-specific assessments to study BN behaviour. For example, one study adapted the Stroop Test to include craving-specific food images as interference stimuli and found that BN individuals performed with lower accuracy than HCs [79]. Another study [80] revealed that women with BN used both health and taste ratings in making uncontrolled food choices, whereas HCs only used tastiness in their food choices. This finding suggests that binge-related food choices in BN are more calculated and less impulsive than previously thought.

In another study [71] using a computerized version of the Race Game modified to include food images designed to provoke cravings, BN individuals also demonstrated superior planning ability based on backward reasoning compared to HCs, which challenges the simplistic view of BN as a purely impulsive disorder. The authors postulated that planning, which was induced in this experiment, may work to reduce cravings for binge foods and extend binge refractory periods. This finding is especially relevant since some

BN individuals deliberately plan for binge episodes in advance, and binge anticipation may decrease the motivation to attempt other coping strategies, resulting in negative reinforcement eating expectancies (i.e., the belief that eating will help mitigate distress) [81].

Thus, therapeutic strategies for BN may benefit from considering the duality of impulsivity co-existing alongside possible goal-oriented binge planning. This nuanced understanding will help inform interventions that add to existing urge surfing strategies, a technique that forms a part of cognitive behaviour therapy (CBT) for EDs and advocates "riding out" impulses by observing them instead of acting on them [82]. By identifying triggers that precede impulses and binge planning, these strategies can better target "at-risk" periods of the binge–purge cycle and inform alternative coping mechanisms that weaken negative reinforcement eating expectancies [83].

4.4. Emotional Processing Difficulties

Emotional processing difficulties have been revealed in individuals with BN. Some research has shown that participants with BN self-report significantly more emotion regulation difficulties than HCs, but do not exhibit difficulties in recognizing emotions [46]. A recent meta-analysis by Mourilhe et al. (2021) [84] reported a positive correlation between the amount of food ingested during a binge eating episode and depressive symptoms in BN individuals. Similarly, Davis and Smith (2023) [85] reported that positive urgency (i.e., the tendency to act impulsively in response to distress or extremely positive emotions) was associated with a greater amount of ingested food during a binge eating episode during an ad-lib meal test among women with BN. These findings may be explained by the fact that foods typically eaten during a binge eating episode are highly palatable and rewarding. Thus, the loss of control during binge episodes may be driven by the instantaneous feelings of the reward related to food consumption [86].

Additionally, individuals with BN often report heightened emotional reactivity, including difficulty managing distressing emotions, which may fuel the urge to binge eat as a form of self-soothing [87]. According to Smyth et al. (2007) [88], negative mood states such as anxiety and sadness commonly precede binge eating episodes, suggesting that binge eating may serve as an emotional escape strategy. Complementing this theory, Fischer et al. (2018) [89] found that individuals with BN are more likely to binge after experiencing negative social interactions, pointing to a connection between interpersonal stress and binge eating urges. Collectively, the evidence supports the view that BN behaviours are intertwined with a maladaptive cycle of affect regulation, where binge eating serves as a temporary escape from negative emotions.

In summary, BN is characterized by dysregulated reward processing, with heightened sensitivity to food rewards, suggesting that the immediate pleasure of binge eating plays a significant role in the loss of control. Additionally, there is some evidence to suggest that individuals with BN may struggle with emotional processing difficulties and that these difficulties drive binge eating behaviours as coping mechanisms for stress.

5. Binge Eating Disorder

According to the DSM-5 [4,5], BED is characterized by recurrent episodes of binge eating, accompanied by a lack of control and overeating during these episodes. Individuals with BED often eat more rapidly than usual, continue eating despite feeling uncomfortably full, eat large amounts without hunger, and may feel distress, guilt, or shame afterward [4,5]. Unlike BN, BED does not involve regular compensatory behaviours (e.g., purging) to counteract the binge episodes [4,5]. Recent research has shed light on the cognitive factors associated with BED in clinical populations [22] and non-clinical community populations [90], which may help inform our understanding of the processes involved in BED.

5.1. Cognitive Flexibility

Cognitive flexibility has been investigated in a small number of studies and found to be consistently impaired in individuals with BED compared to HCs [22,91–95]. These investigations reveal that individuals with BED struggle to adapt their behaviour and cognitive strategies when faced with changing contingencies or rules [22,95]. Moreover, compared to patients with AN, the cognitive profile of BED has been shown to be characterized by poorer cognitive flexibility [22]. Notably, research suggests that cognitive rigidity is not merely a static trait but a dynamic process that can evolve over time. For instance, Messer et al. (2024) [96] demonstrated a significant longitudinal pathway where higher shape and weight overvaluation predicted an increased inflexible adherence to food rules, which subsequently predicted increased binge eating symptoms over a 6-month period. Complementing these findings, early childhood studies by Steegers et al. (2021) [97] revealed that set-shifting difficulties are observable even before the typical onset of EDs.

Cognitive rigidity in BED may contribute to the persistence of maladaptive eating patterns by hindering their ability to engage in adaptive problem solving [61] such as modifying established habits and routines surrounding food and eating. Particularly compelling is the "escape from awareness" theory [98], which provides a nuanced framework for understanding binge eating behaviours. This theoretical approach proposes that binge eating emerges as a complex coping mechanism, whereby individuals attempt to draw attention away from emotional distress by narrowing their cognitive focus to the immediate environment (food) rather than confronting aversive self-perceptions [99]. Consequently, individuals with BED may find it challenging to shift their focus away from food-related stimuli, resulting in increased preoccupation with food, heightened cravings, and ultimately binge eating episodes.

This perspective suggests that cognitive inflexibility is not just a symptom, but a potentially adaptive (albeit maladaptive in the long term) response to underlying emotional distress. Specific intervention strategies might include cognitive rigidity and meta-cognitive training, which helps individuals recognize and modify rigid thinking patterns [100], and acceptance-based therapies that teach individuals to experience emotions without resorting to binge eating as an avoidance mechanism [82].

5.2. Impulsivity

Impulsivity, particularly impaired response inhibition, has been consistently and robustly observed in individuals with BED (for reviews see [101–103]). Longitudinal research provides critical insights into the developmental trajectory of impulsivity in EDs. For instance, Evans et al. (2019) [104] demonstrated that higher levels of impulsivity predicted the development of disordered eating attitudes over time, suggesting impulsivity may be a dynamic risk factor rather than a static trait. Pearson et al. (2015) [105] further illuminated this relationship, revealing that negative urgency and negative affect in children can predict early binge eating engagement through distinct pathways.

The Go/No-Go Task and the Stop Signal Reaction Time Task are commonly used to assess response inhibition. Studies have found that individuals with BED exhibit increased commission errors on the Go/No-Go task and longer stop signal reaction times on the Stop Signal Reaction Time Task [101–103]. These errors and poor reaction times are indicative of impulsivity and poor response inhibition. An impaired ability to inhibit pre-potent responses may contribute to the difficulty in resisting the urge to binge eat, particularly in the presence of tempting or palatable stimuli. This automatic tendency to consume foods despite the individual's awareness of the potential adverse outcomes may result in the initiation or continuation of binge eating episodes [101–103].

To summarize, the literature has shown that impulsivity is a complex, developmentally informed process that interacts with emotional and cognitive mechanisms to potentially maintain binge eating behaviours. Future research should continue to explore the longitudinal pathways and potential intervention points in these developmental trajectories.

5.3. Emotional Processing Difficulties

Emotional processing difficulties have been implicated in the onset and maintenance of BED [106], with research consistently demonstrating greater emotion-related difficulties in BED patients compared to HCs (for a review, see [3]). Longitudinal research provides crucial insights into the dynamic nature of these emotional processing difficulties, revealing that emotion regulation is not a static trait but a fluid process that interacts with ED symptoms [107].

The aforementioned "escape from awareness" theory offers a nuanced framework for understanding this relationship, proposing that binge eating serves as a cognitive mechanism to avoid confronting overwhelming emotional experiences [98,99]. Specifically, individuals with BED may use food and binge eating as a strategic method of emotional avoidance, narrowing their cognitive focus to the immediate sensory experience of eating. This process is believed to block out emotional distress, providing temporary psychological relief [98]. Negative emotions, coupled with an inability to effectively process these feelings, may trigger binge eating as a maladaptive form of emotional regulation—a means of escaping awareness of underlying psychological discomfort [98,106]. The theory explains why individuals often report feeling "numb" or "disconnected" during binge episodes, highlighting binge eating not as a simple lack of self-control, but as a complex coping mechanism for managing emotional distress. Importantly, Bodell et al.'s (2019) [107] research suggests that emotional processing difficulties in BED are dynamic, context-dependent processes that can fluctuate over time and potentially be modified through targeted, momentary interventions.

In summary, deficits in cognitive flexibility and response inhibition and emotional processing difficulties have been consistently observed in people diagnosed with BED. These cognitive impairments may contribute to the persistence of maladaptive eating patterns and the difficulty in regulating eating behaviour by hindering the ability to modify established habits, redirect attention away from food-related cues, and resist the urge to binge eat.

6. Otherwise Specified Feeding or Eating Disorders

OSFEDs encompass a range of disordered eating behaviours that do not fully meet the criteria for AN, BN, or BED. This category is important as it captures the experiences of many individuals who struggle with significant eating and body image disturbances but do not fit neatly into established diagnostic categories. Among the subtypes of OSFEDs, five prominent forms include: atypical anorexia nervosa (AAN), purging disorder (PD), night eating syndrome (NES), and BN and BED of low frequency and/or duration (sub-BN and sub-BED) [4,5].

Most research on OSFEDs has assessed the disorder as an overall OSFED group, treating it as a single entity despite its heterogeneous nature. This approach overlooks the possibility that distinct neurocognitive profiles may exist within OSFED's specific subtypes. Because studies on neurocognitive experimental tasks specific to the OSFED subtypes are limited, we also include neuroimaging findings in the subsequent section, which offer valuable insights into the neural underpinnings of these cognitive processes [108,109]. Neuroimaging studies allow us to examine the activation patterns in brain regions related to reward processing, cognitive control, and emotional regulation, providing a more comprehensive understanding of the neurocognitive characteristics of OSFEDs [31].

6.1. Overall OSFED

The investigation of neurocognitive factors in OSFEDs remains limited, as evidenced by a review focusing on socio-cognitive factors and EDs in young people that found that only four out of the thirty-eight studies included were on OSFEDs [110]. Two studies highlighted that individuals with OSFED exhibited hyperactivation in reward, attention, and visual processing regions in response to high-calorie food cues, while showing hypoactivation in cognitive control areas, indicating difficulties in regulating responses to food-related stimuli [111,112]. However, it needs to be acknowledged that while the study by Bartholdy et al. (2019) [112] assessed a binge purging presentation, the study by Wang et al. (2016) [111] comprised a restrictive OSFED sample. Given the heterogeneous OSFED presentations in these two studies and the small number of participants, drawing clear conclusions on neurocognition in OSFEDs is challenging.

A further finding of the Prince et al. (2022) [110] review was that OSFED participants demonstrated increased neural responses in the prefrontal circuitry and cerebellum when exposed to food images, correlating with heightened obsessive–compulsive symptoms. Finally, Bodell et al. (2018) [113], also included in the Prince et al. (2022) [110] review, found that alterations in reward-related neural circuitry were concurrently and prospectively associated with binge eating in a community-based sample of adolescent girls presenting with OSFED. It should be noted that, while promising, these findings must be interpreted cautiously due to the limited sample sizes and methodological heterogeneity across neuroimaging studies, which constrain the generalizability and robustness of current conclusions.

Taken together, these findings suggest that individuals with OSFED may experience unique cognitive and emotional responses to food cues, which could impact treatment approaches and necessitate further research to develop targeted interventions.

Finally, a recent study by Wang et al. (2021) [114], not included in the Prince et al. (2022) [110] review, assessed female adolescents in a residential ED programme who had been diagnosed with AN, BN, or OSFED. Findings showed that, in comparison to a historical sample of adolescent HCs, adolescents with EDs had significantly greater levels of cognitive rigidity and attention to detail, with both findings presenting large effect sizes. Even after adjusting for age, length of illness, and BMI, there was still a substantial correlation between these neurocognitive deficits and the severity of the EDs (assessed through a clinical ED screening tool). However, in this study, the OSFED sample was very small and not separated from the other EDs. Given these limitations, the findings of Wang et al. (2021) [114] should be interpreted with caution.

Translation from Neuroimaging Findings to Neurocognitive Processes

The observed hyperactivation in reward, attention, and visual processing regions, coupled with hypo-activation in cognitive control areas, underscores a potential vulnerability in individuals with OSFED to food-related stimuli, potentially contributing to disordered eating behaviours. Clinically, these findings suggest that interventions targeting cognitive control processes, such as CRT [31], could help enhance regulatory responses to food cues in OSFEDs.

Similarly, the heightened prefrontal and cerebellar activity observed in response to food images, alongside obsessive–compulsive tendencies, may indicate that treatments addressing obsessive–compulsive symptoms, such as exposure and response prevention (ERP) [115], could be beneficial for certain OSFED presentations.

Finally, alterations in reward-related neural circuitry associated with binge eating symptoms in the OSFED subtypes displaying these symptoms may suggest that approaches aimed at modulating reward sensitivity—such as mindfulness-based interventions [116] or reward restructuring therapies [117]—could mitigate binge eating behaviours by helping individuals develop healthier reward mechanisms.

Future research should focus on validating these neuroimaging findings in larger, more diverse OSFED samples to refine our understanding of these neural mechanisms and their functional implications. Upcoming research should also further explore OSFED subtype-specific neurocognitive traits and compare them to the more-established profiles observed in AN, BN, and BED to enhance diagnostic precision and tailored interventions.

6.2. AAN

AAN is characterized by the same behavioural patterns and cognitive features as AN, but individuals diagnosed with this ED maintain a weight within or above the normal range [4,5]. Often, people with AAN are initially at a higher weight when they develop their ED. Although they may experience a dramatic weight loss, they do not drop to a BMI below 18 and are not classified as underweight [108,109].

People with AAN often experience severe cognitive distortions related to body image, including a pervasive fear of gaining weight and a preoccupation with food and dieting [118]. It is likely that cognitive rigidity and central coherence deficiencies are prevalent in this group, mirroring those observed in individuals with threshold AN. However, research that has assessed neurocognition in AAN and compared ANN to AN and/or other EDs or other comparison groups is currently lacking.

One study [119] found that in a sample of female adolescents with AAN and HCs, there was evidence for increased functional connectivity within the somatosensory network in response to food images in the AAN group. In addition, there was evidence for decreased functional connectivity in the ANN group in the brain networks linked with salience, attention, and inhibitory control and areas of the brain involved in food cue processing and appetite regulation [119]. The findings suggest that high-caloric food is associated with increased somatosensory processing in AAN, but low-caloric food is given greater salience and is considered more engaging [119]. This connectivity pattern may play a key role in the unique challenges AAN individuals face regarding food reward processing [119].

Conversely, another study by the same author found that AAN in newly diagnosed adolescents was not associated with structural changes in the brain [120]. That is, adolescents with AAN and HCs did not significantly differ in brain grey matter volume [120]. This finding contrasts with similar work in adult and adolescent AN (for a review, see [121]), often showing alterations in brain volume and structure, possibly due to factors like malnutrition and prolonged illness. Future research is required to disentangle these findings to clarify whether AAN may or may not involve similar or distinct neurobiological impacts on brain structure as seen in AN.

6.3. PD

PD refers to individuals who engage in purging behaviours—such as self-induced vomiting or excessive exercise—without the binge eating episodes characteristic of BN [4,5]. Negative urgency—the propensity to act impulsively when experiencing negative emotions—along with other dimensions of impulsivity, has been investigated in individuals with PD. A study by Davis et al. (2020) [122] found that individuals with PD exhibited significantly higher levels of negative urgency compared to HC, although these levels were lower than those observed in individuals with BN. However, no significant differences were detected between the PD and HC groups or between the PD and BN groups on additional impulsivity traits, including lack of premeditation, lack of perseverance, and sensation seeking [122].

Consistent with these findings, a more recent study examining a larger sample of individuals with PD reported no significant differences in sensation seeking compared to controls. Furthermore, individuals with PD were characterized by lower reward dependence and novelty seeking but exhibited higher persistence scores compared to those with BN and BED [123]. It is possible that people with PD have a tendency toward impulsive actions under emotional distress, which may reinforce the use of purging behaviours as a maladaptive coping strategy, complicating symptom management and intervention approaches for PD [122]. However, the currently limited and contradictory findings in the literature need to be clarified before such conclusions can be made.

6.4. NES

NES, another subtype of OSFED, involves recurrent episodes of significant food intake after the evening meal or during nighttime awakenings, often causing distress [4,5]. Though neurocognitive research is sparse, individuals with NES may have altered reward sensitivity and emotional regulation difficulties, potentially exacerbating night eating and leading to weight gain [124,125]. Like the other OSFEDs, NES also appears to be influenced by emotional fluctuations, with some individuals using night eating as a temporary coping mechanism for stress, which disrupts circadian rhythms and further heightens distress [126,127]. It is also possible that impulsivity may increase susceptibility to night binge eating episodes by weakening self-control, though this theory requires further investigation. Further research is needed to clarify the neurocognitive underpinnings of NES and its relationship with impulsivity, emotional regulation, and circadian disruptions, which could inform targeted interventions for this understudied OSFED subtype.

6.5. Sub-BN/BED

Sub-BN involves recurrent binge eating episodes followed by compensatory behaviours occurring less than once a week or for less than three months, while sub-BED features binge eating episodes with distress that occur less frequently than what is required for a full BED diagnosis [4,5]. In a study by Darcy et al. (2012) [128], neurocognitive assessments in adolescents with BN, sub-BN, and HCs revealed no significant group differences in set-shifting abilities, with small effect sizes. Neurocognitive factors in sub-BED have also been assessed [129,130]. For instance, Manasse et al. (2015) [129] found that individuals with sub-BED exhibited similar deficits in inhibitory control as those with full-threshold BED.

Overall, these observations suggest that neurocognitive factors may play a role in the development and maintenance of binge eating and purging behaviours along a continuum, rather than being specific to the clinical BN/BED diagnosis. These cognitive impairments may contribute to the perpetuation of maladaptive eating patterns and the potential escalation of binge eating/purging behaviours over time.

Despite the emergence of research on neurocognitive factors associated with specific OSFED subtypes, the literature remains limited compared to that of AN, BN, and BED. The heterogeneity of OSFEDs presents challenges in establishing consistent neurocognitive profiles. Factors such as varying symptomatology, comorbid conditions, and developmental influences further complicate the analysis of cognitive impairments across the different OSFED subtypes [108]. Moreover, the lack of standardized diagnostic assessment tools specifically designed for OSFEDs [109] restricts our understanding of cognitive functioning in this population. Future studies should prioritize examining cognitive and emotional processes across various OSFED subtypes to inform tailored interventions, ultimately improving treatment outcomes for this underrepresented population.

7. Higher Weight

Neurocognitive profiles of HW individuals highlight deficiencies in executive function, reward processing, and reward sensitivity, alongside marked changes in neuroplasticity and cognitive function in brain regions modulating reward, learning, and decision-making [10,131]. HW and neurocognitive alterations (such as impulsivity and cognitive rigidity) have been found to exhibit a bi-directional relationship; neurocognitive patterns are suggested to influence the susceptibility to overconsumption and, reciprocally, weight status and diet-elicited HW promotes changes in the prefrontal cortex structure and functionality, worsening executive functions and episodic memory [132–134]. For instance, in a longitudinal study spanning 9 years, HW was negatively correlated with episodic memory without any changes in executive function [135]. However, the same study found that improved executive function over time corresponded to a decline in HW. Other research has shown that executive function deficits dysregulate eating behaviours and impair physical activity functioning as risk factors for HW [136]. These findings highlight the critical role of neurocognitive processes in shaping the risk and maintenance of HW, offering potential targets for intervention.

7.1. Cognitive Flexibility

Cognitive flexibility has been assessed in those with HW and a meta-analysis of 25 studies found that cognitive flexibility was significantly poorer in HW participants compared to HCs [137]. Supporting this meta-analysis, a recent study also found significantly poorer flexibility in patients with HW compared to HCs [8]. Given these consistent findings, Testa et al. (2021) [8] suggested that cognitive rigidity may contribute to the persistence of unhealthy eating habits and difficulties in behaviour change. In a cognitive control task, HW participants were found to perform significantly poorer than HCs for food stimuli but not neutral stimuli (flowers) [138]. This result could indicate an impairment in cognitive flexibility, with greater cognitive resource demands in response to food stimuli [138].

7.2. Impulsivity

Impulsivity has been suggested to be elevated in those at a HW. A meta-analysis by Yang et al. (2018) [137] revealed that HW participants performed worse than HCs on inhibition tasks and decision-making tasks. Another systematic review by Lavagnino et al. (2016) [102] concluded that HW participants exhibit decreased inhibitory response performance in tasks when compared to HCs. Contrarily, Testa et al. (2021) [8] found greater impulsivity in participants with both HW and Type 2 Diabetes compared to HCs but no significant difference in impulsivity in those with HW compared to HCs. In a more recent study by Reyes et al. (2024) [10], BMI was correlated with task performance such that a higher BMI was associated with lower inhibitory control. The literature suggests that HW individuals tend to prioritize immediate rewards over potential future consequences, which is linked to difficulties in maintaining self-control and regulating responses to reward and punishment [8,139].

7.3. Reward Processing

Reward processing, the appraisal of reward and the subsequent capacity to inhibit gratification, is believed to guide individual eating behaviours in HW individuals [140]. People at an HW appear to show marked changes in reward sensitivity to food cues [141]. In a study comparing HW women to HCs, HW participants were shown to be more likely to choose immediate reward and gratification and forgo future gains, i.e., participants with an HW displayed lower delay discounting compared to HCs [9]. This low delay discounting is proposed to reflect the eating habits of HW individuals, whereby individuals may preferentially elect for immediate reward over a greater potential future benefit of improved health [9].

7.4. Emotional Processing Difficulties

Emotional processing difficulties have been implicated in the development of maladaptive eating behaviours contributing to HW, with a common trend of low levels of recognition, self-reporting, and emotion regulation [11,142]. In a systematic review and meta-analysis, Fernandes et al. (2018) [11] found that compared to HCs, participants at a HW had greater difficulty in identifying emotions, higher alexithymia, lower emotional awareness, and greater difficulties using emotion regulation strategies. However, there was no research to support a hypothesis that people at a HW exhibited an impaired ability to recognize the emotions of others or express their emotions [11]. Although further research is required, it appears that emotion processing in HW is nuanced and that HW is not characterized by a general emotion processing deficit [11].

Emotional factors and subsequent emotional regulation have also been found to underscore HW development. Brain regions such as the limbic system and frontal cortex, which play key roles in modulating emotions, have been revealed to contribute to the overriding of homeostatic mechanisms of feeding in HW [143]. The cortico-limbic system is believed to drive effector mechanisms in the absence of repletion signals—physiological cues indicating satiety or fullness, such as hormonal and neural signals that suppress appetite—but in the presence of potential hedonic reward signals, which promote eating for pleasure rather than need [136,144].

It should also be noted that psychological distress and emotional regulation difficulties are key risk factors for HW. Overeating often emerges as an affective response to anxiety, sadness, or stress, reflecting maladaptive coping strategies when individuals struggle to regulate emotions [145]. Impaired self-regulation and ruminative thinking can drive emotional eating, where food is used to manage negative emotions. The "escape from awareness" theory [98] suggests that individuals overeat to avoid distressing thoughts or aversive self-awareness by focusing on immediate sensory experiences, such as the taste of food. Physiologically, chronic stress and abnormal cortisol secretion can stimulate appetite, promoting cravings for high-calorie, fatty, and sweet foods by activating brain reward systems and suppressing stress response pathways [145,146]. Additionally, emotional regulation challenges may contribute to other HW risk factors, such as sedentary behaviour and sleep disturbances, further exacerbating weight gain [146].

Collectively, these findings highlight the critical interplay between psychological stress, impaired emotional regulation, physiological responses, and neurocognitive factors, such as deficiencies in cognitive flexibility, impulsivity, reward processing, and emotion regulation difficulties, driving maladaptive eating behaviours and contributing to overeating and weight gain in people at an HW.

8. Clinical Implications

8.1. Classification

Neurocognitive knowledge can significantly enhance the classification of EDs by identifying cognitive profiles that differentiate these conditions beyond the DSM-5 [4,5] or ICD-11 [28] diagnostic criteria. The variations in cognitive flexibility, central coherence, attentional biases, emotional processing, and reward processes/impulsivity outlined above across the different ED subtypes and HW (see Table 1 for an overview) can aid in refining diagnostic boundaries, offering a more granular classification system that accounts for cognitive profiles alongside behavioural symptoms (e.g., binge eating behaviour, restriction) [147]. Importantly, some of these neurocognitive factors, such as cognitive flexibility, appear to be transdiagnostic, meaning they may be present across multiple ED subtypes.

Table 1. Neurocognitive processes across eating disorders and higher weight.

Neurocognitive Process	Anorexia * Nervosa (AN)	Bulimia Nervosa (BN)	Binge Eating Disorder (BED)	Higher Weight (HW)
Cognitive Flexibility	↓ (consistently impaired; rigid food rules)	↓ (impaired; cognitive rigidity evident in binge–purge cycles)—evidence lacking	↓ (impaired, particularly in food contexts)	↓ (mild impairment, especially for food-related stimuli)
Impulsivity	↑ (increased inhibitory control during restriction; difficulty modulating impulsivity in binge–purge episodes)	↑ (elevated impulsivity, exacerbated by negative affect and emotional triggers)	↑ (high impulsivity; difficulty resisting binge urges; impaired response inhibition for palatable stimuli)	↑ (low inhibitory control, particularly for food stimuli; associated with BMI and immediate gratification)
Emotional Processing	↓ (greater difficulty identifying and processing emotions; alexithymia noted)	↓ (emotional dysregulation; binge–purge cycles as avoidance)	↓ (heightened emotional dysregulation; bingeing used as emotional avoidance)	↔ or ↓ (context-dependent; alexithymia and emotional challenges present in some individuals)
Reward Processing	↓ (low reward sensitivity and rigid adherence to rules)	↑ (heightened sensitivity to food-related rewards)	↑ (preference for immediate food rewards over delayed benefits)	↑ (greater preference for immediate gratification at the expense of long-term outcomes)

↑: increased/elevated; ↓: decreased; ↔: mixed or context-dependent. * Results might differ between AN-Restrictive and AN-Binge Purging Subtype. OSFEDs have been omitted from the table due to lacking research.

By incorporating these cognitive traits into future classification models, we can enhance the identification of distinct subtypes within and across different EDs. This approach would shift towards a dimensional framework that emphasizes underlying neurocognitive features, rather than relying solely on traditional diagnostic categories [8,75]. This model does not imply collapsing all ED diagnoses into a single group but rather focusing on the neurocognitive profiles that might cut across different ED subtypes, helping to tailor treatment based on individual cognitive characteristics.

8.2. Treatment

An important question in understanding neurocognitive factors in EDs is whether potential deficits in cognitive functioning represent stable traits or whether they are state factors associated with the illness. Are these deficits likely to remit on their own with recovery, or do they require targeted intervention [148]? Addressing this issue is crucial for developing effective treatment strategies. While some cognitive impairments may improve as individuals recover from the disorder, others may persist and need to be specifically targeted in treatment to optimize outcomes. Understanding the nature of these deficits—whether trait-like or state-dependent—can help clinicians decide whether to focus on cognitive remediation as part of the therapeutic process or whether to simply monitor cognitive functioning throughout recovery [148]. Presently, it remains unclear if neurocognitive impairments in EDs are traits or state factors and further research is needed to understand this issue.

Understanding the neurocognitive profiles in individuals with AN, BN, BED, OSFED, and HW is crucial for developing effective treatment interventions. In a very recent Delphi consensus paper [149], improving cognitive flexibility and impulse control were identified by researchers, clinicians, careers, and those with lived experience as key targets for ED treatments. In AN, potential deficits in cognitive flexibility, attentional biases, and emotional processing difficulties reveal specific targets for therapy. CRT (e.g., [31]) has been developed to help patients improve cognitive flexibility and central coherence, in addition to preparing patients to participate in other therapies [150].

However, a recent meta-analysis of randomized controlled trials on CRT for AN showed no significant improvement in central coherence over control treatments at the end of treatment, but this finding was based on only three studies [151]. Cognitive Remediation and Emotion Skills Training (CREST) builds on CRT by integrating cognitive training with emotion skills training. This combination has shown promising results in AN patients, with significant improvements in social anhedonia, emotional labelling, and patients' confidence in their capacity for change [152]. Finally, it is also worth noting that there are aspects of traditional CBT that encourage adaptive and flexible thinking [153]. Additional research is therefore required to further improve CRT/CREST and develop additional treatments that can target poor cognitive flexibility across the different ED subtypes.

To address attentional biases in AN, exposure-based therapies can gradually desensitize ED individuals to anxiety-provoking food cues [115]. For instance, through repeated exposure to food-related scenarios, patients can learn to tolerate these cues without resorting to avoidance or restrictive behaviours. Furthermore, emotional processing challenges can be tackled using emotion regulation training, such as dialectical behaviour therapy (DBT) [154], which teaches ED patients to identify and manage their emotions more effectively. Skills like mindfulness [155] and distress tolerance training [156] can also enhance emotional resilience in ED individuals, potentially lowering the risk of relapse.

In BN and BED, cognitive rigidity and attentional biases may manifest in food preoccupations and impulsive behaviours. Recently, Transdiagnostic Cognitive Remediation Therapy (TCRT), a new adaptation of CRT for EDs, has been developed, which addresses common cognitive difficulties across ED diagnoses (i.e., cognitive flexibility, central coherence, and impulsivity). A recent qualitative study of thirteen patients with restrictive or binge–purge EDs and concurrent cognitive difficulties examined the impact of TCRT through semi-structured interviews [157]. Eleven participants viewed the treatment favourably, highlighting its relevance and the insights it provided into their thinking styles. Seven participants noted TCRT as a foundation for initiating changes and adopting new strategies. Engagement appeared to be enhanced by experiencing challenges directly related to their cognitive difficulties.

Other treatment modalities to consider for BN and BED, similar to AN, include attentional bias modification/training techniques, which may redirect attention away from food stimuli, helping to decrease cravings and impulsivity associated with binge episodes [35]. ERP techniques, adapted from anxiety treatments, can help BN/BED patients build a tolerance to high-craving environments [115]. Finally, adapted DPT interventions, such as DBTfor BED(DBT-BED) [158], aim to reduce binge eating by improving adaptive emotion-regulation skills and have been found to also help BED patients improve their emotion regulation difficulties.

For OSFEDs, the diverse presentations necessitate flexible and integrative interventions, as research on its classification, subtypes, and effective treatments is still in its infancy. This diagnostic category includes various symptom patterns that do not fully align with the other EDs, requiring approaches that address both the cognitive and emotional challenges specific to each presentation in addition to ED symptoms [108,109]. Combining elements from CRT/CREST, broader emotion regulation training and attentional bias modification may effectively target these unique needs. As our understanding of OSFEDs develops, refining such targeted interventions will be essential for enhancing treatment outcomes and providing tailored support.

Finally, in HW populations, impulsivity, reward processing difficulties, and emotional processing difficulties may perpetuate cycles of overeating and negatively impact body image. Mindfulness-based exercises can enhance focus and control over food-related impulses [159], while strategies from acceptance and commitment therapy and DBT [160] can help individuals reframe their relationship with food. Acceptance and commitment therapy encourages the acceptance of cravings without acting on them, fostering healthier responses to food cues and reducing binge eating behaviour [161]. Together, these interventions can foster a more adaptive relationship with food; reduce the impact of impulsivity, reward processing difficulties, and emotional biases; and enhance overall well-being.

However, it needs to be outlined that the practical implementation of these treatments requires careful consideration of their feasibility, scalability, and cultural adaptability. CRT and its adaptations (e.g., CREST and TCRT) can be delivered in both individual and group formats, increasing scalability [162]. Incorporating digital platforms or app-based interventions may further enhance accessibility, particularly for remote or underserved populations. Emotion regulation therapies, such as DBT and its adaptations (e.g., DBT-BED), have demonstrated efficacy [158], but their intensive training requirements for clinicians could pose barriers to broader implementation. Simplified versions or modular approaches might improve scalability.

Cultural adaptability is also critical. Treatments should account for variations in cultural attitudes toward food, weight, and body image, ensuring that interventions resonate with the diverse experiences of individuals across different cultural and ethnic backgrounds. Co-designing therapies with input from culturally diverse individuals with lived experience may enhance relevance and acceptability. Further research is needed to refine these approaches to ensure equitable access and culturally sensitive care for all individuals affected by EDs and HW.

8.2.1. Virtual Reality

Emerging treatment modalities, such as virtual reality (VR) [163] interventions, offer innovative approaches to targeting neurocognitive deficiencies in EDs and HW populations, addressing challenges like cognitive inflexibility, attentional biases, and emotional dysregulation [163]. For attentional biases, VR can offer controlled, immersive environments where exposure-based therapies are more precisely tailored and engaging [164]. For instance, VR exposure sessions can simulate real-life food-related scenarios, allowing patients to practice exposure techniques in a safe, yet realistic setting. By engaging with these VR-based scenarios, patients could incrementally increase their tolerance for anxiety-provoking cues without using avoidance or restrictive behaviours and coping mechanisms, leading to sustained desensitization [163].

In addressing emotional processing challenges, VR can complement emotion regulation training [165] and enhance interventions like DBT [166]. By replicating challenging social or emotional contexts, VR scenarios could help individuals practice distress tolerance and mindfulness in simulated situations that they might find stressful in real life. The immersive nature of VR allows for an experiential form of learning, where patients can safely explore emotional responses, develop resilience, and refine coping skills [165,166]. This integration could lower the risk of relapse by fostering emotional resilience and enhancing self-regulation skills that are essential for recovery. In addition, given the widespread adoption of VR technologies, these skills could be practised by patients in their homes outside of medical appointments with clinicians.

8.2.2. Brain Stimulation

Different brain stimulation techniques can also offer a promising approach to improving cognitive deficiencies in individuals with EDs and those with HW by directly targeting the neural circuits associated with cognitive flexibility, emotional regulation, and/or impulse control. Techniques such as transcranial magnetic stimulation [167] and transcranial direct current stimulation [168,169] can modulate neural activity in areas of the brain implicated in these cognitive domains, potentially enhancing the effectiveness of traditional therapies.

Cognitive flexibility has largely been associated with functioning in the prefrontal cortex [170], the anterior cingulate cortex [171], and the orbitofrontal cortex [172]. Stimulating these areas may increase activity in these brain regions, neural pathways, and neural plasticity, potentially improving cognitive flexibility and reducing rigid, rule-bound thinking. Similarly, individuals with BN and BED, who may exhibit heightened impulsivity and attentional biases toward food cues, could benefit from brain stimulation targeting the dorsolateral prefrontal cortex to improve inhibitory control and reduce impulsive behaviours [173,174].

In individuals with HW, brain stimulation may address impairments in reward processing and executive function, which are often associated with challenges in regulating food intake. Stimulating or inhibiting activity in the prefrontal cortex could enhance impulse control and support better decision-making in food-related contexts, potentially leading to healthier eating patterns [175,176].

9. Limitations

While our narrative review encompasses a broad range of studies examining neurocognitive and related factors in EDs and HW individuals, it may not be comprehensive. We recognize the necessity for additional structured systematic reviews and/or meta-analyses to further explore this topic, as these approaches would provide a more rigorous synthesis of the literature, including standardized inclusion criteria and quantitative pooling of results. The decision to conduct a narrative review, rather than a systematic review, was based on the exploratory nature of this topic and the need to provide a broad overview of diverse studies across multiple domains of neurocognitive processes. A narrative review allows for a more flexible and comprehensive discussion of varied study designs, methodologies, and findings, which may be less feasible in the structured format of a systematic review. Another limitation of this review is the exclusion of studies on ARFID and other EDsin childhood [4,5]. This decision is in line with previous reviews [89] given that these disorders typically develop in early childhood and are clinically distinct in presentation to AN, BN, BED, and OSFED [4,5].

Omitting ARFID from the review limits the comprehensiveness of understanding neurocognitive factors across the full spectrum of EDs. It overlooks unique developmental and neurocognitive challenges associated with early-onset disorders, such as sensory sensitivities and anxiety-related behaviours, which differ from those observed in other EDs [4,5]. Future research may wish to include ARFID to ensure a more comprehensive understanding of neurocognitive factors across the full spectrum of EDs, including early-onset disorders, which may present unique developmental and cognitive challenges.

There are also various limitations within the reviewed studies that need to be considered. First, the study of neurocognitive profiles in EDs and HW populations is constrained by several methodological limitations. A significant challenge lies in the diversity of cognitive assessment tools utilized across studies. This variability in tasks designed to evaluate key domains such as cognitive flexibility, attentional bias, and emotion regulation complicates cross-study comparisons and hinders the identification of shared or disorder-specific impairments. For instance, while some studies use standardized neurocognitive tests, others employ experimental paradigms or self-report measures, each with varying levels of reliability and ecological validity.

Second, many studies lack uniformity in the operational definitions and measurement of neurocognitive constructs, leading to inconsistent results. Small and non-representative sample sizes are another limitation, often reducing the generalizability of findings to broader clinical populations. Few studies stratify their samples using important demographic or clinical factors, such as age, gender, comorbidities, or the duration of the illness/condition, which may influence neurocognitive functioning.

Third, theoretical limitations also warrant consideration. Many studies fail to clearly differentiate between trait-like neurocognitive deficits that may predispose individuals to EDs and HW conditions and state-like impairments that emerge as consequences of these disorders or associated factors such as malnutrition or weight changes. This lack of theoretical clarity complicates the interpretation of findings and the development of targeted interventions. Furthermore, it remains unclear which cognitive factors are inherent traits, which exist premorbidly, which are scar effects, and which are symptoms of the ED illness and HW, underscoring the need for more nuanced research in this area.

Fourth, the reliance on cross-sectional studies restricts the understanding of how neurocognitive deficits develop and progress across different stages of ED, recovery, and in people with an HW. The limited amount of longitudinal research available on EDs and cognition restricts insights into whether neurocognitive impairments endure over time or improve with treatment and recovery. For example, longitudinal tracking of cognitive flexibility in AN could help clarify whether such deficits improve with weight restoration and recovery or if they persist as chronic features of the disorder. Similarly, observing attentional biases in BN and BED across treatment phases could reveal whether these biases diminish as part of recovery or if they remain stable, potentially contributing to relapse risk.

Fifth, it is important to acknowledge the influence of weight and nutritional status on neurocognitive function and highlight that BMI alone is insufficient to capture the full scope of malnutrition and starvation and the impact that they might have on cognition. For instance, cognitive flexibility difficulties have been found in AN, yet BMI does not account for this complexity in understanding the neurocognitive profile of AN (for a review, see [20]).

Sixth, the variability in ED subtypes and illness stages among participants, which may affect neurocognitive findings across disorders, complicates the comparison of studies. AN-R and AN-BP present with different characteristics [4,5], yet most studies have lumped the two groups into one overall AN group due to small sample sizes. The transdiagnostic nature of ED symptoms further blurs the lines between disorders, as features like impulsivity and reward sensitivity, commonly observed in AN-BP, BN and BED, may represent transdiagnostic vulnerabilities rather than disorder-specific traits. Additionally, there is likely substantial heterogeneity in cognitive deficits across EDs and within cognitive domains—some deficits may be more prominent in one ED subtype than another, reflecting variability in the nature and intensity of these impairments.

Finally, as outlined in the current review, OSFEDs are underrepresented in the literature, and this lack of data makes it difficult to determine whether their neurocognitive profile aligns with other EDs or HW individuals.

10. Future Research Directions

Future research should focus on refining our understanding of neurocognitive profiles in AN, BN, BED, OSFED, and HW through detailed longitudinal studies. Longitudinal studies are needed to track cognitive changes over time and capture the dynamic nature of these disorders and their recovery phases. However, the challenges of such research need to be addressed. The key challenges include maintaining participant engagement over extended periods, managing attrition rates, and the need for sophisticated methodologies to assess cognitive changes reliably. Specific testable hypotheses for future studies should include the following question: are the observed neurocognitive deficits in these disorders temporarily associated with the current illness stage or severity, or are they stable traits that persist beyond weight restoration? It would also be important to further assess how specific neurocognitive traits predict recovery trajectories or relapse risks in EDs and HW. Future studies could, for instance, assess the following hypothesis: "Do deficits in cognitive flexibility and impulse control at the start of treatment predict poorer recovery trajectories in AN patients?" Such concrete research questions will help guide future studies in identifying predictors of treatment success and relapse, thus informing more personalized and effective intervention strategies.

Incorporating neuroimaging data can further refine this understanding. Neuroimaging studies, such as functional magnetic resonance imaging (fMRI), can elucidate changes in brain activity related to cognitive flexibility, reward processing, and other executive functions in these populations. Integrating neuroimaging with biomarkers could lead to a more comprehensive understanding of the biological underpinnings of cognitive impairments in these populations and help in designing targeted interventions that address both nutritional and cognitive deficits effectively.

Furthermore, the inclusion of different OSFED presentations and ARFID in future research is essential for comprehensively assessing the full range of cognitive impairments and their connection to emotional and behavioural patterns in individuals with disordered eating. By expanding the research focus to encompass OSFEDs, we can better understand how individuals with these illnesses navigate their cognitive challenges and develop targeted interventions that address their unique needs.

Finally, there is a need for further interdisciplinary collaborations to investigate neurocognitive profiles in EDs and HW populations. These collaborations will enable the integration of diverse expertise, including psychology, neuroscience, nutrition, and clinical treatment strategies, to develop a holistic understanding of the complex interplay between neurocognitive functioning, physiological markers, and behavioural data. Such an approach will be essential in advancing personalized treatment approaches that are responsive to the unique needs of individuals with EDs and HW.

11. Conclusions

To conclude, the unique contributions of the current review include its wide coverage of the most up-to-date literature on neurocognitive factors across EDs and HW, providing a comprehensive synthesis of the existing research in this area. It highlights the significance of poor cognitive flexibility and attentional biases in AN, underscoring the need for tailored interventions to address these specific cognitive patterns, such as CRT/CREST and CBT strategies. For BN and BED, this review discusses how poor cognitive flexibility, emotional processing difficulties, and heightened reward sensitivity contribute to binge eating and purging behaviours, suggesting the need for therapeutic approaches that manage these complex relationships, such as DBT-BED. Finally, individuals with HW face neurocognitive challenges like impaired decision-making and executive function, further emphasizing the need for individualized, transdiagnostic treatment strategies. Given that research on OSFED subtypes is still in its infancy, conclusions regarding OSFEDs remain preliminary and highlight the need for further investigation to better understand these subtypes and their unique cognitive challenges. Future research should prioritize longitudinal studies to explore the evolution of these neurocognitive profiles over time, conduct further neuroimaging, consider biomarkers, and collaborate with other fields. Such research will ensure the development of effective, tailored interventions that improve recovery outcomes across diverse ED and HW populations.

Author Contributions: I.K.—Conceptualization, original draft preparation, review and editing; A.B.D.—writing part on anorexia nervosa; E.L.—writing part on HW; W.L.O.—writing part on BN; J.P.—writing part on BED; S.M.—original draft preparation, review, editing. All authors have read and agreed to the published version of the manuscript.

Funding: This research received no external funding.

Conflicts of Interest: The authors declare no conflicts of interest.

References

1. Howard, M.; Gregertsen, E.C.; Hindocha, C.; Serpell, L. Impulsivity and compulsivity in anorexia and bulimia nervosa: A systematic review. *Psychiatry Res.* **2020**, *293*, 113354. [CrossRef]
2. Miles, S.; Gnatt, I.; Phillipou, A.; Nedeljkovic, M. Cognitive flexibility in acute anorexia nervosa and after recovery: A systematic review. *Clin. Psychol. Rev.* **2020**, *81*, 101905. [CrossRef]
3. Kittel, R.; Brauhardt, A.; Hilbert, A. Cognitive and emotional functioning in binge-eating disorder: A systematic review. *Int. J. Eat. Disord.* **2015**, *48*, 535–554. [CrossRef] [PubMed]
4. American Psychiatric Association. *Diagnostic and Statistical Manual of Mental Disorders*; American Psychiatric Association: Wahington, DC, USA, 2013.
5. American Psychiatric Association. *Diagnostic and Statistical Manual of Mental Disorders*, 5th ed.; Text Revision (DSM-5-TR); American Psychiatric Association: Washington, DC, USA, 2022. [CrossRef]
6. Lim, Y.; Boster, J. Obesity and Comorbid Conditions. In *StatPearls*; StatPearls Publishing: Treasure Island, FL, USA, 2024.
7. Villarejo, C.; Fernandez-Aranda, F.; Jimenez-Murcia, S.; Penas-Lledo, E.; Granero, R.; Penelo, E.; Tinahones, F.J.; Sancho, C.; Vilarrasa, N.; Montserrat-Gil de Bernabe, M.; et al. Lifetime obesity in patients with eating disorders: Increasing prevalence, clinical and personality correlates. *Eur. Eat. Disord. Rev.* **2012**, *20*, 250–254. [CrossRef] [PubMed]
8. Testa, G.; Mora-Maltas, B.; Camacho-Barcia, L.; Granero, R.; Lucas, I.; Aguera, Z.; Jimenez-Murcia, S.; Banos, R.; Bertaina-Anglade, V.; Botella, C.; et al. Transdiagnostic perspective of impulsivity and compulsivity in obesity: From cognitive profile to self-reported dimensions in clinical samples with and without Diabetes. *Nutrients* **2021**, *13*, 4426. [CrossRef]
9. Miranda-Olivos, R.; Steward, T.; Martinez-Zalacain, I.; Mestre-Bach, G.; Juaneda-Segui, A.; Jimenez-Murcia, S.; Fernandez-Formoso, J.A.; Vilarrasa, N.; Veciana de Las Heras, M.; Custal, N.; et al. The neural correlates of delay discounting in obesity and binge eating disorder. *J. Behav. Addict.* **2021**, *10*, 498–507. [CrossRef] [PubMed]
10. Reyes, S.; Peirano, P.; Gahagan, S.; Blanco, E.; Algarin, C. Neurocognitive factors predicting BMI changes from adolescence to young adulthood. *Obesity* **2024**, *32*, 768–777. [CrossRef]
11. Fernandes, J.; Ferreira-Santos, F.; Miller, K.; Torres, S. Emotional processing in obesity: A systematic review and exploratory meta-analysis. *Obes. Rev.* **2018**, *19*, 111–120. [CrossRef]
12. Ralph, A.F.; Brennan, L.; Byrne, S.; Caldwell, B.; Farmer, J.; Hart, L.M.; Heruc, G.A.; Maguire, S.; Piya, M.K.; Quin, J.; et al. Management of eating disorders for people with higher weight: Clinical practice guideline. *J. Eat. Disord.* **2022**, *10*, 121. [CrossRef]
13. Hubbard, V.S. Defining overweight and obesity: What are the issues? *Am. J. Clin. Nutr.* **2000**, *72*, 1067–1068. [CrossRef]
14. Fulton, M.; Dadana, S.; Srinivasan, V.N. Obesity, Stigma, and Discrimination. In *StatPearls*; StatPearls Publishing: Treasure Island, FL, USA, 2024.
15. Page, M.J.; McKenzie, J.E.; Bossuyt, P.M.; Boutron, I.; Hoffmann, T.C.; Mulrow, C.D.; Shamseer, L.; Tetzlaff, J.M.; Akl, E.A.; Brennan, S.E.; et al. The PRISMA 2020 statement: An updated guideline for reporting systematic reviews. *BMJ* **2021**, *372*, n71. [CrossRef] [PubMed]
16. Keski-Rahkonen, A.; Mustelin, L. Epidemiology of eating disorders in Europe: Prevalence, incidence, comorbidity, course, consequences, and risk factors. *Curr. Opin. Psychiatry* **2016**, *29*, 340–345. [CrossRef]
17. Baenas, I.; Etxandi, M.; Fernandez-Aranda, F. Medical complications in anorexia and bulimia nervosa. *Med. Clin.* **2024**, *162*, 67–72. [CrossRef]
18. Stedal, K.; Broomfield, C.; Hay, P.; Touyz, S.; Scherer, R. Neuropsychological functioning in adult anorexia nervosa: A meta-analysis. *Neurosci. Biobehav. Rev.* **2021**, *130*, 214–226. [CrossRef]
19. Phillipou, A.; Rossell, S.L.; Castle, D.J. Anorexia nervosa or starvation? *Eur. J. Neurosci.* **2018**, *48*, 3317–3318. [CrossRef] [PubMed]
20. Fuglset, T.S. Is set-shifting and central coherence in anorexia nervosa influenced by body mass index, anxiety or depression? A systematic review. *BMC Psychiatry* **2021**, *21*, 137. [CrossRef]
21. Patel, K.; Tchanturia, K.; Harrison, A. An exploration of social functioning in young people with eating disorders: A qualitative study. *PLoS ONE* **2016**, *11*, e0159910. [CrossRef]
22. Aloi, M.; Rania, M.; Caroleo, M.; Bruni, A.; Palmieri, A.; Cauteruccio, M.A.; De Fazio, P.; Segura-Garcia, C. Decision making, central coherence and set-shifting: A comparison between binge eating disorder, anorexia nervosa and healthy controls. *BMC Psychiatry* **2015**, *15*, 6. [CrossRef]
23. Nakazato, M.; Hashimoto, K.; Schmidt, U.; Tchanturia, K.; Campbell, I.C.; Collier, D.A.; Iyo, M.; Treasure, J. Serum glutamine, set-shifting ability and anorexia nervosa. *Ann. Gen. Psychiatry* **2010**, *9*, 29. [CrossRef]
24. Buzzichelli, S.; Marzola, E.; Amianto, F.; Fassino, S.; Abbate-Daga, G. Perfectionism and cognitive rigidity in anorexia nervosa: Is there an association? *Eur. Eat. Disord. Rev.* **2018**, *26*, 360–366. [CrossRef]

25. Castro, T.F.; Miller, K.; Araujo, M.X.; Brandao, I.; Torres, S. Emotional processing in recovered anorexia nervosa patients: A 15 year longitudinal study. *Eur. Eat. Disord. Rev.* **2021**, *29*, 955–968. [CrossRef] [PubMed]
26. Giel, K.E.; Wittorf, A.; Wolkenstein, L.; Klingberg, S.; Drimmer, E.; Schonenberg, M.; Rapp, A.M.; Fallgatter, A.J.; Hautzinger, M.; Zipfel, S. Is impaired set-shifting a feature of "pure" anorexia nervosa? Investigating the role of depression in set-shifting ability in anorexia nervosa and unipolar depression. *Psychiatry Res.* **2012**, *200*, 538–543. [CrossRef]
27. Konstantakopoulos, G.; Tchanturia, K.; Surguladze, S.A.; David, A.S. Insight in eating disorders: Clinical and cognitive correlates. *Psychol. Med.* **2011**, *41*, 1951–1961. [CrossRef] [PubMed]
28. World Health Organization. ICD-11: International Classification of Diseases 2022. Available online: https://icd.who.int/ (accessed on 17 December 2024).
29. Dougherty, E.N.; Bottera, A.R.; Forester, G.; Schaefer, L.M.; Forbes, E.E.; Wildes, J.E. Prospective associations between cognitive flexibility and eating disorder symptoms in anorexia nervosa and bulimia nervosa. *Psychiatry Res.* **2024**, *332*, 115717. [CrossRef] [PubMed]
30. Hemmingsen, S.D.; Daugaard, N.; Sjogren, M.; Lichtenstein, M.B.; Gudex, C.; Piil, F.; Stoving, R.K. Cognitive flexibility in hospitalized patients with severe or extreme anorexia nervosa: A case-control study. *J. Pers. Med.* **2023**, *13*, 1000. [CrossRef] [PubMed]
31. Tchanturia, K.; Lloyd, S.; Lang, K. Cognitive remediation therapy for anorexia nervosa: Current evidence and future research directions. *Int. J. Eat. Disord.* **2013**, *46*, 492–495. [CrossRef] [PubMed]
32. Keegan, E.; Tchanturia, K.; Wade, T.D. Central coherence and set-shifting between nonunderweight eating disorders and anorexia nervosa: A systematic review and meta-analysis. *Int. J. Eat. Disord.* **2021**, *54*, 229–243. [CrossRef] [PubMed]
33. Lopez, C.; Tchanturia, K.; Stahl, D.; Booth, R.; Holliday, J.; Treasure, J. An examination of the concept of central coherence in women with anorexia nervosa. *Int. J. Eat. Disord.* **2008**, *41*, 143–152. [CrossRef]
34. Herbrich, L.; Kappel, V.; van Noort, B.M.; Winter, S. Differences in set-shifting and central coherence across anorexia nervosa subtypes in children and adolescents. *Eur. Eat. Disord. Rev.* **2018**, *26*, 499–507. [CrossRef]
35. Stott, N.; Fox, J.R.E.; Williams, M.O. Attentional bias in eating disorders: A meta-review. *Int. J. Eat. Disord.* **2021**, *54*, 1377–1399. [CrossRef] [PubMed]
36. Werthmann, J.; Simic, M.; Konstantellou, A.; Mansfield, P.; Mercado, D.; van Ens, W.; Schmidt, U. Same, same but different: Attention bias for food cues in adults and adolescents with anorexia nervosa. *Int. J. Eat. Disord.* **2019**, *52*, 681–690. [CrossRef] [PubMed]
37. Garcia-Burgos, D.; Wilhelm, P.; Vogele, C.; Munsch, S. Food restriction in anorexia nervosa in the light of modern learning theory: A narrative review. *Behav. Sci.* **2023**, *13*, 96. [CrossRef]
38. Gilon Mann, T.; Hamdan, S.; Bar-Haim, Y.; Lazarov, A.; Enoch-Levy, A.; Dubnov-Raz, G.; Treasure, J.; Stein, D. Different attention bias patterns in anorexia nervosa restricting and binge/purge types. *Eur. Eat. Disord. Rev.* **2018**, *26*, 293–301. [CrossRef]
39. Moeller, F.G.; Barratt, E.S.; Dougherty, D.M.; Schmitz, J.M.; Swann, A.C. Psychiatric aspects of impulsivity. *Am. J. Psychiatry* **2001**, *158*, 1783–1793. [CrossRef]
40. Waxman, S.E. A systematic review of impulsivity in eating disorders. *Eur. Eat. Disord. Rev.* **2009**, *17*, 408–425. [CrossRef]
41. Claes, L.; Nederkoorn, C.; Vandereycken, W.; Guerrieri, R.; Vertommen, H. Impulsiveness and lack of inhibitory control in eating disorders. *Eat. Behav.* **2006**, *7*, 196–203. [CrossRef]
42. Steward, T.; Mestre-Bach, G.; Vintro-Alcaraz, C.; Aguera, Z.; Jimenez-Murcia, S.; Granero, R.; Fernandez-Aranda, F. Delay discounting of reward and impulsivity in eating disorders: From anorexia nervosa to binge eating disorder. *Eur. Eat. Disord. Rev.* **2017**, *25*, 601–606. [CrossRef] [PubMed]
43. Miyamoto, E.; Okumura, Y.; Maruo, K.; Kitani, S. Shoplifting behavior among patients with an eating disorder at a medical correctional center in Japan: A cross-sectional study. *Front. Psychiatry* **2022**, *13*, 767170. [CrossRef]
44. Hatch, A.; Madden, S.; Kohn, M.R.; Clarke, S.; Touyz, S.; Gordon, E.; Williams, L.M. In first presentation adolescent anorexia nervosa, do cognitive markers of underweight status change with weight gain following a refeeding intervention? *Int. J. Eat. Disord.* **2010**, *43*, 295–306. [CrossRef] [PubMed]
45. Oldershaw, A.; DeJong, H.; Hambrook, D.; Broadbent, H.; Tchanturia, K.; Treasure, J.; Schmidt, U. Emotional processing following recovery from anorexia nervosa. *Eur. Eat. Disord. Rev.* **2012**, *20*, 502–509. [CrossRef]
46. Harrison, A.; Sullivan, S.; Tchanturia, K.; Treasure, J. Emotional functioning in eating disorders: Attentional bias, emotion recognition and emotion regulation. *Psychol. Med.* **2010**, *40*, 1887–1897. [CrossRef] [PubMed]
47. Saure, E.; Raevuori, A.; Laasonen, M.; Lepisto-Paisley, T. Emotion recognition, alexithymia, empathy, and emotion regulation in women with anorexia nervosa. *Eat. Weight. Disord.* **2022**, *27*, 3587–3597. [CrossRef]
48. Caglar-Nazali, H.P.; Corfield, F.; Cardi, V.; Ambwani, S.; Leppanen, J.; Olabintan, O.; Deriziotis, S.; Hadjimichalis, A.; Scognamiglio, P.; Eshkevari, E.; et al. A systematic review and meta-analysis of 'Systems for Social Processes' in eating disorders. *Neurosci. Biobehav. Rev.* **2014**, *42*, 55–92. [CrossRef] [PubMed]
49. Oldershaw, A.; Hambrook, D.; Stahl, D.; Tchanturia, K.; Treasure, J.; Schmidt, U. The socio-emotional processing stream in Anorexia Nervosa. *Neurosci. Biobehav. Rev.* **2011**, *35*, 970–988. [CrossRef] [PubMed]
50. Racine, S.E.; Wildes, J.E. Dynamic longitudinal relations between emotion regulation difficulties and anorexia nervosa symptoms over the year following intensive treatment. *J. Consult. Clin. Psychol.* **2015**, *83*, 785–795. [CrossRef] [PubMed]

51. Brockmeyer, T.; Febry, H.; Leiteritz-Rausch, A.; Wunsch-Leiteritz, W.; Leiteritz, A.; Friederich, H.C. Cognitive flexibility, central coherence, and quality of life in anorexia nervosa. *J. Eat. Disord.* **2022**, *10*, 22. [CrossRef]
52. Nowakowski, M.E.; McFarlane, T.; Cassin, S. Alexithymia and eating disorders: A critical review of the literature. *J. Eat. Disord.* **2013**, *1*, 21. [CrossRef]
53. Westwood, H.; Kerr-Gaffney, J.; Stahl, D.; Tchanturia, K. Alexithymia in eating disorders: Systematic review and meta-analyses of studies using the Toronto Alexithymia Scale. *J. Psychosom. Res.* **2017**, *99*, 66–81. [CrossRef]
54. Haynos, A.F.; Utzinger, L.M.; Lavender, J.M.; Crosby, R.D.; Cao, L.; Peterson, C.B.; Crow, S.J.; Wonderlich, S.A.; Engel, S.G.; Mitchell, J.E.; et al. Subtypes of adaptive and maladaptive perfectionism in anorexia nervosa: Associations with eating Disorder and affective symptoms. *J. Psychopathol. Behav. Assess.* **2018**, *40*, 691–700. [CrossRef]
55. Henderson, Z.B.; Fox, J.R.E.; Trayner, P.; Wittkowski, A. Emotional development in eating disorders: A qualitative metasynthesis. *Clin. Psychol. Psychother.* **2019**, *26*, 440–457. [CrossRef]
56. Skunde, M.; Walther, S.; Simon, J.J.; Wu, M.; Bendszus, M.; Herzog, W.; Friederich, H.C. Neural signature of behavioural inhibition in women with bulimia nervosa. *J. Psychiatry Neurosci.* **2016**, *41*, E69–E78. [CrossRef] [PubMed]
57. Liao, P.C.; Uher, R.; Lawrence, N.; Treasure, J.; Schmidt, U.; Campbell, I.C.; Collier, D.A.; Tchanturia, K. An examination of decision making in bulimia nervosa. *J. Clin. Exp. Neuropsychol.* **2009**, *31*, 455–461. [CrossRef]
58. Boeka, A.G.; Lokken, K.L. The Iowa gambling task as a measure of decision making in women with bulimia nervosa. *J. Int. Neuropsychol. Soc.* **2006**, *12*, 741–745. [CrossRef] [PubMed]
59. Brand, M.; Franke-Sievert, C.; Jacoby, G.E.; Markowitsch, H.J.; Tuschen-Caffier, B. Neuropsychological correlates of decision making in patients with bulimia nervosa. *Neuropsychology* **2007**, *21*, 742–750. [CrossRef] [PubMed]
60. Matsumoto, J.; Hirano, Y.; Numata, N.; Matzuzawa, D.; Murano, S.; Yokote, K.; Iyo, M.; Shimizu, E.; Nakazato, M. Comparison in decision-making between bulimia nervosa, anorexia nervosa, and healthy women: Influence of mood status and pathological eating concerns. *J. Eat. Disord.* **2015**, *3*, 14. [CrossRef]
61. Roberts, M.E.; Tchanturia, K.; Stahl, D.; Southgate, L.; Treasure, J. A systematic review and meta-analysis of set-shifting ability in eating disorders. *Psychol. Med.* **2007**, *37*, 1075–1084. [CrossRef]
62. Tchanturia, K.; Anderluh, M.B.; Morris, R.G.; Rabe-Hesketh, S.; Collier, D.A.; Sanchez, P.; Treasure, J.L. Cognitive flexibility in anorexia nervosa and bulimia nervosa. *J. Int. Neuropsychol. Soc.* **2004**, *10*, 513–520. [CrossRef]
63. Tchanturia, K.; Davies, H.; Roberts, M.; Harrison, A.; Nakazato, M.; Schmidt, U.; Treasure, J.; Morris, R. Poor cognitive flexibility in eating disorders: Examining the evidence using the Wisconsin Card Sorting Task. *PLoS ONE* **2012**, *7*, e28331. [CrossRef]
64. Vall, E.; Wade, T.D. Trail making task performance in inpatients with anorexia nervosa and bulimia nervosa. *Eur. Eat. Disord. Rev.* **2015**, *23*, 304–311. [CrossRef]
65. Galimberti, E.; Martoni, R.M.; Cavallini, M.C.; Erzegovesi, S.; Bellodi, L. Motor inhibition and cognitive flexibility in eating disorder subtypes. *Prog. Neuropsychopharmacol. Biol. Psychiatry* **2012**, *36*, 307–312. [CrossRef]
66. Nusslock, R.; Alloy, L.B. Reward processing and mood-related symptoms: An RDoC and translational neuroscience perspective. *J. Affect. Disord.* **2017**, *216*, 3–16. [CrossRef]
67. Hofmann, W.; Friese, M.; Strack, F. Impulse and Self-Control from a Dual-Systems Perspective. *Perspect. Psychol. Sci.* **2009**, *4*, 162–176. [CrossRef]
68. Leslie, M.; Lambert, E.; Treasure, J. Towards a translational approach to food addiction: Implications for bulimia nervosa. *Curr. Addict. Rep.* **2019**, *6*, 258–265. [CrossRef]
69. Harrison, A.; O'Brien, N.; Lopez, C.; Treasure, J. Sensitivity to reward and punishment in eating disorders. *Psychiatry Res.* **2010**, *177*, 1–11. [CrossRef]
70. Matta, A.D.; Gonçalves, F.L.; Bizarro, L. Delay discounting: Concepts and measures. *Psychol. Neurosci.* **2012**, *5*, 135–146. [CrossRef]
71. Neveu, R.; Neveu, D.; Barsumian, F.; Fouragnan, E.; Carrier, E.; Lai, M.; Sultan, J.; Nicolas, A.; Coricelli, G. Improved planning abilities in binge eating. *PLoS ONE* **2014**, *9*, e105657. [CrossRef]
72. Kekic, M.; Bartholdy, S.; Cheng, J.; McClelland, J.; Boysen, E.; Musiat, P.; O'Daly, O.G.; Campbell, I.C.; Schmidt, U. Increased temporal discounting in bulimia nervosa. *Int. J. Eat. Disord.* **2016**, *49*, 1077–1081. [CrossRef] [PubMed]
73. Bartholdy, S.; Rennalls, S.; Danby, H.; Jacques, C.; Campbell, I.C.; Schmidt, U.; O'Daly, O.G. Temporal discounting and the tendency to delay gratification across the eating disorder spectrum. *Eur. Eat. Disord. Rev.* **2017**, *25*, 344–350. [CrossRef] [PubMed]
74. Hagan, K.E.; Jarmolowicz, D.P.; Forbush, K.T. Reconsidering delay discounting in bulimia nervosa. *Eat. Behav.* **2021**, *41*, 101506. [CrossRef]
75. Amlung, M.; Marsden, E.; Holshausen, K.; Morris, V.; Patel, H.; Vedelago, L.; Naish, K.R.; Reed, D.D.; McCabe, R.E. Delay discounting as a transdiagnostic process in psychiatric disorders: A meta-analysis. *JAMA Psychiatry* **2019**, *76*, 1176–1186. [CrossRef]
76. Rosval, L.; Steiger, H.; Bruce, K.; Israel, M.; Richardson, J.; Aubut, M. Impulsivity in women with eating disorders: Problem of response inhibition, planning, or attention? *Int. J. Eat. Disord.* **2006**, *39*, 590–593. [CrossRef] [PubMed]
77. Van den Eynde, F.; Samarawickrema, N.; Kenyon, M.; DeJong, H.; Lavender, A.; Startup, H.; Schmidt, U. A study of neurocognition in bulimia nervosa and eating disorder not otherwise specified-bulimia type. *J. Clin. Exp. Neuropsychol.* **2012**, *34*, 67–77. [CrossRef]
78. Kemps, E.; Wilsdon, A. Preliminary evidence for a role for impulsivity in cognitive disinhibition in bulimia nervosa. *J. Clin. Exp. Neuropsychol.* **2010**, *32*, 515–521. [CrossRef] [PubMed]

79. Lee, J.E.; Namkoong, K.; Jung, Y.C. Impaired prefrontal cognitive control over interference by food images in binge-eating disorder and bulimia nervosa. *Neurosci. Lett.* **2017**, *651*, 95–101. [CrossRef] [PubMed]
80. Neveu, R.; Neveu, D.; Carrier, E.; Gay, A.; Nicolas, A.; Coricelli, G. Goal directed and self-control systems in bulimia nervosa: An fMRI Study. *EBioMedicine* **2018**, *34*, 214–222. [CrossRef]
81. Manasse, S.M.; Murray, H.B.; Parker, M.; Forman, E.M.; Juarascio, A.S. A characterization of binge planning behavior in individuals with binge-spectrum eating disorders. *Eat. Weight. Disord.* **2020**, *25*, 1099–1103. [CrossRef]
82. Juarascio, A.S.; Manasse, S.M.; Schumacher, L.; Espel, H.; Forman, E.M. Developing an acceptance-based behavioral treatment for binge eating disorder: Rationale and challenges. *Cogn. Behav. Pract.* **2017**, *24*, 1–13. [CrossRef]
83. Murphy, R.; Straebler, S.; Cooper, Z.; Fairburn, C.G. Cognitive behavioral therapy for eating disorders. *Psychiatr. Clin. N. Am.* **2010**, *33*, 611–627. [CrossRef] [PubMed]
84. Mourilhe, C.; Moraes, C.E.; Veiga, G.D.; Da Luz, F.Q.; Pompeu, A.; Nazar, B.P.; Coutinho, E.S.F.; Hay, P.; Appolinario, J.C. An evaluation of binge eating characteristics in individuals with eating disorders: A systematic review and meta-analysis. *Appetite* **2021**, *162*, 105176. [CrossRef]
85. Davis, H.A.; Smith, G.T. Examining the role of urgency in predicting binge size in bulimia nervosa. *Front. Psychol.* **2023**, *14*, 1166119. [CrossRef]
86. Donnelly, B.; Touyz, S.; Hay, P.; Burton, A.; Russell, J.; Caterson, I. Neuroimaging in bulimia nervosa and binge eating disorder: A systematic review. *J. Eat. Disord.* **2018**, *6*, 3. [CrossRef]
87. MacDonald, D.E.; Solomon-Krakus, S.; Jewett, R.; Liebman, R.E.; Trottier, K. Emotion regulation in bulimia nervosa and purging disorder. In *Eating Disorders*; Springer International Publishing: Cham, Switzerland, 2023.
88. Smyth, J.M.; Wonderlich, S.A.; Heron, K.E.; Sliwinski, M.J.; Crosby, R.D.; Mitchell, J.E.; Engel, S.G. Daily and momentary mood and stress are associated with binge eating and vomiting in bulimia nervosa patients in the natural environment. *J. Consult. Clin. Psychol.* **2007**, *75*, 629–638. [CrossRef] [PubMed]
89. Fischer, S.; Wonderlich, J.; Breithaupt, L.; Byrne, C.; Engel, S. Negative urgency and expectancies increase vulnerability to binge eating in bulimia nervosa. *Eat. Disord.* **2018**, *26*, 39–51. [CrossRef] [PubMed]
90. Carr, M.M.; Wiedemann, A.A.; Macdonald-Gagnon, G.; Potenza, M.N. Impulsivity and compulsivity in binge eating disorder: A systematic review of behavioral studies. *Prog. Neuropsychopharmacol Biol. Psychiatry* **2021**, *110*, 110318. [CrossRef]
91. Banca, P.; Harrison, N.A.; Voon, V. Compulsivity across the pathological misuse of drug and non-drug rewards. *Front. Behav. Neurosci.* **2016**, *10*, 154. [CrossRef]
92. Dingemans, A.E.; Vanhaelen, C.B.; Aardoom, J.J.; van Furth, E.F. The influence of depressive symptoms on executive functioning in binge eating disorder: A comparison of patients and non-obese healthy controls. *Psychiatry Res.* **2019**, *274*, 138–145. [CrossRef]
93. Kittel, R.; Schmidt, R.; Hilbert, A. Executive functions in adolescents with binge-eating disorder and obesity. *Int. J. Eat. Disord.* **2017**, *50*, 933–941. [CrossRef]
94. Kollei, I.; Rustemeier, M.; Schroeder, S.; Jongen, S.; Herpertz, S.; Loeber, S. Cognitive control functions in individuals with obesity with and without binge-eating disorder. *Int. J. Eat. Disord.* **2018**, *51*, 233–240. [CrossRef] [PubMed]
95. Mobbs, O.; Iglesias, K.; Golay, A.; Van der Linden, M. Cognitive deficits in obese persons with and without binge eating disorder. Investigation using a mental flexibility task. *Appetite* **2011**, *57*, 263–271. [CrossRef]
96. Messer, M.; Eckley, T.; Milesi, M.; Storey, L.; Linardon, J. An inflexible adherence to food rules mediates the longitudinal association between shape/weight overvaluation and binge eating. *J. Psychiatr. Res.* **2024**, *169*, 378–381. [CrossRef]
97. Steegers, C.; Dieleman, G.; Moskalenko, V.; Santos, S.; Hillegers, M.; White, T.; Jansen, P.W. The longitudinal relationship between set-shifting at 4 years of age and eating disorder related features at 9 years of age in the general pediatric population. *Int. J. Eat. Disord.* **2021**, *54*, 2180–2191. [CrossRef] [PubMed]
98. Heatherton, T.F.; Baumeister, R.F. Binge eating as escape from self-awareness. *Psychol. Bull.* **1991**, *110*, 86–108. [CrossRef]
99. Dingemans, A.E.; Visser, H.; Paul, L.; van Furth, E.F. Set-shifting abilities, mood and loss of control over eating in binge eating disorder: An experimental study. *Psychiatry Res.* **2015**, *230*, 242–248. [CrossRef]
100. Giel, K.E.; Bulik, C.M.; Fernandez-Aranda, F.; Hay, P.; Keski-Rahkonen, A.; Schag, K.; Schmidt, U.; Zipfel, S. Binge eating disorder. *Nat. Rev. Dis. Primers* **2022**, *8*, 16. [CrossRef]
101. Giel, K.E.; Teufel, M.; Junne, F.; Zipfel, S.; Schag, K. Food-related impulsivity in obesity and binge eating disorder—A Systematic update of the evidence. *Nutrients* **2017**, *9*, 1170. [CrossRef] [PubMed]
102. Lavagnino, L.; Arnone, D.; Cao, B.; Soares, J.C.; Selvaraj, S. Inhibitory control in obesity and binge eating disorder: A systematic review and meta-analysis of neurocognitive and neuroimaging studies. *Neurosci. Biobehav. Rev.* **2016**, *68*, 714–726. [CrossRef]
103. Schag, K.; Schonleber, J.; Teufel, M.; Zipfel, S.; Giel, K.E. Food-related impulsivity in obesity and binge eating disorder—A systematic review. *Obes. Rev.* **2013**, *14*, 477–495. [CrossRef]
104. Evans, B.C.; Felton, J.W.; Lagacey, M.A.; Manasse, S.M.; Lejuez, C.W.; Juarascio, A.S. Impulsivity and affect reactivity prospectively predict disordered eating attitudes in adolescents: A 6-year longitudinal study. *Eur. Child. Adolesc. Psychiatry* **2019**, *28*, 1193–1202. [CrossRef] [PubMed]
105. Pearson, C.M.; Zapolski, T.C.; Smith, G.T. A longitudinal test of impulsivity and depression pathways to early binge eating onset. *Int. J. Eat. Disord.* **2015**, *48*, 230–237. [CrossRef]
106. Gianini, L.M.; White, M.A.; Masheb, R.M. Eating pathology, emotion regulation, and emotional overeating in obese adults with binge eating disorder. *Eat. Behav.* **2013**, *14*, 309–313. [CrossRef]

107. Bodell, L.P.; Pearson, C.M.; Smith, K.E.; Cao, L.; Crosby, R.D.; Peterson, C.B.; Crow, S.J.; Berg, K.C. Longitudinal associations between emotion regulation skills, negative affect, and eating disorder symptoms in a clinical sample of individuals with binge eating. *Eat. Behav.* **2019**, *32*, 69–73. [CrossRef] [PubMed]
108. Dang, T.B.; Hughes, E.K.; Dang, A.B.; Lai, H.Y.; Lee, J.; Liu, S.; Portingale, J.; Fuller-Tyszkiewicz, M.; Krug, I. Taking a deeper dive into OSFED subtypes: A meta-analysis and systematic review. *Int. J. Eat. Disord.* **2024**, *57*, 2006–2040. [CrossRef]
109. Krug, I.; Dang, A.B.; Hughes, E.K. There is nothing as inconsistent as the OSFED diagnostic criteria. *Trends Mol. Med.* **2024**, *30*, 403–415. [CrossRef] [PubMed]
110. Prince, T.; McLoughlin, L.; Lagopoulos, J.; Elwyn, R.; Hermens, D.F. The neural correlates of socio-cognitive factors and eating disorders in young people: A systematic review. *J. Psychiatr. Res.* **2022**, *156*, 647–659. [CrossRef] [PubMed]
111. Wang, Y.; Dong, D.; Todd, J.; Du, J.; Yang, Z.; Lu, H.; Chen, H. Neural correlates of restrained eaters' high susceptibility to food cues: An fMRI study. *Neurosci. Lett.* **2016**, *631*, 56–62. [CrossRef]
112. Bartholdy, S.; O'Daly, O.G.; Campbell, I.C.; Banaschewski, T.; Barker, G.; Bokde, A.L.W.; Bromberg, U.; Buchel, C.; Quinlan, E.B.; Desrivieres, S.; et al. Neural correlates of failed inhibitory control as an early marker of disordered eating in adolescents. *Biol. Psychiatry* **2019**, *85*, 956–965. [CrossRef]
113. Bodell, L.P.; Wildes, J.E.; Goldschmidt, A.B.; Lepage, R.; Keenan, K.E.; Guyer, A.E.; Hipwell, A.E.; Stepp, S.D.; Forbes, E.E. Associations between neural reward processing and binge eating among adolescent girls. *J. Adolesc. Health* **2018**, *62*, 107–113. [CrossRef] [PubMed]
114. Wang, S.B.; Gray, E.K.; Coniglio, K.A.; Murray, H.B.; Stone, M.; Becker, K.R.; Thomas, J.J.; Eddy, K.T. Cognitive rigidity and heightened attention to detail occur transdiagnostically in adolescents with eating disorders. *Eat. Disord.* **2021**, *29*, 408–420. [CrossRef] [PubMed]
115. Koskina, A.; Campbell, I.C.; Schmidt, U. Exposure therapy in eating disorders revisited. *Neurosci. Biobehav. Rev.* **2013**, *37*, 193–208. [CrossRef]
116. Dikmeer, N.; Ersoz Alan, B.; Foto Ozdemir, D. The role of mindfulness on the psychological aspects of anorexia nervosa. *Clin. Child. Psychol. Psychiatry* **2024**, *29*, 15–29. [CrossRef]
117. Monteleone, A.M.; Castellini, G.; Volpe, U.; Ricca, V.; Lelli, L.; Monteleone, P.; Maj, M. Neuroendocrinology and brain imaging of reward in eating disorders: A possible key to the treatment of anorexia nervosa and bulimia nervosa. *Prog. Neuropsychopharmacol. Biol. Psychiatry* **2018**, *80*, 132–142. [CrossRef] [PubMed]
118. Johnson-Munguia, S.; Negi, S.; Chen, Y.; Thomeczek, M.L.; Forbush, K.T. Eating disorder psychopathology, psychiatric impairment, and symptom frequency of atypical anorexia nervosa versus anorexia nervosa: A systematic review and meta-analysis. *Int. J. Eat. Disord.* **2024**, *57*, 761–779. [CrossRef]
119. Olivo, G.; Zhukovsky, C.; Salonen-Ros, H.; Larsson, E.M.; Brooks, S.; Schioth, H.B. Functional connectivity underlying hedonic response to food in female adolescents with atypical AN: The role of somatosensory and salience networks. *Transl. Psychiatry* **2019**, *9*, 276. [CrossRef]
120. Olivo, G.; Solstrand Dahlberg, L.; Wiemerslage, L.; Swenne, I.; Zhukovsky, C.; Salonen-Ros, H.; Larsson, E.M.; Gaudio, S.; Brooks, S.J.; Schioth, H.B. Atypical anorexia nervosa is not related to brain structural changes in newly diagnosed adolescent patients. *Int. J. Eat. Disord.* **2018**, *51*, 39–45. [CrossRef]
121. Seitz, J.; Herpertz-Dahlmann, B.; Konrad, K. Brain morphological changes in adolescent and adult patients with anorexia nervosa. *J. Neural. Trans.* **2016**, *123*, 949–959. [CrossRef]
122. Davis, H.A.; Smith, G.T.; Keel, P.K. An examination of negative urgency and other impulsigenic traits in purging disorder. *Eat. Behav.* **2020**, *36*, 101365. [CrossRef]
123. Krug, I.; Giles, S.E.; Granero, R.; Aguera, Z.; Sanchez, I.; Sanchez-Gonzalez, J.; Jimenez-Murcia, S.; Fernandez-Aranda, F. Where does purging disorder lie on the symptomatologic and personality continuum when compared to other eating disorder subtypes? Implications for the DSM. *Eur. Eat. Disord. Rev.* **2022**, *30*, 36–49. [CrossRef] [PubMed]
124. Cleator, J.; Abbott, J.; Judd, P.; Sutton, C.; Wilding, J.P. Night eating syndrome: Implications for severe obesity. *Nutr. Diabetes* **2012**, *2*, e44. [CrossRef]
125. Kaur, J.; Dang, A.B.; Gan, J.; An, Z.; Krug, I. Night eating syndrome in patients with obesity and binge eating disorder: A systematic review. *Front. Psychol.* **2021**, *12*, 766827. [CrossRef] [PubMed]
126. Lavery, M.E.; Frum-Vassallo, D. An updated review of night eating syndrome: An under-represented eating disorder. *Curr. Obes. Rep.* **2022**, *11*, 395–404. [CrossRef]
127. Bargagna, M.; Casu, M. Night Eating Syndrome: A review of etiology, assessment, and suggestions for clinical treatment. *Psychiatry Int.* **2024**, *5*, 289–304. [CrossRef]
128. Darcy, A.M.; Fitzpatrick, K.K.; Colborn, D.; Manasse, S.; Datta, N.; Aspen, V.; Shields, C.S.; Le Grange, D.; Lock, J. Set-shifting among adolescents with bulimic spectrum eating disorders. *Psychosom. Med.* **2012**, *74*, 869–872. [CrossRef]
129. Manasse, S.M.; Forman, E.M.; Ruocco, A.C.; Butryn, M.L.; Juarascio, A.S.; Fitzpatrick, K.K. Do executive functioning deficits underpin binge eating disorder? A comparison of overweight women with and without binge eating pathology. *Int. J. Eat. Disord.* **2015**, *48*, 677–683. [CrossRef] [PubMed]
130. Oliva, R.; Morys, F.; Horstmann, A.; Castiello, U.; Begliomini, C. The impulsive brain: Neural underpinnings of binge eating behavior in normal-weight adults. *Appetite* **2019**, *136*, 33–49. [CrossRef] [PubMed]

131. Mattavelli, G.; Gorrino, I.; Tornaghi, D.; Canessa, N. Cognitive and motor impulsivity in the healthy brain, and implications for eating disorders and obesity: A coordinate-based meta-analysis and systematic review. *Cortex* **2024**, *171*, 90–112. [CrossRef]
132. Lane, J.M.; Wright, R.O.; Eggers, S. The interconnection between obesity and executive function in adolescence: The role of the gut microbiome. *Neurosci. Biobehav. Rev.* **2023**, *153*, 105337. [CrossRef]
133. Sakib, M.N.; Best, J.R.; Hall, P.A. Bidirectional associations between adiposity and cognitive function and mediation by brain morphology in the ABCD Study. *JAMA Netw. Open* **2023**, *6*, e2255631. [CrossRef] [PubMed]
134. Sui, S.X.; Pasco, J.A. Obesity and brain function: The brain-body crosstalk. *Medicina* **2020**, *56*, 499. [CrossRef]
135. Hartanto, A.; Yong, J.C.; Toh, W.X. Bidirectional associations between obesity and cognitive function in midlife adults: A longitudinal study. *Nutrients* **2019**, *11*, 2343. [CrossRef]
136. Dallman, M.F. Stress-induced obesity and the emotional nervous system. *Trends Endocrinol. Metab.* **2010**, *21*, 159–165. [CrossRef]
137. Yang, Y.; Shields, G.S.; Guo, C.; Liu, Y. Executive function performance in obesity and overweight individuals: A meta-analysis and review. *Neurosci. Biobehav. Rev.* **2018**, *84*, 225–244. [CrossRef] [PubMed]
138. Song, S.; Li, Q.; Jiang, Y.; Liu, Y.; Xu, A.; Liu, X.; Chen, H. Do overweight people have worse cognitive flexibility? Cues-triggered food craving may have a greater impact. *Nutrients* **2022**, *14*, 240. [CrossRef] [PubMed]
139. Fagundo, A.B.; de la Torre, R.; Jimenez-Murcia, S.; Aguera, Z.; Granero, R.; Tarrega, S.; Botella, C.; Banos, R.; Fernandez-Real, J.M.; Rodriguez, R.; et al. Executive functions profile in extreme eating/weight conditions: From anorexia nervosa to obesity. *PLoS ONE* **2012**, *7*, e43382. [CrossRef]
140. Volkow, N.D.; Wang, G.J.; Baler, R.D. Reward, dopamine and the control of food intake: Implications for obesity. *Trends Cogn. Sci.* **2011**, *15*, 37–46. [CrossRef]
141. Belfort-DeAguiar, R.; Seo, D. Food cues and obesity: Overpowering hormones and energy balance regulation. *Curr. Obes. Rep.* **2018**, *7*, 122–129. [CrossRef]
142. Kass, A.E.; Wildes, J.E.; Coccaro, E.F. Identification and regulation of emotions in adults of varying weight statuses. *J. Health Psychol.* **2019**, *24*, 941–952. [CrossRef] [PubMed]
143. Berthoud, H.R.; Munzberg, H.; Morrison, C.D. Blaming the brain for obesity: Integration of hedonic and homeostatic mechanisms. *Gastroenterology* **2017**, *152*, 1728–1738. [CrossRef] [PubMed]
144. Zheng, H.; Lenard, N.R.; Shin, A.C.; Berthoud, H.R. Appetite control and energy balance regulation in the modern world: Reward-driven brain overrides repletion signals. *Int. J. Obes.* **2009**, *33*, S8–S13. [CrossRef]
145. Micanti, F.; Iasevoli, F.; Cucciniello, C.; Costabile, R.; Loiarro, G.; Pecoraro, G.; Pasanisi, F.; Rossetti, G.; Galletta, D. The relationship between emotional regulation and eating behaviour: A multidimensional analysis of obesity psychopathology. *Eat. Weight. Disord.* **2017**, *22*, 105–115. [CrossRef]
146. Aparicio, E.; Canals, J.; Arija, V.; De Henauw, S.; Michels, N. The role of emotion regulation in childhood obesity: Implications for prevention and treatment. *Nutr. Res. Rev.* **2016**, *29*, 17–29. [CrossRef]
147. McGorry, P.; Keshavan, M.; Goldstone, S.; Amminger, P.; Allott, K.; Berk, M.; Lavoie, S.; Pantelis, C.; Yung, A.; Wood, S.; et al. Biomarkers and clinical staging in psychiatry. *World Psychiatry* **2014**, *13*, 211–223. [CrossRef] [PubMed]
148. Harrison, A.; Tchanturia, K.; Treasure, J. Attentional bias, emotion recognition, and emotion regulation in anorexia: State or trait? *Biol. Psychiatry* **2010**, *68*, 755–761. [CrossRef]
149. Hanegraaf, L.; Anderson, A.; Neill, E.; Giddens, E.; Boon, E.; Bryant, E.; Calvert, S.; Carroll, B.; Fernandez-Aranda, F.; Ikin, S.; et al. Treatment targets and strategies for eating disorders recovery: A Delphi consensus with lived experience, carers, researchers, and clinicians. *Int. J. Eat. Disord.* **2024**, *57*, 2494–2507. [CrossRef] [PubMed]
150. Fonville, L.; Giampietro, V.; Williams, S.C.; Simmons, A.; Tchanturia, K. Alterations in brain structure in adults with anorexia nervosa and the impact of illness duration. *Psychol. Med.* **2014**, *44*, 1965–1975. [CrossRef]
151. Hagan, K.E.; Christensen, K.A.; Forbush, K.T. A preliminary systematic review and meta-analysis of randomized-controlled trials of cognitive remediation therapy for anorexia nervosa. *Eat. Behav.* **2020**, *37*, 101391. [CrossRef]
152. Tchanturia, K.; Doris, E.; Mountford, V.; Fleming, C. Cognitive remediation and emotion skills training (CREST) for anorexia nervosa in individual format: Self-reported outcomes. *BMC Psychiatry* **2015**, *15*, 53. [CrossRef] [PubMed]
153. Beck, A.T.; Dozois, D.J. Cognitive therapy: Current status and future directions. *Annu. Rev. Med.* **2011**, *62*, 397–409. [CrossRef]
154. Brown, T.A.; Wisniewski, L.; Anderson, L.K. Dialectical behavior therapy for eating disorders: State of the research and new directions. *Eat. Disord.* **2020**, *28*, 97–100. [CrossRef]
155. Sala, M.; Shankar Ram, S.; Vanzhula, I.A.; Levinson, C.A. Mindfulness and eating disorder psychopathology: A meta-analysis. *Int. J. Eat. Disord.* **2020**, *53*, 834–851. [CrossRef] [PubMed]
156. Mattingley, S.; Youssef, G.J.; Manning, V.; Graeme, L.; Hall, K. Distress tolerance across substance use, eating, and borderline personality disorders: A meta-analysis. *J. Affect. Disord.* **2022**, *300*, 492–504. [CrossRef] [PubMed]
157. Thorsrud, T.; Bang, M.A.; Dahlgren, C.L.; Nordfjaern, T.; Weider, S. Cognitive remediation therapy for patients with eating disorders: A qualitative study. *J. Eat. Disord.* **2024**, *12*, 142. [CrossRef]
158. Telch, C.F.; Agras, W.S.; Linehan, M.M. Dialectical behavior therapy for binge eating disorder. *J. Consult. Clin. Psychol.* **2001**, *69*, 1061–1065. [CrossRef]
159. Keck-Kester, T.; Huerta-Saenz, L.; Spotts, R.; Duda, L.; Raja-Khan, N. Do mindfulness interventions improve obesity rates in children and adolescents: A review of the evidence. *Diabetes Metab. Syndr. Obes.* **2021**, *14*, 4621–4629. [CrossRef] [PubMed]

160. Braden, A.; Redondo, R.; Ferrell, E.; Anderson, L.; Weinandy, J.G.; Watford, T.; Barnhart, W.R. An open trial examining dialectical behavior therapy skills and behavioral weight loss for adults with emotional eating and overweight/obesity. *Behav. Ther.* **2022**, *53*, 614–627. [CrossRef]
161. Chew, H.S.J.; Chng, S.; Rajasegaran, N.N.; Choy, K.H.; Chong, Y.Y. Effectiveness of acceptance and commitment therapy on weight, eating behaviours and psychological outcomes: A systematic review and meta-analysis. *Eat. Weight. Disord.* **2023**, *28*, 6. [CrossRef] [PubMed]
162. Tchanturia, K.; Larsson, E.; Brown, A. Benefits of group cognitive remediation therapy in anorexia nervosa: Case series. *Neuropsychiatrie* **2016**, *30*, 42–49. [CrossRef] [PubMed]
163. Di Natale, A.F.; Pizzoli, S.F.M.; Brizzi, G.; Di Lernia, D.; Frisone, F.; Gaggioli, A.; Rabarbari, E.; Oasi, O.; Repetto, C.; Rossi, C.; et al. Harnessing immersive virtual reality: A comprehensive scoping review of its applications in assessing, understanding, and treating eating disorders. *Curr. Psychiatry Rep.* **2024**, *26*, 470–486. [CrossRef]
164. Riva, G.; Malighetti, C.; Serino, S. Virtual reality in the treatment of eating disorders. *Clin. Psychol. Psychother.* **2021**, *28*, 477–488. [CrossRef] [PubMed]
165. Montana, J.I.; Matamala-Gomez, M.; Maisto, M.; Mavrodiev, P.A.; Cavalera, C.M.; Diana, B.; Mantovani, F.; Realdon, O. The benefits of emotion regulation interventions in virtual reality for the improvement of wellbeing in adults and older adults: A systematic review. *J. Clin. Med.* **2020**, *9*, 500. [CrossRef] [PubMed]
166. Navarro-Haro, M.V.; Modrego-Alarcon, M.; Hoffman, H.G.; Lopez-Montoyo, A.; Navarro-Gil, M.; Montero-Marin, J.; Garcia-Palacios, A.; Borao, L.; Garcia-Campayo, J. Evaluation of a mindfulness-based intervention with and without virtual reality dialectical behavior therapy® mindfulness skills training for the treatment of generalized anxiety disorder in primary care: A pilot study. *Front. Psychol.* **2019**, *10*, 55. [CrossRef]
167. Marcolini, F.; Ravaglia, A.; Tempia Valenta, S.; Bosco, G.; Marconi, G.; De Ronchi, D.; Atti, A.R. Severe enduring anorexia nervosa (SE-AN) treatment options and their effectiveness: A review of literature. *J. Eat. Disord.* **2024**, *12*, 48. [CrossRef] [PubMed]
168. Chmiel, J.; Kurpas, D.; Rybakowski, F.; Leszek, J. The effectiveness of transcranial direct current stimulation (tDCS) in binge eating disorder (BED)—Review and insight into the mechanisms of action. *Nutrients* **2024**, *16*, 1521. [CrossRef] [PubMed]
169. Duriez, P.; Bou Khalil, R.; Chamoun, Y.; Maatoug, R.; Strumila, R.; Seneque, M.; Gorwood, P.; Courtet, P.; Guillaume, S. Brain stimulation in eating disorders: State of the art and future perspectives. *J. Clin. Med.* **2020**, *9*, 2358. [CrossRef] [PubMed]
170. Sato, Y.; Saito, N.; Utsumi, A.; Aizawa, E.; Shoji, T.; Izumiyama, M.; Mushiake, H.; Hongo, M.; Fukudo, S. Neural basis of impaired cognitive flexibility in patients with anorexia nervosa. *PLoS ONE* **2013**, *8*, e61108. [CrossRef]
171. Friederich, H.C.; Walther, S.; Bendszus, M.; Biller, A.; Thomann, P.; Zeigermann, S.; Katus, T.; Brunner, R.; Zastrow, A.; Herzog, W. Grey matter abnormalities within cortico-limbic-striatal circuits in acute and weight-restored anorexia nervosa patients. *Neuroimage* **2012**, *59*, 1106–1113. [CrossRef] [PubMed]
172. Kaye, W.H.; Fudge, J.L.; Paulus, M. New insights into symptoms and neurocircuit function of anorexia nervosa. *Nat. Rev. Neurosci.* **2009**, *10*, 573–584. [CrossRef]
173. Lee, D.J.; Elias, G.J.B.; Lozano, A.M. Neuromodulation for the treatment of eating disorders and obesity. *Ther. Adv. Psychopharmacol.* **2018**, *8*, 73–92. [CrossRef]
174. Gallop, L.; Flynn, M.; Campbell, I.C.; Schmidt, U. Neuromodulation and eating disorders. *Curr. Psychiatry Rep.* **2022**, *24*, 61–69. [CrossRef] [PubMed]
175. Formolo, D.A.; Gaspar, J.M.; Melo, H.M.; Eichwald, T.; Zepeda, R.J.; Latini, A.; Okun, M.S.; Walz, R. Deep brain stimulation for obesity: A review and future directions. *Front. Neurosci.* **2019**, *13*, 323. [CrossRef] [PubMed]
176. Gouveia, F.V.; Silk, E.; Davidson, B.; Pople, C.B.; Abrahao, A.; Hamilton, J.; Ibrahim, G.M.; Muller, D.J.; Giacobbe, P.; Lipsman, N.; et al. A systematic review on neuromodulation therapies for reducing body weight in patients with obesity. *Obes. Rev.* **2021**, *22*, e13309. [CrossRef]

nutrients

MDPI

Article

Yeast Beta-Glucan Supplementation with Multivitamins Attenuates Cognitive Impairments in Individuals with Myalgic Encephalomyelitis/Chronic Fatigue Syndrome: A Randomized, Double-Blind, Placebo-Controlled Trial

Marcos Lacasa [1,†], Jose Alegre-Martin [2], Ramon Sanmartin Sentañes [2], Luisa Varela-Sende [3], Joanna Jurek [2,†] and Jesus Castro-Marrero [2,*,†]

[1] E-Health Center, Universitat Oberta de Catalunya, 08018 Barcelona, Spain; mlacasaca@uoc.edu
[2] Myalgic Encephalomyelitis/Chronic Fatigue Syndrome Research Unit, Division of Rheumatology, Vall d´Hebron University Hospital Research Institute, Universitat Autònoma de Barcelona, 08035 Barcelona, Spain; jose.alegre@vallhebron.cat (J.A.-M.); ramon.sanmartin@vallhebron.cat (R.S.S.); joanna.michalina.jurek@gmail.com (J.J.)
[3] Clinical Research Department, VITAE Health Innovation, Montmeló, 08160 Barcelona, Spain; lvarela@vitae.es
* Correspondence: jesus.castro@vhir.org; Tel.: +34-93-4893000 (ext. 3753)
† These authors contributed equally to this work.

Abstract: This research aimed to examine the potential alleviative effects of beta-glucan administration on fatigue, unrefreshing sleep, anxiety/depression symptoms and health-related quality of life in ME/CFS. A 36-week unicenter, randomized, double-blind, placebo-controlled trial was conducted in 65 ME/CFS patients, who were randomly allocated to one of two arms to receive four capsules each one of 250 mg beta-glucan, 3.75 µg vitamin D3, 1.05 mg vitamin B6, and 7.5 mg zinc (n = 35), or matching placebo including only microcrystalline cellulose as an excipient (n = 30) once daily. The findings showed that the beta-glucan supplementation significantly improved cognitive fatigue (assessed with FIS-40 scores) after the 36-week treatment compared to the baseline ($p = 0.0338$). Taken together, this study presents the novel finding that yeast-derived beta-glucan may alleviate cognitive fatigue symptoms in ME/CFS. Thus, it offers valuable scientific insights into the potential use of yeast beta-glucan as a nutritional supplement and/or functional food to prevent or reduce cognitive dysfunction in patients with ME/CFS. Further interventions are warranted to validate these findings and also to delve deeper into the possible immunometabolic pathomechanisms of beta-glucans in ME/CFS.

Keywords: chronic fatigue syndrome; beta-glucan; zinc; vitamin D_3; vitamin B_6; myalgic encephalomyelitis; mitochondria; non-restorative sleep; quality of life

Citation: Lacasa, M.; Alegre-Martin, J.; Sentañes, R.S.; Varela-Sende, L.; Jurek, J.; Castro-Marrero, J. Yeast Beta-Glucan Supplementation with Multivitamins Attenuates Cognitive Impairments in Individuals with Myalgic Encephalomyelitis/Chronic Fatigue Syndrome: A Randomized, Double-Blind, Placebo-Controlled Trial. *Nutrients* **2023**, *15*, 4504. https://doi.org/10.3390/nu15214504

Academic Editors: Roser Granero and Gemma Guillazo-Blanch

Received: 3 October 2023
Revised: 18 October 2023
Accepted: 23 October 2023
Published: 24 October 2023

1. Introduction

Myalgic encephalomyelitis or chronic fatigue syndrome (ME/CFS) is a complex debilitating disorder affecting approximately 17 million people worldwide with a prevalence ranging between 0.2 and 2.6% [1] and a higher frequency in women [2]. ME/CFS is characterized by unexplained and persistent post-exertional fatigue lasting for at least six months, which worsens with physical or mental activity and is not relieved by rest or sleep [3]. ME/CFS is often accompanied by a cluster of other symptoms such as cognitive impairments, impaired immune function, neuroendocrine alterations, and autonomic dysfunction [4]. The condition represents a considerable public health problem and is a cause of severe disability in society, with a marked impact on professional activities and on social and personal relationships [5,6]. All these symptoms can significantly compromise the quality of life of sufferers, as they limit the ability of ME/CFS patients to perform daily tasks [7,8].

In addition, the sleep disturbances commonly reported in ME/CFS patients have been shown to exaggerate these cognitive symptoms and make them more difficult to control [9,10]. At present, there are no specific tests for diagnosing ME/CFS, and so a comprehensive clinical assessment is essential, especially when evaluating the impact of fatigue, quality of life, anxiety/depression symptoms, and health-related quality of life; this assessment should include consultation of medical records, physical examination, laboratory testing, and neuroimaging techniques, along with validated neuropsychiatric tools [11,12]. Although the exact pathophysiological mechanisms underlying cognitive dysfunction are not yet fully understood, alterations in the autonomic nervous system and cerebral blood flow have been proposed as possible causes [13]. In addition, poor sleep quality in ME/CFS has been shown to worsen mental and muscular fatigue, causing intolerance to physical exercise and presenting clinically as myalgia and insufficient/poor blood flow to the brain with additional disturbances in energy production [10].

Functional alterations of redox metabolism, gene expression, and mitochondrial biomarkers in peripheral blood mononuclear cells (PBMC), aerobic oxidative metabolism, decreased aerobic activity, and deconditioning after physical exercise have also been described in ME/CFS [4,14]. High levels of pro-inflammatory cytokines, such as interleukin-1 (IL-1), tumor necrosis factor (TNF-α), and elastase, as well as high oxidative and nitrosative stress, may have multiple effects; they can inhibit mitochondrial respiration, decrease electron transport chain activity and change mitochondrial membrane potential, increase the mitochondrial membrane permeability, and interfere with the ATP production, finally leading to mitochondrial inactivation [15]. Along with morning fatigue, exercise intolerance, and alterations in concentration and memory, sleep disturbances is a particular salient feature of ME/CFS, in the form of unrefreshing sleep, insomnia, hypersomnia, presence of nightmares and/or bad dreams, restless leg syndrome, and sleep apnea syndrome [16].

In addition, many individuals with ME/CFS report gastrointestinal complaints such as irritable bowel syndrome (IBS), a common functional disorder of the gastrointestinal tract, characterized by abdominal pain or discomfort and altered bowel habit. Although the exact mechanism of the gut disturbances in ME/CFS needs to be explored further, the high frequency of IBS diagnoses in ME/CFS patients suggests that impaired composition of intestinal microbiota along with immune dysfunction and increased inflammation beyond the gut may play a role in the onset and development of the illness [17]. The involvement of a bidirectional link between the gut and the central nervous system (CNS) in ME/CFS, known as the gut–brain axis, was supported by studies showing improvements of various symptoms, including anxiety/depression, sleep quality, and neurocognitive impairments after probiotic supplementation interventions [18,19]. Moreover, the dysbiosis of the gut microbiome observed in ME/CFS was linked to the elevated levels of circulating inflammatory mediators, possibly due to an increase in intestinal permeability that allowed for bacterial translocation [20].

Studies investigating the role of short-chain fatty acids (SCFA) in ME/CFS pathogenesis have suggested that SCFA deficiency, in particular butyrate-producing bacteria, is associated with fatigue severity in these individuals [21], as well in other chronic comorbidity conditions, including IBS [22], cancer [23], multiple sclerosis [24], and type 1 diabetes [25]. In view of these early findings, enhancing butyrate production in the gut may have a beneficial therapeutic effect in ME/CFS. One way to increase SCFA levels is through the supplementation of prebiotics, in form of non-digestible polysaccharides (NPS), which upon fermentation, can selectively stimulate the growth and/or activity of anti-inflammatory bacteria in the gut [25]. Beta-glucan, an example of an NPS found as glucose polymers in yeast, fungi, algae, and cereals, such as oats and barley, can promote the growth of probiotic bacteria and increase the production of SCFA, in particularly butyrate [26,27].

Although many studies have investigated the health benefits of beta-glucan, including the prevention and treatment of chronic gut inflammation and conditions related to metabolic disturbances and neurodegeneration, its use in ME/CFS is still under investigation [26,28,29]. Experimental pre-clinical studies using murine models have shown that beta-glucan supplementation can reduce microbial translocation, restore immune homeostasis, and decrease fatigue [30]; these early findings are now under investigation in clinical trials (https://clinicaltrials.gov, accessed on 11 May 2023; NCT05726435 and NCT05524688). The accompanying synergistic improvements in terms of blood pressure, decreased confusion, and improved mood can also help to reduce perceived fatigue [30,31].

Furthermore, by promoting the activity of the desired intestinal microbiota and limiting the growth of pathogens, beta-glucan can play an important role in maintaining proper gut function and thus prevent chronic inflammation. For example, the use of a yeast-derived beta-glucan was effective in reducing hyperpermeability in ileal specimens from patients with Crohn's disease [32], and it also reduced chronic abdominal pain associated with altered bowel habits in an experimental IBS murine model [33]. Similar improvements in bloating, flatulence, and abdominal pain were also observed in a clinical intervention with a mixture of beta-glucan, inositol, and digestive enzymes in IBS patients [34]. This finding may be of particular importance in ME/CFS, as the gastrointestinal issues frequently reported by these patients are often associated with psychological distress and increased release of corticotrophin-releasing hormone, which is known to be involved in the stimulation the hypothalamic–pituitary–adrenal (HPA) axis and is associated with major depression and IBS [35,36].

Thus, beta-glucan supplementation is associated with numerous health benefits including improved gut health, enhanced immune function, and reduced fatigue, and may provide a potential therapeutic advantage for ME/CFS. The present randomized placebo-controlled trial aimed to assess the effect of ImmunoVita®, a dietary supplement composed of yeast-derived beta-glucan combined with vitamin D3, vitamin B6, and zinc on fatigue, sleep problems, anxiety/depression, and health-related quality of life in ME/CFS.

2. Materials and Methods

2.1. Participants

This study was conducted in 67 Caucasian ME/CFS patients consecutively recruited from a single outpatient tertiary referral center (ME/CFS Clinical Unit, Vall d'Hebron University Hospital, Barcelona, Spain) from September 2021 to December 2022. Figure 1 shows a flowchart of the participants prior to analysis. Patients were potentially eligible for the study if they were female, aged 18 years or older, and had a confirmed diagnosis of ME/CFS according to the 1994 CDC/Fukuda case definition [37].

Exclusion criteria comprised participation in another intervention within 30 days prior to study inclusion; inability (in the opinion of the investigator) to follow the instructions or to complete the treatment satisfactorily; failure to provide signed informed consent; consumption of certain drugs/supplements that might influence outcome measures in the last 90 days or whose withdrawal might be a relevant problem, anticoagulant treatment, pregnancy or breast-feeding, smoking, alcohol intake or substance abuse, BMI $\geq$ 25 kg/m^2, and hypersensitivity to any of the components of treatments. Patients with missing data from the follow-up visits were considered to have dropped out. The participants signed an informed consent form prior to the study.

2.2. Intervention Protocol

Of the 67 eligible ME/CFS participants screened, two were excluded. The remaining 65 participants were allocated to treatment by an independent investigator not otherwise involved in the intervention, using a list of random numbers generated by a computer program. The participants were randomly assigned in a double-blind fashion in a 1:1 ratio to receive either active treatment (n = 35) or a matching placebo (n = 30) in the form of four capsules daily for nine months. They were instructed to ingest the capsules on an empty stomach, 30 minutes before breakfast and dinner, only with water. The intervention comprised the intake of a food supplement containing beta-glucan, vitamin D3, vitamin

B6, and zinc. The placebo group received the same food supplement containing only microcrystalline cellulose instead of active ingredients.

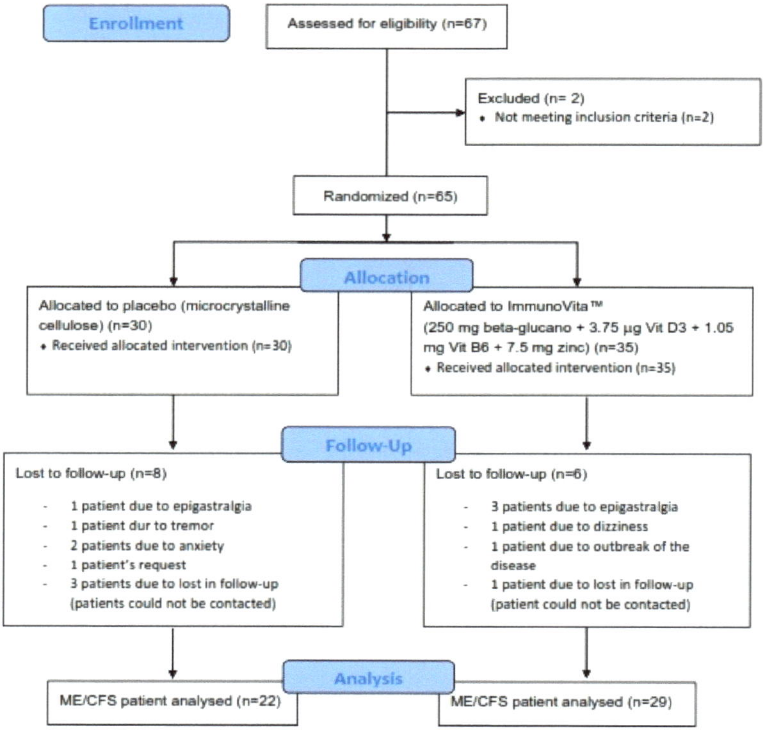

Figure 1. Consolidated Standards of Reporting Trials (CONSORT) flow diagram illustrating the steps of screening, enrollment, assignment, and follow-up of the study participants.

Safety information recorded at all study visits included data on adverse events, vital signs, and the results of the general physical examination. Adverse events, including serious ones, were reviewed throughout the trial by the independent medical monitor, the steering committee, and the independent data and safety monitoring board. Provision was made for investigator-initiated temporary or permanent dose reductions or suspensions due to adverse effects.

During the study, nine subjects dropped out due to adverse events, specifically five in the intervention group (three epigastralgias, one dizziness, and one outbreak of the disease) and four in the placebo group (one epigastralgia, one tremor, and two anxiety episodes). Four patients were lost to follow-up (one in the intervention group and three in the placebo group). Finally, one patient in the placebo group was withdrawn at her own request. The remaining 51 cases of ME/CFS (78%, 22 in the placebo group and 29 in the intervention group) completed all the study protocol procedures and were included in the overall analysis of outcome measures as displayed in Figure 1.

2.3. *Testing of Dietary Supplements*

Patients randomized to the intervention's experimental group received a daily dose of four capsules composed of 250 mg beta-glucan, 3.75 µg vitamin D3, 1.05 mg vitamin B6, and 7.5 mg zinc, plus microcrystalline cellulose and plant capsule as excipients. The placebo composition was the same capsule with microcrystalline cellulose without any active ingredients. The treatments were identical in terms of size, color, opacity, shape, presentation, and packaging. All capsules were manufactured and donated by Vitae Health Innovation S.L. (Montmeló, Barcelona, Spain). The study pharmacist recorded all treatments supplied on the medication-dispensing forms along with their original prescription.

2.4. Study Design and Procedures

The trial was a 36-week long, single-center, randomized, double-blind, placebo-controlled study. Clinical visits and trial design of both groups are detailed in Figure 2. After an oral explanation of the study, all participants provided their written consent prior to the commencement of the study, and they received no compensation for their participation.

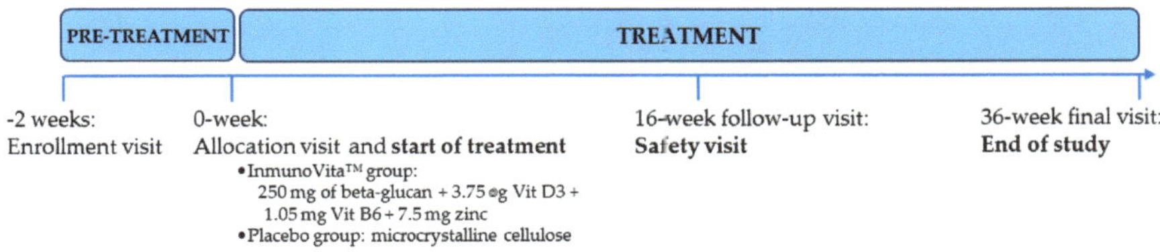

Figure 2. Summary of the study schedule at each visit during the clinical trial.

Patients were evaluated at baseline, at a 16-week follow-up (safety) visit, and then at a 36-week visit by the site investigator. Changes in symptoms were assessed through validated self-report questionnaires completed by participants under the supervision of two trained investigators (J.C.-M. and J.A.). Compliance was checked through medication logs. The use of concomitant medications was tracked at the 36-week visit. The study protocol was reviewed and approved by the local IRB at the participating site (Clinical Research Ethics Committee, Vall d'Hebron University Hospital, Barcelona, Spain, under protocol reference InmunoVitaME-PR(AG)-447-2019, approved on 28 February 2019).

The study protocol was conducted in accordance with the guidelines of the Declaration of Helsinki, the current Spanish regulations on clinical research, and the standards of good clinical practice of the European Union. It also followed the Consolidated Standards of Reporting Trials (CONSORT) guidelines. The current clinical trial was registered on https://clinicaltrials.gov as NCT04301609.

2.5. Primary Endpoint

Fatigue Perception

The primary endpoint was the change in self-reported fatigue perception assessed by using the validated Fatigue Impact Scale (FIS-40) questionnaire from the baseline to the final (week 36) study visit. Briefly, the FIS-40 comprises 40 items divided into three domains that describe how perceived fatigue impacts on cognitive (10 items), physical (10 items), and psychosocial functioning (20 items) over the previous four weeks. Each item is scored from 0 (no fatigue) to 4 (severe fatigue). The total score is calculated by adding together responses from the 40 questions (score range 0–160). Higher scores indicate more functional limitations due to severe fatigue [38].

2.6. Secondary Endpoints

The secondary outcome measures included changes in sleep disturbance, anxiety/depression symptoms, and health-related quality of life (HRQoL) on the validated self-reported questionnaires.

2.6.1. Sleep Quality

Sleep quality was assessed using the self-administered 19-item Pittsburgh Sleep Quality Index (PSQI) questionnaire. Scores are obtained on each of seven domains of sleep quality: subjective sleep quality, sleep latency, sleep duration, habitual sleep efficiency, sleep perturbations, use of sleeping medication, and daytime dysfunction. Each component is scored from 0 to 3 (0 = no sleep problems and 3 = severe sleep problems). The global PSQI score ranges from 0 to 21 points, with scores of >5 indicating poorer sleep quality [39].

2.6.2. Anxiety and Depression

Severity of anxiety/depression symptoms was assessed using the Hospital Anxiety and Depression Scale (HADS), a validated self-reported tool composed of 14 items (seven related to anxiety symptoms and seven to depression). Each item on the HADS questionnaire is scored from 0–3, and so scores range from 0 to 21; scores of 0–7 are interpreted as normal, 8–10 as mild, 11–14 as moderate, and 15–21 as severe for either anxiety or depression. The total HADS score ranges from 0 (no anxiety or depression) to 42 (severe anxiety and depression) [40].

2.6.3. Health-Related Quality of Life

The 36-item Short Form Health Survey (SF-36) was used to assess HRQoL. The SF-36 is a broadly based self-reported survey of health-related physical and mental functioning statuses. It assesses functioning on eight subscales including domains of physical functioning, physical role, bodily pain, general health, social functioning, vitality, emotional role, and mental health, and two general subscales covering the physical and mental health domains rated on a scale from 0–100. Lower scores indicate a more negative impact on health and daily functioning [41].

2.7. Sample Size Estimation and Power Analysis

This trial was the first exploratory, population-based proof-of-concept study in people with ME/CFS. Sixty participants were enrolled with 30 patients being randomly allocated to each arm.

2.8. Compliance Monitoring and Adverse Events

All participants were asked to return any remaining study products after the intervention. Adherence was measured by calculating all remaining capsules for all patients, including withdrawals. Participants who did not take the supplement for more than two days (either consecutive or non-consecutive) were considered non-compliant (n = 0). All adverse events following administration and intake of the study product were monitored until the end of the study.

2.9. Statistical Analysis

A total of 51 patients were analyzed, divided into two groups: active (n = 29) and placebo (n = 22). The variables were evaluated (1) at different times (questionnaire domains) and (2) at the time of inclusion (demographic and clinical characteristics). For the purpose of questionnaire analysis, a total of 23 numerical values corresponding to subscales of the FIS-40, PSQI, HADS, and SF-36 outcome measures were used. For each one, two samples collected at different times were analyzed, as shown in the CONSORT chart. For variables describing demographic and clinical characteristics, such as age, BMI, heart rate, and medication use, a total of four numerical and five dichotomous variables obtained at baseline were analyzed. The normality of the data was evaluated for all numerical variables using the Shapiro–Wilk test, and the statistical value W was calculated using the appropriate formula. For all cases, results were considered significant for an alpha value = 0.05, and the *p*-value was reported with four digits or as indicated if the value was less than 0.001. All statistical analyses were performed using Python package Pingouin (version 0.5.2) for Windows (University of California, Berkeley, CA, USA).

$$W = \frac{\left(\sum_{i=1}^{n} a_i\, x_i\right)^2}{\sum_{i=1}^{n} (x_i - \overline{x})^2}$$

2.9.1. Independent Sample Analysis

The normality of independent samples was analyzed using the Welch–Satterthwaite equation, an approximation of the adjusted degrees of freedom, since the sizes were assumed to be unequal. The formula used was as follows (Delacre, Lakens, and Leys, n.d.):

$$v = \frac{\left(\frac{s_x^2}{n_x} + \frac{s_y^2}{n_y}\right)^2}{\frac{\left(\frac{s_x^2}{n_x}\right)^2}{(n_x - 1)} + \frac{\left(\frac{s_y^2}{n_y}\right)^2}{(n_y - 1)}}$$

The Mann–Whitney U test, a nonparametric test of the null hypothesis in which a value chosen at random from a sample is equally likely to be less than or greater than a random value, was analyzed. A brute force version of the formula from Vargha and Delaney, 2000, was used. For all cases, results were considered significant for an alpha value = 0.05, and the p-value was reported with four digits or as indicated if the value was less than 0.001.

2.9.2. Paired Data Analysis

To analyze paired samples of questionnaires whose values were collected at different times, the paired sample t-test was used to assess the data normality. If data were non-normal, the Wilcoxon signed-rank test was applied.

2.9.3. Categorical Data Analysis

To evaluate the balance of the samples of the two groups, the Chi-squared test of independence was used consisting of a 2 × 2 contingency table, since the variables were dichotomous and the degrees of freedom were 1 in all cases. For all cases, results were considered significant for an alpha value = 0.05, and the p-value was reported with four digits or as indicated if the value was less than 0.001.

3. Results

3.1. Participants' Characteristics

The baseline demographic and clinical features of the participants are displayed in Table 1. In this study, there was no statistically significant differences in participants' demographic and clinical data during the intervention (Table 1). The mean (SD) age of patients was 52.90 (6.47) in the intervention arm and 52.5 (7.48) in the placebo. All participants had a normal BMI with means of 23.58 (3.15) and 22.95 (2.83), for intervention and placebo, respectively. All received medications comprised anticonvulsants, antidepressants, anxiolytics, analgesics, and NSAIDs.

Table 1. Baseline demographic and clinical features for each arm of the study participants.

Variables	Active (n = 29)	Placebo (n = 22)	p-Values
Age (years)	52.90 ± 6.47	52.50 ± 7.48	0.90
BMI (kg/m^2)	23.58 ± 3.15	22.95 ± 2.83	0.39
Heart rate (bpm)	75.27 ± 11.69	74.50 ± 7.71	1.00
Concomitant drugs			
Anticonvulsants	9	6	0.98
Antidepressants	24	16	0.60
Anxiolytics	19	14	0.87
Analgesics	21	13	0.48
NSAIDs	6	5	0.86

Data are expressed as means ± standard deviation (SD) for continuous variables. In both cases, the non-parametric Mann–Whitney U test was used because the samples were not normally distributed. No significant differences were observed in either case, confirming that both samples were derived from the same population. The Chi-squared test of independence was performed with one degree of freedom, and no significant differences in the proportions were observed, so no variable was considered to exert a different influence depending on the group. Abbreviations: BMI, body mass index; NSAIDs, non-steroidal anti-inflammatory drugs.

3.2. Changes in Fatigue Perception

Cognitive fatigue (Table 2), as indicated by the change in the cognitive domain, improved significantly from the baseline at the 36-week visit in the intervention group ($p = 0.0338$). The FIS-40 domain scores evolved in parallel between groups over the course of the study. The actual percentage difference was 5.7%, so the improvement effect could be due to the patient-self-reported interindividual variability and/or synergic effects of beta-glucans plus multivitamins among other potential effects (Figure 3).

Table 2. Changes in the fatigue severity assessed with the FIS-40 score from the baseline to the final assessment (at week 36) in the study participants.

FIS-40 Domains	Baseline	36-Weeks	*p*-Values [1]
Active arm (n = 29)			
Cognitive	33.31 ± 7.03	31.45 ± 9.76	0.0338 *
Psychosocial	61.79 ± 14.59	60.45 ± 16.92	0.3681
Physical functioning	34.52 ± 5.20	33.28 ± 6.78	0.0725
Total FIS-40 score	129.62 ± 25.37	125.17 ± 31.43	0.1070
Placebo (n = 22)			
Cognitive	33.82 ± 5.42	32.73 ± 5.76	0.3725
Psychosocial	64.14 ± 11.79	59.45 ± 12.92	0.1398
Physical functioning	33.73 ± 5.90	32.32 ± 6.95	0.1313
Total FIS-40 score	131.68 ± 21.16	124.50 ± 23.83	0.1375

Data are expressed as means ± SD. [1] The statistical significance of the paired data is analyzed. Statistical significance was set at * $p < 0.05$. The cognitive domain in the active arm presented a slight difference (5.7% from the baseline). Depending on the normality of the data, the test of independence of parametric (*t*-test) or non-parametric (Wilcoxon) paired data was used. There were no significant differences between the groups at baseline. Intervention group was compared with the baseline. Abbreviations: FIS-40, 40-item fatigue impact scale. Lower scores indicate an improvement in fatigue perception. [1] *p*-value for intergroup analysis.

3.3. Changes in Sleep Quality, Anxiety/Depression, and Health-Related Quality of Life

3.3.1. Sleep Quality Assessment

The changes observed in the sleep quality between study groups from the baseline to the final assessment are displayed in Table 3. The intervention with dietary supplements significantly improved daytime dysfunction at the 36-week visit in the active group ($p = 0.0131$ with respect to the baseline) compared to the placebo group. The other PSQI domain scores of the two groups evolved in parallel over the course of the study.

Table 3. Changes in sleep quality assessed using the PSQI questionnaire from the baseline to the final assessment (week 36).

PSQI Domains	Baseline	36 Weeks	*p*-Values [1]
Active arm (n = 29)			
Subjective sleep quality	2.14 ± 0.88	2.17 ± 0.89	0.7389
Sleep latency	2.07 ± 1.03	2.14 ± 1.16	0.5271
Sleep duration	1.69 ± 1.00	1.62 ± 0.98	0.4795
Habitual sleep efficiency	1.93 ± 1.33	1.83 ± 1.20	0.5728
Sleep disturbances	2.10 ± 0.72	2.21 ± 0.73	0.1797
Use of sleeping medication	2.07 ± 1.31	2.00 ± 1.39	0.6256
Daytime dysfunction *	2.31 ± 0.89	2.28 ± 0.75	0.7963
Overall PSQI score	14.31 ± 4.91	14.24 ± 4.93	0.8845

Table 3. *Cont.*

PSQI Domains	Baseline	36 Weeks	*p*-Values [1]
Placebo (n = 22)			
Subjective sleep quality	2.05 ± 0.84	1.68 ± 0.99	0.0588
Sleep latency	2.32 ± 0.78	2.18 ± 0.85	0.3173
Sleep duration	1.41 ± 1.05	1.36 ± 1.09	0.7630
Habitual sleep efficiency	1.77 ± 1.31	1.59 ± 1.40	0.2575
Sleep disturbances	2.09 ± 0.53	1.95 ± 0.58	0.2568
Use of sleeping medication	1.95 ± 1.36	2.14 ± 1.17	0.3795
Daytime dysfunction *	1.59 ± 0.73	1.73 ± 0.83	0.4386
Overall PSQI score	13.18 ± 3.85	12.64 ± 4.70	0.4567

Data are expressed as means ± SD. [1] The statistical significance of the paired data is analyzed. Depending on the normality of the samples, parametric (*t*-test) or non-parametric (Wilcoxon) tests for paired data were used. Baseline data showed no significant differences between the groups, indicating that there was no bias at the baseline between the two groups, (*) except in daytime dysfunction, in which significant differences were found using the Mann–Whitney U test for independence with a *p*-value of 0.0015; therefore, this variable should not be considered.

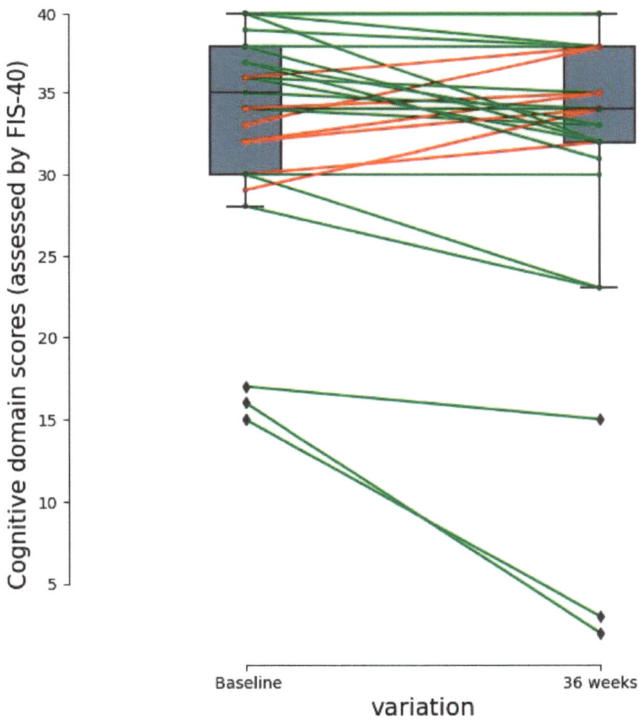

Figure 3. Dot plot of individual paired data of the cognitive fatigue domain (assessed using FIS-40) with significant differences. The differences between the values of the cognitive subscale domain are shown. Each point represents the score of each patient. Bars depict group medians. Lines indicate that cognitive scores belong to the same patient. Green lines depict a decrease in the perceived cognitive fatigue score (better cognitive function), and the red lines indicate an increase in the perceived cognitive fatigue score (poor cognitive function) from the baseline as quantified on the *Y* axis.

3.3.2. Anxiety and Depression

As shown in Table 4, the anxiety and depression symptoms did not present statistical differences between groups over the course of the study.

Table 4. Changes in the anxiety/depression symptoms assessed through the HADS questionnaire from the baseline to the final assessment (at week 36).

FIS-40 Domains	Baseline	36-Weeks	*p*-Values [1]
Active arm (n = 29)			
Anxiety	12.86 ± 5.05	12.76 ± 4.70	0.7940
Depression	11.86 ± 5.11	11.86 ± 5.59	0.5354
Total HADS	24.72 ± 9.60	24.62 ± 9.67	0.6716
Placebo (n = 22)			
Anxiety	11.82 ± 4.55	11.00 ± 4.65	0.1821
Depression	11.59 ± 4.07	10.68 ± 3.98	0.1218
Total HADS	23.41 ± 8.19	21.68 ± 8.20	0.1890

Data are expressed as means ± SD. [1] The statistical significance of the paired data is analyzed. Depending on the normality of the samples, parametric (*t*-test) or non-parametric (Wilcoxon) tests for paired data were used. Baseline data showed no significant differences between the groups, indicating that there was no bias at the baseline between the two groups.

3.3.3. Health-Related Quality of Life

As display in Table 5, social role functioning improved significantly at the 36-week visit compared to the baseline in the placebo group ($p = 0.0131$). The SF-36 domain scores evolved in parallel between groups over the course of the study.

Table 5. Changes in the health-related quality of life evaluated using the SF-36 questionnaire from the baseline to the final assessment (at week 36).

SF-36 Domains	Baseline	36-Weeks	*p*-Values [1]
Active arm (n = 29)			
Physical functioning	38.45 ± 20.49	40.17 ± 22.50	0.8178
Physical role functioning	6.03 ± 16.66	10.34 ± 20.61	0.2020
Bodily pain	15.93 ± 15.58	20.90 ± 18.68	0.1468
General health perception	22.76 ± 14.18	21.90 ± 13.19	0.5683
Vitality	12.24 ± 13.53	16.55 ± 15.93	0.0526
Social role functioning	32.33 ± 26.63	36.64 ± 25.65	0.3344
Emotional role functioning	34.48 ± 46.70	28.74 ± 43.39	0.1695
Mental health status	38.21 ± 21.18	42.07 ± 22.69	0.1393
Placebo (n = 22)			
Physical functioning	39.32 ± 21.17	38.18 ± 20.21	0.9243
Physical role functioning	1.14 ± 5.33	4.55 ± 16.61	0.3287
Bodily pain	20.14 ± 19.22	23.73 ± 15.33	0.1089
General health perception	25.32 ± 14.49	27.36 ± 17.57	0.3225
Vitality	17.27 ± 16.24	15.23 ± 12.77	0.5847
Social role functioning	30.68 ± 20.68	42.05 ± 22.34	0.0131 *
Emotional role functioning	33.33 ± 44.84	37.88 ± 45.19	0.4797
Mental health status	38.73 ± 23.11	44.73 ± 20.01	0.1918

Data are expressed as means ± SD. [1] The statistical significance of the paired data is analyzed. (*) Social role functioning in the placebo group presented a significant difference. Depending on the normality of the samples, parametric (*t*-test) or non-parametric (Wilcoxon) tests for paired data were used. Baseline data were analyzed between the two groups, indicating that there was no bias at the baseline between the two groups.

3.4. Clinical Safety and Intervention Tolerability

No relevant treatment-related adverse events were recorded in the study population. The intervention with dietary supplement containing yeast-derived beta-glucans + vitamin D3 + vitamin B6 + zinc over the period of 9 months was safe and well tolerated by the patients.

4. Discussion

Emerging evidence linking alterations in the gut microbiota composition with the clinical symptoms reported by ME/CFS patients suggests a potential therapeutic role for microbiome-targeted interventions, such as prebiotic supplementation. By restoring intestinal homeostasis, this approach may help alleviate sufferers' health complaints and improve their quality of life. Therefore, to investigate the advantages of the proposed intervention, this clinical trial was designed to evaluate the effect of a food supplement ImmunoVita®, containing yeast-derived beta-glucan, combined with vitamin D3, vitamin B6, and zinc, on fatigue, sleep problems, anxiety/depression, and overall quality of life in ME/CFS patients.

In this study, beta-glucan supplements were administered to individuals with ME/CFS over a prolonged time period (36 weeks). A slight reduction in cognitive fatigue symptoms was reported along with an improvement in self-reported HR-QoL in the active arm of the study participants. Another controlled study assessing the effects of beta-glucan supplementation in ME/CFS patients over a 12-week period showed a significant reduction in patients' self-perceived fatigue and an improvement in their immune function compared to the placebo group [42].

The main findings of this study provide early evidence that administration of beta-glucan may influence certain neurocognitive outcomes related to perceived fatigue in ME/CFS patients after 36 months' treatment. The outcomes are consistent with the growing body of evidence supporting the presence of a two-way hormonal and neural signaling pathway between the gut microbiome–brain axis and its ability to influence metabolism, behavior, and neurocognitive functions through the production of microbial by-products exerting various local and systemic effects on gut hormones, oxidative stress, and inflammation in ME/CFS [21,43–45]. The gut–brain axis is considered to be a key regulator of cognitive function. In the present study, we demonstrated beneficial effects of beta-glucan supplementation on cognitive fatigue in ME/CFS and presented the first evidence of 36 weeks of beta-glucan supplementation improving cognitive impairment, assessed using FIS-40 measures.

Cognitive fatigue became less severe after the 36-week treatment with beta-glucan, as did exhaustion, but the differences with respect to placebo were not significant. The lack of cognitive energy was less severe in the active group compared to the baseline. These results are in line with pre-clinical studies showing that beta-glucan attenuates cognitive impairment via the gut–brain axis in diet-induced obese mice [46–48]. Experimental studies using murine models have shown that beta-glucan treatment can exert significant anti-fatigue effects, as demonstrated by the increased exhaustive swimming time in mice during the forced swimming test [30]. These benefits were attributed to the potential beneficial effects of beta-glucan on energy metabolism and oxidative stress, demonstrated in the form of reduced levels of exercise fatigue and injury-related blood biomarkers, including lactate, blood urea nitrogen (BUN), creatinine kinase (CK), alanine transaminase (ALT), and aspartate transaminase (AST), reduced serum glucose, and improvements in the response to exercise-induced oxidative stress [30].

Evidence from human trials has shown that increasing prebiotic fiber intake can influence perceived fatigue. For example, consuming cereals high in wheat fiber for two weeks reduced fatigue compared to the control in healthy adults [49], whereas a 13-week long supplementation with a prebiotic containing inulin and fru-oligosaccharides reduced exhaustion in elderly subjects when compared to the control [50]. In healthy adults, supplementation with oats (1 g), providing 1.9 g of dietary fiber as beta-glucan, significantly decreased the occurrence of exhaustion and fatigue compared with the baseline ($p < 0.05$). Interestingly, individuals who received beta-glucan had less severe headaches and lower perception of cold than controls. In addition, changes in inflammatory markers, C-reactive-protein (CRP), and oxidized-LDL with gastrointestinal symptom severity were associated with the occurrence and severity of several non-GI symptoms [51]. Furthermore, the results of a phase I/II clinical trial conducted in patients with advanced malignancies receiving chemotherapy indicated that beta-(1,3)-(1,6)-D-glucan administered as an adjunctive therapy may improve white blood cells and platelet counts, and may also raise levels of hemoglobin, which in up to 40% of patients reduces the feeling of fatigue compared with the period before the supplementation [52].

Fatigue is associated with a lack of sleep, an association that may be mediated by increased inflammation [53]. To date, the therapeutic effects of beta-glucans in ME/CFS have not been assessed. Beta-glucans are naturally occurring polysaccharides found in the cell walls of fungi, algae, bacteria, and some cereals. It has been suggested that they may have immunomodulatory and anti-inflammatory effects, which could be beneficial for ME/CFS. Some preliminary studies have shown improvements in ME/CFS patients' perception of fatigue after beta-glucan administration [54].

In relation to sleep disturbances and anxiety/depression, there is limited evidence on the effects of beta-glucan on these symptoms in ME/CFS. Some studies have suggested that beta-glucan may have anxiolytic and antidepressant properties, but further research is required to support these claims and to determine its efficacy in this situation [55]. In a recent study assessing the effects of beta-glucan administration on mental health and HPA axis, reactivity was assessed in ME/CFS, and this approach improved anxiety/depression and HPA axis function [56]. In another study, apparently healthy adults who regularly consume an oats-based supplement containing 1.9 g of dietary fiber like beta-glucan had significantly fewer feelings of anxiety/depression [30].

Another preliminary study found that beta-glucan administration improved mood and vitality among HR-QoL measures in ME/CFS [51]. Overall, while there are some preliminary research studies suggesting possible potential benefits of beta-glucan administration on fatigue, mental health, and quality of life in ME/CFS, the current evidence is limited, and more research is needed to fully evaluate its efficacy and understand the pathophysiological mechanisms after beta-glucan administration in ME/CFS and other chronic post-infectious conditions.

These previous studies suggest that beta-glucans have potential beneficial effects in ME/CFS, including improving quality of life, reducing fatigue, decreasing anxiety/depression, and modulating the immune response. However, research on this topic is still ongoing, and more studies are needed to confirm and extend these findings, and also to determine the different sources, functionality (viscosity, fermentability, solubility, etc.), optimal doses, and duration of beta-glucan treatment that may affect physiological outcomes in ME/CFS.

The current results provide consistent evidence linking increased beta-glucan intake to enhanced cognitive function in ME/CFS. The beneficial effect suggests that the relationship between gut microbiota alteration and cognitive impairment may be causal. In addition to highlighting the adverse impact of western diets on the gut–brain axis, the findings of this study suggest that enhanced consumption of beta-glucan-rich foods is an easily implementable nutritional strategy for attenuating the diet-induced cognitive decline in ME/CFS patients [57].

Strengths and Limitations

This study has several strengths and some limitations that must be considered. To the best of our knowledge, this trial is the first clinical evaluation of the effects of beta-glucan supplementation with multivitamins (including vitamin D3, vitamin B6, and zinc) involved in energy metabolism and immune function enhancement on ME/CFS patients' perceptions of their neurocognitive symptoms, fatigue, sleep quality, and anxiety/depression. It should be noted that a cognition improvement found through percentage differences of 5.7% in active arm is more likely to be due to a real treatment effect using beta-glucans plus multivitamins among the participants. In addition, study participants were assessed according to the ME/CFS case criteria based on the 1994 CDC/Fukuda definition, and a potential gender bias was avoided by restricting the study to females.

The main limitation of this study was the relatively small sample size. In addition, these participants were recruited from a single tertiary referral center, so the results cannot be generalized to other ME/CFS populations. It should also be noted that the primary endpoint, the perception of fatigue assessed with the FIS-40 questionnaire, was a self-reported parameter. Finally, the lack of statistical differences between groups may suggest a placebo effect for microcrystalline cellulose and plant capsule.

In future studies, the doses and follow-up timing of the intervention should be pre-established, so as to ensure appropriate monitoring beyond the intervention. In addition, objective physiological and biological parameters should be used to evaluate beneficial effects of beta-glucan in ME/CFS and other post-viral fatigue syndromes.

5. Conclusions and Future Directions

These findings provide hypothesis-generating evidence that beta-glucan may be beneficial for several affective and physical states in ME/CFS. For example, its positive effect on cognitive function and gut microbiome could be extended and applied in a disease model of cognitive decline. Since information is lacking on the effects on non-GI symptoms in ME/CFS of dietary fibers in general, and of beta-glucan in particular, these results provide potentially useful data for the design of controlled studies required to confirm these observations.

This study provides the first evidence that beta-glucan administration improves indices of cognition function with major beneficial effects all along the gut microbiota–immune–brain axis. Our data suggest that the consumption of 1 g of beta-glucan is an easily implementable nutritional strategy for alleviating the detrimental features of gut–brain dysregulation and for preventing cognitive decline in ME/CFS.

Author Contributions: Conceptualization, J.A.-M., R.S.S., L.V-S. and J.C.-M.; methodology, M.L., J.A.-M. and J.J.; software, M.L.; validation, J.A.-M., L.V.-S. and J.C.-M.; formal analysis, M.L.; investigation, J.C.-M.; resources, L.V.-S.; data curation, M.L. and J.A.-M.; writing—original draft preparation, M.L., J.J. and J.C.-M.; writing—review and editing, M.L., L.V.-S., J.J. and J.C.-M.; supervision, L.V.-S.; project administration, J.A.-M. and L.V.-S.; funding acquisition, J.A.-M. and L.V.-S. All authors have read and agreed to the published version of the manuscript.

Funding: J.C.-M. received financial support and honoraria from Vitae Health Innovation S.L. (Montmeló, Barcelona, Spain). This study was supported by Vitae Health Innovation S.L. (Montmeló, Spain) which supplied both treatments (funding number: 2020-0445).

Institutional Review Board Statement: All study procedures were reviewed and approved by the local Clinical Research Ethics Committee of the Vall d'Hebron University Hospital in Barcelona, Spain (protocol code: InmunoVitaME-PR(AG)-447-2019; approved on 28 February 2019). The study was conducted in accordance with the guidelines of the Declaration of Helsinki, the current Spanish regulations on clinical research, and the EU's standards of Good Clinical Practice. It also followed the Consolidated Standards of Reporting Trials (CONSORT) guidelines.

Informed Consent Statement: Informed consent was obtained from all participants in the study.

Data Availability Statement: All relevant data analyzed during the current trial are included in the article. Access to raw datasets may be shared upon reasonable request to the corresponding author.

Acknowledgments: The authors thank the patients who participated. The authors are grateful to Maria Cleofé Zaragoza for her help in data curation and for her contribution to the paper. We also thank Michael Maudsley for editing and his useful linguistic advice on the updated manuscript.

Conflicts of Interest: L.V. is an employee of VITAE Health Innovation S.L. (Montmeló, Barcelona, Spain). As stated in the author contributions, the funders declare that they had no role in the design, execution, analysis and interpretation, and presentation of data. J.C.-M. received financial support from VITAE Health Innovation S.L. to conduct this intervention study. The rest of the authors declare no conflicts of interest.

References

1. Estevez-Lopez, F.; Mudie, K.; Wang-Steverding, X.; Bakken, I.J.; Ivanovs, A.; Castro-Marrero, J.; Nacul, L.; Alegre, J.; Zalewski, P.; Słomko, J.; et al. Systematic Review of the Epidemiological Burden of Myalgic Encephalomyelitis/Chronic Fatigue Syndrome Across Europe: Current Evidence and EUROMENE Research Recommendations for Epidemiology. *J. Clin. Med.* **2020**, *9*, 1557. [CrossRef] [PubMed]
2. Faro, M.; Saez-Francas, N.; Castro-Marrero, J.; Aliste, L.; Fernandez de Sevilla, T.; Alegre, J. Gender differences in chronic fatigue syndrome. *Reumatol. Clin.* **2016**, *12*, 72–77. [CrossRef]
3. Nacul, L.; Authier, F.J.; Scheibenbogen, C.; Lorusso, L.; Helland, I.B.; Martin, J.A.; Sirbu, C.A.; Mengshoel, A.M.; Polo, O.; Behrends, U.; et al. European Network on Myalgic Encephalomyelitis/Chronic Fatigue Syndrome (EUROMENE): Expert Consensus on the Diagnosis, Service Provision, and Care of People with ME/CFS in Europe. *Medicina* **2021**, *57*, 510. [CrossRef] [PubMed]
4. Cortes Rivera, M.; Mastronardi, C.; Silva-Aldana, C.T.; Arcos-Burgos, M.; Lidbury, B.A. Myalgic Encephalomyelitis/Chronic Fatigue Syndrome: A Comprehensive Review. *Diagnostics* **2019**, *9*, 91. [CrossRef] [PubMed]
5. Castro-Marrero, J.; Saez-Francas, N.; Santillo, D.; Alegre, J. Treatment and management of chronic fatigue syndrome/myalgic encephalomyelitis: All roads lead to Rome. *Br. J. Pharmacol.* **2017**, *174*, 345–369. [CrossRef]
6. Castro-Marrero, J.; Faro, M.; Zaragoza, M.C.; Aliste, L.; de Sevilla, T.F.; Alegre, J. Unemployment and work disability in individuals with chronic fatigue syndrome/myalgic encephalomyelitis: A community-based cross-sectional study from Spain. *BMC Public Health* **2019**, *19*, 840. [CrossRef]
7. Roberts, D. Chronic fatigue syndrome and quality of life. *Patient Relat. Outcome Meas.* **2018**, *9*, 253–262. [CrossRef]
8. Fernandez-Quiros, J.; Lacasa-Cazcarra, M.; Alegre-Martin, J.; Sanmartin-Sentanes, R.; Almirall, M.; Launois-Obregon, P.; Castro-Marrero, J.; Rodríguez-Urrutia, A.; Navarro-Sanchis, J.A.; Ramos-Quiroga, J.A. The Conners Continuous Performance Test CPT3^{TM}: Is it a reliable marker to predict neurocognitive dysfunction in Myalgic encephalomyelitis/chronic fatigue syndrome? *Front. Psychol.* **2023**, *14*, 1127193. [CrossRef]
9. Jain, V.; Arunkumar, A.; Kingdon, C.; Lacerda, E.; Nacul, L. Prevalence of and risk factors for severe cognitive and sleep symptoms in ME/CFS and MS. *BMC Neurol.* **2017**, *17*, 117. [CrossRef]
10. Wirth, K.J.; Scheibenbogen, C.; Paul, F. An attempt to explain the neurological symptoms of Myalgic Encephalomyelitis/Chronic Fatigue Syndrome. *J. Transl. Med.* **2021**, *19*, 471. [CrossRef]
11. Carruthers, B.M.; van de Sande, M.I.; De Meirleir, K.L.; Klimas, N.G.; Broderick, G.; Mitchell, T.; Staines, D.; Powles, A.P.; Speight, N.; Vallings, R.; et al. Myalgic encephalomyelitis: International Consensus Criteria. *J. Intern. Med.* **2011**, *270*, 327–338. [CrossRef]
12. What's in a name? Systemic exertion intolerance disease. *Lancet* **2015**, *385*, 663. [CrossRef] [PubMed]
13. Cvejic, E.; Birch, R.C.; Vollmer-Conna, U. Cognitive Dysfunction in Chronic Fatigue Syndrome: A Review of Recent Evidence. *Curr. Rheumatol. Rep.* **2016**, *18*, 24. [CrossRef] [PubMed]
14. Castro-Marrero, J.; Saez-Francas, N.; Segundo, M.J.; Calvo, N.; Faro, M.; Aliste, L.; de Sevilla, T.F.; Alegre, J. Effect of coenzyme Q10 plus nicotinamide adenine dinucleotide supplementation on maximum heart rate after exercise testing in chronic fatigue syndrome—A randomized, controlled, double-blind trial. *Clin. Nutr.* **2016**, *35*, 826–834. [CrossRef] [PubMed]
15. Maes, M.; Twisk, F.N. Why myalgic encephalomyelitis/chronic fatigue syndrome (ME/CFS) may kill you: Disorders in the inflammatory and oxidative and nitrosative stress (IO&NS) pathways may explain cardiovascular disorders in ME/CFS. *Neuroendocrinol. Lett.* **2009**, *30*, 677–693.
16. Castro-Marrero, J.; Zaragoza, M.C.; Gonzalez-Garcia, S.; Aliste, L.; Saez-Francas, N.; Romero, O.; Ferré, A.; Fernandez de Sevilla, T.; Alegre, J. Poor self-reported sleep quality and health-related quality of life in patients with chronic fatigue syndrome/myalgic encephalomyelitis. *J. Sleep Res.* **2018**, *27*, e12703. [CrossRef]
17. Lakhan, S.E.; Kirchgessner, A. Gut inflammation in chronic fatigue syndrome. *Nutr. Metab.* **2010**, *7*, 79. [CrossRef]
18. Rao, A.V.; Bested, A.C.; Beaulne, T.M.; Katzman, M.A.; Iorio, C.; Berardi, J.M.; Logan, A.C. A randomized, double-blind, placebo-controlled pilot study of a probiotic in emotional symptoms of chronic fatigue syndrome. *Gut Pathog.* **2009**, *1*, 6. [CrossRef]
19. Wallis, A.; Ball, M.; Butt, H.; Lewis, D.P.; McKechnie, S.; Paull, P.; Jaa-Kwee, A.; Bruck, D. Open-label pilot for treatment targeting gut dysbiosis in myalgic encephalomyelitis/chronic fatigue syndrome: Neuropsychological symptoms and sex comparisons. *J. Transl. Med.* **2018**, *16*, 24. [CrossRef]
20. Martin, F.; Blanco-Suarez, M.; Zambrano, P.; Caceres, O.; Almirall, M.; Alegre-Martin, J.; Lobo, B.; González-Castro, A.M.; Santos, J.; Domingo, J.C.; et al. Increased gut permeability and bacterial translocation are associated with fibromyalgia and myalgic encephalomyelitis/chronic fatigue syndrome: Implications for disease-related biomarker discovery. *Front. Immunol.* **2023**, *14*, 1253121. [CrossRef]
21. Guo, C.; Che, X.; Briese, T.; Ranjan, A.; Allicock, O.; Yates, R.A.; Cheng, A.; March, D.; Hornig, M.; Komaroff, A.L.; et al. Deficient butyrate-producing capacity in the gut microbiome is associated with bacterial network disturbances and fatigue symptoms in ME/CFS. *Cell Host Microbe* **2023**, *31*, 288–304.e288. [CrossRef] [PubMed]
22. Borren, N.Z.; Plichta, D.; Joshi, A.D.; Bonilla, G.; Peng, V.; Colizzo, F.P.; Luther, J.; Khalili, H.; Garber, J.J.; van der Woude, C.J.; et al. Alterations in Fecal Microbiomes and Serum Metabolomes of Fatigued Patients With Quiescent Inflammatory Bowel Diseases. *Clin. Gastroenterol. Hepatol.* **2021**, *19*, 519–527.e5. [CrossRef] [PubMed]

23. Xiao, C.; Fedirko, V.; Beitler, J.; Bai, J.; Peng, G.; Zhou, C.; Gu, J.; Zhao, H.; Lin, I.H.; Chico, C.E.; et al. The role of the gut microbiome in cancer-related fatigue: Pilot study on epigenetic mechanisms. *Support. Care Cancer* **2021**, *29*, 3173–3182. [CrossRef] [PubMed]
24. Miyake, S.; Kim, S.; Suda, W.; Oshima, K.; Nakamura, M.; Matsuoka, T.; Chihara, N.; Tomita, A.; Sato, W.; Kim, S.W.; et al. Dysbiosis in the Gut Microbiota of Patients with Multiple Sclerosis, with a Striking Depletion of Species Belonging to Clostridia XIVa and IV Clusters. *PLoS ONE* **2015**, *10*, e0137429. [CrossRef]
25. Leiva-Gea, I.; Sanchez-Alcoholado, L.; Martin-Tejedor, B.; Castellano-Castillo, D.; Moreno-Indias, I.; Urda-Cardona, A.; Tinahones, F.J.; Fernández-García, J.C.; Queipo-Ortuño, M.I. Gut Microbiota Differs in Composition and Functionality Between Children With Type 1 Diabetes and MODY2 and Healthy Control Subjects: A Case-Control Study. *Diabetes Care* **2018**, *41*, 2385–2395. [CrossRef]
26. Singh, R.P.; Bhardwaj, A. beta-glucans: A potential source for maintaining gut microbiota and the immune system. *Front. Nutr.* **2023**, *10*, 1143682. [CrossRef]
27. Hughes, S.A.; Shewry, P.R.; Gibson, G.R.; McCleary, B.V.; Rastall, R.A. In vitro fermentation of oat and barley derived beta-glucans by human faecal microbiota. *FEMS Microbiol. Ecol.* **2008**, *64*, 482–493. [CrossRef]
28. Varesi, A.; Deumer, U.S.; Ananth, S.; Ricevuti, G. The Emerging Role of Gut Microbiota in Myalgic Encephalomyelitis/Chronic Fatigue Syndrome (ME/CFS): Current Evidence and Potential Therapeutic Applications. *J. Clin. Med.* **2021**, *10*, 5077. [CrossRef]
29. Konig, R.S.; Albrich, W.C.; Kahlert, C.R.; Bahr, L.S.; Lober, U.; Vernazza, P.; Scheibenbogen, C.; Forslund, S.K. The Gut Microbiome in Myalgic Encephalomyelitis (ME)/Chronic Fatigue Syndrome (CFS). *Front. Immunol.* **2021**, *12*, 628741. [CrossRef]
30. Xu, X.; Ding, Y.; Yang, Y.; Gao, Y.; Sun, Q.; Liu, J.; Yang, X.; Wang, J.; Zhang, J. beta-glucan Salecan Improves Exercise Performance and Displays Anti-Fatigue Effects through Regulating Energy Metabolism and Oxidative Stress in Mice. *Nutrients* **2018**, *10*, 858. [CrossRef]
31. Dharsono, T.; Rudnicka, K.; Wilhelm, M.; Schoen, C. Effects of Yeast (1,3)-(1,6)-Beta-Glucan on Severity of Upper Respiratory Tract Infections: A Double-Blind, Randomized, Placebo-Controlled Study in Healthy Subjects. *J. Am. Coll. Nutr.* **2019**, *38*, 40–50. [CrossRef] [PubMed]
32. Ganda Mall, J.P.; Casado-Bedmar, M.; Winberg, M.E.; Brummer, R.J.; Schoultz, I.; Keita, A.V. A beta-Glucan-Based Dietary Fiber Reduces Mast Cell-Induced Hyperpermeability in Ileum From Patients With Crohn's Disease and Control Subjects. *Inflamm. Bowel Dis.* **2017**, *24*, 166–178. [CrossRef] [PubMed]
33. Asano, T.; Tanaka, K.; Suemasu, S.; Ishihara, T.; Tahara, K.; Suzuki, T.; Suzuki, H.; Fukudo, S.; Mizushima, T. Effects of beta-(1,3-1,6)-D-glucan on irritable bowel syndrome-related colonic hypersensitivity. *Biochem. Biophys. Res. Commun.* **2012**, *420*, 444–449. [CrossRef]
34. Ciacci, C.; Franceschi, F.; Purchiaroni, F.; Capone, P.; Buccelletti, F.; Iacomini, P.; Ranaudo, A.; Andreozzi, P.; Tondi, P.; Gentiloni Siveri, N.; et al. Effect of beta-glucan, inositol and digestive enzymes in GI symptoms of patients with IBS. *Eur. Rev. Med. Pharmacol. Sci.* **2011**, *15*, 637–643.
35. Glynn, L.M.; Sandman, C.A. Evaluation of the association between placental corticotrophin-releasing hormone and postpartum depressive symptoms. *Psychosom. Med.* **2014**, *76*, 355–362. [CrossRef] [PubMed]
36. Kano, M.; Muratsubaki, T.; Van Oudenhove, L.; Morishita, J.; Yoshizawa, M.; Kohno, K.; Yagihashi, M.; Tanaka, Y.; Mugikura, S.; Dupont, P.; et al. Altered brain and gut responses to corticotropin-releasing hormone (CRH) in patients with irritable bowel syndrome. *Sci. Rep.* **2017**, *7*, 12425. [CrossRef]
37. Fukuda, K.; Straus, S.E.; Hickie, I.; Sharpe, M.C.; Dobbins, J.G.; Komaroff, A. The chronic fatigue syndrome: A comprehensive approach to its definition and study. International Chronic Fatigue Syndrome Study Group. *Ann. Intern. Med.* **1994**, *121*, 953–959. [CrossRef]
38. Fisk, J.D.; Ritvo, P.G.; Ross, L.; Haase, D.A.; Marrie, T.J.; Schlech, W.F. Measuring the functional impact of fatigue: Initial validation of the fatigue impact scale. *Clin. Infect. Dis.* **1994**, *18* (Suppl. S1), S79–S83. [CrossRef]
39. Buysse, D.J.; Reynolds, C.F., 3rd; Monk, T.H.; Berman, S.R.; Kupfer, D.J. The Pittsburgh Sleep Quality Index: A new instrument for psychiatric practice and research. *Psychiatry Res.* **1989**, *28*, 193–213. [CrossRef]
40. Herrero, M.J.; Blanch, J.; Peri, J.M.; De Pablo, J.; Pintor, L.; Bulbena, A. A validation study of the hospital anxiety and depression scale (HADS) in a Spanish population. *Gen. Hosp. Psychiatry* **2003**, *25*, 277–283. [CrossRef]
41. Alonso, J.; Prieto, L.; Anto, J.M. The Spanish version of the SF-36 Health Survey (the SF-36 health questionnaire): An instrument for measuring clinical results. *Med. Clin.* **1995**, *104*, 771–776.
42. Davis, J.M.; Murphy, E.A.; Brown, A.S.; Carmichael, M.D.; Ghaffar, A.; Mayer, E.P. Effects of oat beta-glucan on innate immunity and infection after exercise stress. *Med. Sci. Sport. Exerc.* **2004**, *36*, 1321–1327. [CrossRef] [PubMed]
43. Wachsmuth, H.R.; Weninger, S.N.; Duca, F.A. Role of the gut-brain axis in energy and glucose metabolism. *Exp. Mol. Med.* **2022**, *54*, 377–392. [CrossRef] [PubMed]
44. Marano, G.; Mazza, M.; Lisci, F.M.; Ciliberto, M.; Traversi, G.; Kotzalidis, G.D.; De Berardis, D.; Laterza, L.; Sani, G.; Gasbarrini, A.; et al. The Microbiota-Gut-Brain Axis: Psychoneuroimmunological Insights. *Nutrients* **2023**, *15*, 1496. [CrossRef] [PubMed]
45. Xiong, R.; Gunter, C.; Fleming, E.; Vernon, S.D.; Bateman, L.; Unutmaz, D.; Oh, J. Multi-'omics of gut microbiome-host interactions in short- and long-term myalgic encephalomyelitis/chronic fatigue syndrome patients. *Cell Host Microbe* **2023**, *31*, 273–287.e275. [CrossRef]
46. Tornero-Aguilera, J.F.; Jimenez-Morcillo, J.; Rubio-Zarapuz, A.; Clemente-Suarez, V.J. Central and Peripheral Fatigue in Physical Exercise Explained: A Narrative Review. *Int. J. Environ. Res. Public. Health* **2022**, *19*, 3909. [CrossRef]

47. Germain, A.; Giloteaux, L.; Moore, G.E.; Levine, S.M.; Chia, J.K.; Keller, B.A.; Stevens, J.; Franconi, C.J.; Mao, X.; Shungu, D.C.; et al. Plasma metabolomics reveals disrupted response and recovery following maximal exercise in myalgic encephalomyelitis/chronic fatigue syndrome. *JCI Insight* **2022**, *7*, e157621. [CrossRef]
48. Joseph, P.; Singh, I.; Oliveira, R.; Capone, C.A.; Mullen, M.P.; Cook, D.B.; Stovall, M.C.; Squires, J.; Madsen, K.; Waxman, A.B.; et al. Exercise Pathophysiology in Myalgic Encephalomyelitis/Chronic Fatigue Syndrome and Postacute Sequelae of SARS-CoV-2: More in Common Than Not? *Chest* **2023**, *164*, 717–726. [CrossRef]
49. Smith, A.; Bazzoni, C.; Beale, J.; Elliott-Smith, J.; Tiley, M. High fibre breakfast cereals reduce fatigue. *Appetite* **2001**, *37*, 249–250. [CrossRef]
50. Buigues, C.; Fernandez-Garrido, J.; Pruimboom, L.; Hoogland, A.J.; Navarro-Martinez, R.; Martinez-Martinez, M.; Verdejo, Y.; Mascarós, M.C.; Peris, C.; Cauli, O. Effect of a Prebiotic Formulation on Frailty Syndrome: A Randomized, Double-Blind Clinical Trial. *Int. J. Mol. Sci.* **2016**, *17*, 932. [CrossRef]
51. Wolever, T.M.S.; Rahn, M.; Dioum, E.H.; Jenkins, A.L.; Ezatagha, A.; Campbell, J.E.; Chu, Y. Effect of Oat beta-Glucan on Affective and Physical Feeling States in Healthy Adults: Evidence for Reduced Headache, Fatigue, Anxiety and Limb/Joint Pains. *Nutrients* **2021**, *13*, 1534. [CrossRef] [PubMed]
52. Weitberg, A.B. A phase I/II trial of beta-(1,3)/(1,6) D-glucan in the treatment of patients with advanced malignancies receiving chemotherapy. *J. Exp. Clin. Cancer Res.* **2008**, *27*, 40. [CrossRef] [PubMed]
53. Thomas, K.S.; Motivala, S.; Olmstead, R.; Irwin, M.R. Sleep depth and fatigue: Role of cellular inflammatory activation. *Brain Behav. Immun.* **2011**, *25*, 53–58. [CrossRef] [PubMed]
54. Vetvicka, V.; Vannucci, L.; Sima, P.; Richter, J. Beta Glucan: Supplement or Drug? From Laboratory to Clinical Trials. *Molecules* **2019**, *24*, 1251. [CrossRef] [PubMed]
55. Murphy, E.J.; Rezoagli, E.; Major, I.; Rowan, N.J.; Laffey, J.G. beta-Glucan Metabolic and Immunomodulatory Properties and Potential for Clinical Application. *J. Fungi* **2020**, *6*, 356. [CrossRef]
56. Cryan, J.F.; O'Riordan, K.J.; Cowan, C.S.M.; Sandhu, K.V.; Bastiaanssen, T.F.S.; Boehme, M.; Codagnone, M.G.; Cussotto, S.; Fulling, C.; Golubeva, A.V.; et al. The Microbiota-Gut-Brain Axis. *Physiol. Rev.* **2019**, *99*, 1877–2013. [CrossRef]
57. Hu, M.; Zhang, P.; Wang, R.; Zhou, M.; Pang, N.; Cui, X.; Ge, X.; Liu, X.; Huang, X.F.; Yu, Y. Three Different Types of beta-Glucans Enhance Cognition: The Role of the Gut-Brain Axis. *Front. Nutr.* **2022**, *9*, 848930. [CrossRef]

nutrients

MDPI

Article

The Effects of Polyphenol Supplementation on BDNF, Cytokines and Cognition in Trained Male Cyclists following Acute Ozone Exposure during High-Intensity Cycling

Lillian Morton [1,*], Carl Paton [2] and Andrea Braakhuis [1]

[1] Department of Nutrition, Faculty of Medical & Health Science, The University of Auckland, Auckland 1023, New Zealand; a.braakhuis@auckland.ac.nz

[2] School of Health and Sport Science, The Eastern Institute of Technology, Napier 4142, New Zealand; cpaton@eit.ac.nz

* Correspondence: lillian.morton@auckland.ac.nz

Abstract: The neurotoxic effects of ozone exposure are related to neuroinflammation and increases in reactive oxygen species (ROS). This study aimed to assess inflammation, Brain-Derived Neurotrophic Factor (BDNF), and cognition in healthy male cyclists following polyphenol supplementation and exercise in an ozone-polluted environment. Ten male cyclists initially completed a maximal incremental test and maximal effort 4 km time trial in ambient air. Cyclists then completed two trials in an ozone-polluted environment (0.25 ppm) following 7 days of supplementation with either polyphenol (POLY) or placebo (PL). Experimental trials consisted of a three-stage submaximal test followed by a 4 km time trial. Blood samples were drawn pre- and post-exercise, and analyzed for BDNF, interleukin 6 (IL-6), interleukin 10 (IL-10) and tumor necrosis factor (TNF-α). The Stroop test and serial subtraction task were performed before ozone exposure and again after the 4 km TT. Serum BDNF increased post-exercise ($p < 0.0001$), and positive differences were observed post-exercise in the ozone POLY group relative to PL ($p = 0.013$). Plasma IL-6 increased post-exercise ($p = 0.0015$), and TNF-α increased post-ozone exposure ($p = 0.0018$). There were no differences in Stroop or serial subtraction tasks pre- or post-exercise. Exercise increases BDNF in ozone.

Keywords: BDNF; cognition; polyphenols; exercise; ozone

Citation: Morton, L.; Paton, C.; Braakhuis, A. The Effects of Polyphenol Supplementation on BDNF, Cytokines and Cognition in Trained Male Cyclists following Acute Ozone Exposure during High-Intensity Cycling. *Nutrients* **2024**, *16*, 233. https://doi.org/10.3390/nu16020233

Academic Editor: Maria Digiacomo

Received: 28 November 2023
Revised: 2 January 2024
Accepted: 9 January 2024
Published: 11 January 2024

1. Introduction

Tropospheric ozone is an environmental component of urban air pollution. It is generated photochemically with hydrocarbons, nitrogen oxides, and volatile organic compounds (VOCs) [1,2]. Ozone is a highly reactive oxidizing molecule linked to dysfunction of the respiratory and cardiovascular systems [3–7]. The adverse effects of ozone exposure on the central nervous system (CNS) have been described, and ozone exposure is associated with neurological disorders such as Alzheimer's and Parkinson's disease [7,8], cognitive impairment [9,10], dementia [11], and neuroinflammation [12].

The neurotoxic effects of ozone exposure on the CNS have been established in both human and animal studies. Animal models suggest that ozone significantly interferes with neural physiology by increasing lipid peroxidation, reducing dopaminergic neurons, increasing interleukin-6 (IL-6) and tumor necrosis factor α (TNF-α), and accumulating amyloid-b and a-synuclein, which are pathologic proteins in Alzheimer's and Parkinson's disease respectively [7,12–15]. Compared to other structures, the hippocampus is differentially sensitive to the oxidative effects of ozone [6] and is the first region to be affected by acute ozone exposure [7], due to the connection of the olfactory bulbs and nerves to the hippocampus, the varying antioxidant capacity of brain regions, or a combination of these [7].

Brain-derived neurotrophic factor (BDNF) is found throughout the brain and abundantly in the hippocampus [16]. BDNF plays a role in neuronal growth, differentiation, neuronal survival, synaptic plasticity, and memory and learning processes [16,17]. Human and animal studies have demonstrated that acute exercise bouts stimulate neuronal function, brain vascularization, and neurogenesis, improve mood, and enhance learning [18,19] via the elevation of BDNF [18–23]. Conversely, exercise in polluted air has been shown to inhibit the acute exercise-induced increase in BDNF secretion typically seen following exercise bouts, suggesting that exposure to air pollution blunts the improvement in cognitive health and CNS plasticity [18–20].

Epidemiological and randomized control trials have shown that an increased intake of polyphenols can be linked to neuroprotective effects and improved cognitive function [24–33], as well as reduced inflammation in the respiratory system [34–42]. Phenolic acids and phenolic compounds have also been reported to have a beneficial effect on BDNF levels [25].

Controlled trials examining the acute effects of exercise on BDNF with ozone exposure in human subjects are lacking, particularly in the context of using a nutritional intervention to augment the effects. This study therefore investigated whether supplementation with a functional blend of phytonutrients containing blackcurrant, L-theanine, and pine bark extract has a neuroprotective effect and affects cognitive processes following high-intensity interval exercise performed during ozone exposure.

2. Materials and Methods

2.1. Participants

Ten healthy male cyclists gave written informed consent prior to participation in the study (mean ± SD: age, 43.8 ± 12.38 years; height, 177.8 ± 7.1 cm; weight, 76.03 ± 7.88 kg; $\dot{V}O_{2max}$ 4.12 ± 0.72 L·min^{-1}). Participants were required to avoid strenuous training and activity in the 24 h preceding testing, but light activity or training was allowed. Dietary intakes over a 24 h period were recorded by participants before the first trial. Physical activity, light training, and nutrition were replicated prior to each testing session. Participants refrained from eating and drank only plain water in the two hours before the commencement of each testing session. All trials were attended at the same time of day (±90 min) to control for any potential diurnal variations. The study was conducted according to the guidelines of the Declaration of Helsinki, approved by the Northern Health and Disability Ethics Committee (ref 21/NTB/68, 19 April 2021), and registered with the Australia New Zealand Clinical Trial Registry (ACTRN12622001198718).

2.2. Experimental Design

The study was a randomized, double-blind, placebo-controlled, crossover design. Participants visited the laboratory on three separate occasions. An initial visit to determine maximal oxygen consumption ($\dot{V}O_{2max}$) and peak power output, and familiarize the participants with the cognitive testing procedures and equipment, and was completed in ambient air. Following this, participants reported to the laboratory for two trials performed in an ozone-polluted environment after 7 d of supplementation with either polyphenol (POLY + ozone) or placebo (PL + ozone). A washout period of 14 d occurred between each supplementation period. The same researcher supervised all trials and was blinded to the experimental conditions. A summary of the study design is shown in Figure 1.

2.3. Ozone Exposure

An ozone concentration of 0.25 ppm was generated by a silent discharge method using an ozone generator (N50-C Ozone Generator). An ozone concentration within ±10% of 0.25 ppm was automatically maintained by a relay sensor (airQual, SM-70, Novozone, Auckland, New Zealand).

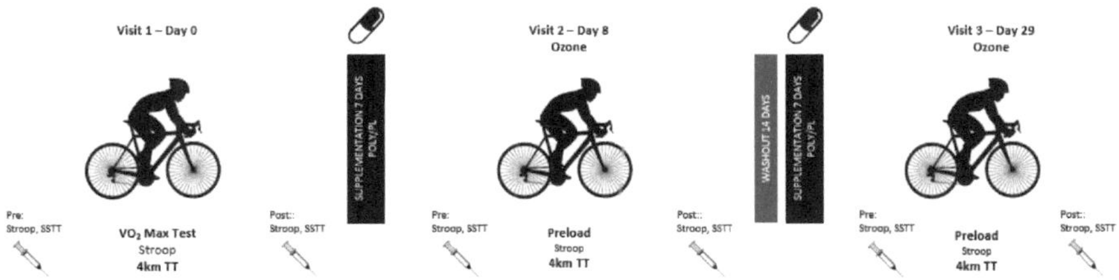

Figure 1. Study design and data collection points.

2.4. Experimental Trial

Full details of the exercise testing regimes and exercise endpoints have been reported elsewhere [43]. In brief, subjects were randomly assigned in a double-blind crossover design to receive either PL or POLY for 7 days prior to exercise and cognitive testing. The POLY supplement was a commercially available combination of freeze-dried NZ blackcurrant (94%; Delphinidin-3-0-Glucoside, 176 mg/5 g, Delphinidin-3-0-Rutinoside, 752 mg/5 g, Cyanidin-3-0-Glucoside, 84 mg/5 g, Cyanidin-3-0-Rutinoside, 722 mg/5 g, Total Anthocyanins, 1733.5 mg/5 g), L-theanine (3%), and Pinus radiata extract (3%) (Ārepa™), and was prescribed as a relative dose of 4.3 mg anthocyanins/kg^{-1}. A berry-flavored powder that contained no vitamin C, active ingredients, or phenolics was used as the PL [43]. The POLY and PL were equivalent in energy and carbohydrate content (per 5 g—POLY: 15 cal, carbohydrate 3 g, PL: 16 cal, carbohydrate 3.6 g). Both the POLY and PL were encapsulated into purple, berry-flavored gelatin capsules and delivered in opaque unmarked bottles to maintain the integrity of the anthocyanins. An independent person gave either POLY or PL to the researcher on the day of testing for distribution to participants. To determine adherence to the supplementation protocol, participants were oversupplied with capsules and a manual countback of returned capsules was completed.

Following 7 days of supplementation, participants completed the experimental protocol [43]. Participants were weighed when they arrived at the laboratory, and blood samples were drawn. Participants then completed the Stroop test and serial 3 and serial 7 subtraction tasks and fitted with measurement equipment. All cycling trials were performed on a calibrated Velotron Dynafit Pro cycle ergometer (RacerMate Inc., Seattle, WA, USA) using the company's associated software package. Participants performed a warm-up for 5 min before completing a cycling protocol consisting of 10 min at 50% peak power output (PPO), 10 min at 60% PPO, and 5 min at 70% PPO. PPO was determined at the participant's initial visit. The cycling load was automatically controlled by the ergometer. A 10 min rest followed the cycling protocol, and participants completed the Stroop test in a seated position within the chamber during the rest period. Participants were then required to complete a maximal effort 4-km TT in the shortest time possible. After completion of the 4-km TT, participants dismounted the ergometer. In a seated position within the chamber, a blood sample was drawn, and participants then completed the Stroop test and serial 3's and 7's subtraction task. Participants were permitted to drink water ad libitum in the rest period and after the 4-km TT.

2.5. Blood Sampling

Venous blood samples were drawn from an antecubital vein 30 min before exercise and 5 min after the completion of the 4-km TT, as BDNF levels have been shown to return to baseline levels within 20 min after exercise [44]. At each sampling point, 5 mL of blood was drawn into a coagulant-free serum separator tube (SST Tube), and 5 mL was drawn into a vacutainer containing ethylenediaminetetraacetic acid (EDTA) (Becton, Dickinson and Company, Franklin Lakes, NJ, USA). Blood samples were left to clot at room temperature for 20 min and then centrifuged at 1000× g for 10 min to separate serum and plasma. The resulting supernatant was then aliquoted into Eppendorf tubes and stored at −20 °C until analysis.

2.6. Sample Analysis

2.6.1. BDNF

BDNF levels were determined from serum using a quantitative sandwich enzyme-linked immunosorbent assay (ELISA) kit (Quantikine Human Free BDNF ELISA, R&D Systems, Biotechne, Minneapolis, MN, USA) according to the manufacturer's protocol. All samples were diluted 20x prior to analysis (10 µL of sample to 190 µL of calibrator Diluent RD6P). The coefficients of variation for BDNF were 7.37% at low levels (233 ± 17.18 pg/mL), 2.04% at medium levels (896 ± 18.24 pg/mL) and 5.23% at high levels (1946 ± 101.82 pg/mL) of control material.

2.6.2. IL-6, IL-10 and tnf-α

Plasma cytokine IL-6, IL-10 and TNF-α levels were assessed using the multiplex bead-based immunoassay Luminex system using the Milliplex® MAP Human Cytokine/Chemokine/Growth Factor panel (EMD Millipore, Billerica, MA, USA) according to the manufacturers' protocol. Analytes included IL-6, IL-10, and TNF-α. Twenty-five microliters of neat plasma sample was used in the wells, and the plate was sealed and incubated with agitation on a plate shaker overnight (16–18 h) at 2–8 °C. Data were analyzed using Luminex xPonent 3.1 software. The average CVs of quality control were 6.30 ± 4.26% for IL-6, 13.57 ± 15.68% for IL-10 and 8.03 ± 2.71% for TNF-α.

2.7. Cognitive Tests

Participants completed a Stroop test and serial 3's (SST3) and serial 7's subtraction task (SST7) pre- and post-exercise. The pre-test was completed before entry into the ozone chamber in a quiet room with no distractions. Post-testing was completed 15 min post-exercise and conducted in the ozone chamber.

2.7.1. Stroop Test

The Stroop test was administered on an iPad using a validated app-based version (EncephelApp), which has been shown to have high test-retest reliability with an intraclass coefficient of 0.83 [45]. The task has an easier 'OFF' state where subjects selected the appropriate color of hashtag symbols (###) presented in one of four colors 'RED', 'GREEN', 'BLUE' 'YELLOW' as fast as possible by selecting the matching color of the stimulus at the bottom of the screen. Subjects performed one training run and one trial of 10 stimuli presentations. If an incorrect color was selected, the run was stopped and restarted. In the 'ON' state of the test, incongruent stimuli are presented in 9 of the 10 stimuli. Words describing one of four colors were randomly presented where the word and font were different colors (i.e., the word 'RED' is displayed in blue). Subjects had to select the correct color of the word, not the name (i.e., selecting blue in the preceding example), by selecting the correct color at the bottom of the screen as fast as possible. Subjects completed one practice run and three trials of 10 stimuli presentations. Both the stimuli and the response buttons were randomized and not fixed in their respective positions each time. The average reaction time and error rate for each trial were calculated.

2.7.2. Serial Subtraction Task (3's and 7's)

Serial 3's and 7's subtraction tasks are used to assess attention or working memory function [46]. In brief, participants were required to sequentially subtract 7 from 100 and continue subtracting 7 from their answer within a given time. The serial 3's are similar in nature but start at 50. The protocols used in the present study are based on those of Bistow et al. [46], where subjects had 20 s to complete as many answers as possible. To minimize any potential learning effect, the serial 3 start numbers in the pre-test were 60 and 51 post-exercise in trial 1, and 80 and 76 pre- and post-exercise respectively in trial 2. The start numbers for the serial 7 numbers were 71 pre-trial and 82 post-exercise in trial 1 and 130 and 110 in trial 2.

The examiner read the following instructions to the participant:

> "I want you to perform a mental, cognitive task that requires subtracting. I am going to say a number and I would like you to subtract 3/7 from that number and continue to subtract 3/7 from your answer until I tell you to stop. Work as quickly as you can and try not to make any mis-takes. Any questions? Ready? Here is the number XX".

The responses of the participant were recorded by the researcher. Correct calculations of 3 or 7 were scored as a correct response. If another number other than 3 or 7 was given, it was recorded as an error. The total number of correct responses and number of errors were used for data analysis.

2.8. Data Analysis Procedures and Statistical Analysis

Statistical analyses were conducted using GraphPad Prism version 9.3.0 for Windows (GraphPad Software, San Diego, CA, USA). The normality of data residuals was confirmed using the Shapiro–Wilk test prior to all analyses. Where normality was violated, data were log-transformed. Differences between treatments (treatment × time) were determined using a two-way repeated measures analysis of variance (ANOVA), and Šídák's multiple comparisons test post hoc analysis was used where significance was detected to compare differences between treatments. Given the potential for learning effects, the data from Stroop and serial subtraction tasks in the familiarization trials were excluded from analysis.

Due to technical issues with blood samples, six samples were missing from a total of 40 samples under ozone exposure. Plasma cytokine analyses were therefore analyzed using a restricted maximum likelihood (REML) mixed-effects model to account for the missing values. To determine the goodness of fit of the REML model, visual assessment of the residual QQ plots was undertaken to check for deviations. The fixed effects (type III) in the model were time, treatment, and time × treatment. Statistical significance was defined as $p \leq 0.05$. Šídák's multiple comparisons test post hoc analysis was used to compare differences between treatments. The magnitudes of the standardized effects for the test measures were determined using the Cohen effect size (d). Thresholds of 0.2, 0.5, and 0.8 for small, moderate, and large effects, respectively, were used in accordance with the recommendations of Cohen [47]. ES values < 0.2 were deemed trivial differences. Simple group statistics are shown as the means ± SDs, unless otherwise stated. Percentage (%) differences between treatments are reported as the mean ± 95% confidence intervals (CI).

3. Results

3.1. BDNF

BDNF levels increased in both the PL and POLY treatment arms following exercise in an ozone-polluted environment (main time effect $p < 0.0001$). A main treatment effect was observed in BDNF levels between PL and POLY ($p = 0.013$). Šídák's post hoc analysis revealed a significant difference and a small effect ($p = 0.019$, −3523 95% CI −6479 to −566.9, d = 0.25) between PL (34,732.50 ± 7833.30 8263.92 pg/mL) and POLY (36,638.70 ± 7493.77 pg/mL) post-exercise (Figure 2).

3.2. IL-6, IL-10 and TNF-α

There was a significant main effect for time in plasma IL-6 levels ($p = 0.0015$, $F_{(1, 9)} = 21.94$). IL-6 increased post-exercise (PL: 1.33 ± 2.01 to 4.32 ± 2.42 pg/mL, $p = 0.001$, POLY: 1.41 ± 1.39 to 4.87 ± 2.17 pg/mL, $p = 0.019$) regardless of supplementation (Figure 3A). A significant time effect ($p = 0.0018$, $F_{(1, 7)} = 23.65$) was observed in plasma TNF-α (Figure 3B). Post hoc analysis revealed significantly higher TNF-α levels post exercise in ozone. TNF-α levels increased from 29.03 ± 10.24 to 40.34 ± 20.78 pg/mL in the PL arm ($p = 0.005$), and 33.74 ± 15.16 to 49.72 ± 23.58 pg/mL following POLY supplementation ($p = 0.016$). No statistical differences were observed between PL and POLY TNF-α levels, however small effects were seen for POLY treatment both pre (d = 0.36) and post (d = 0.42) exercise. No significant changes in plasma IL-10 were observed between treatments ($p = 0.89$), but a significant main effect for time was observed ($p = 0.016$). Plasma IL-10 increased post exercise in both PL (pre: 5.56 ± 3.78, post: 7.33 ± 3.66, $p = 0.06$) and POLY (pre: 4.99 ± 2.90, post: 9.05 ± 5.61 pg/mL, $p = 0.016$).

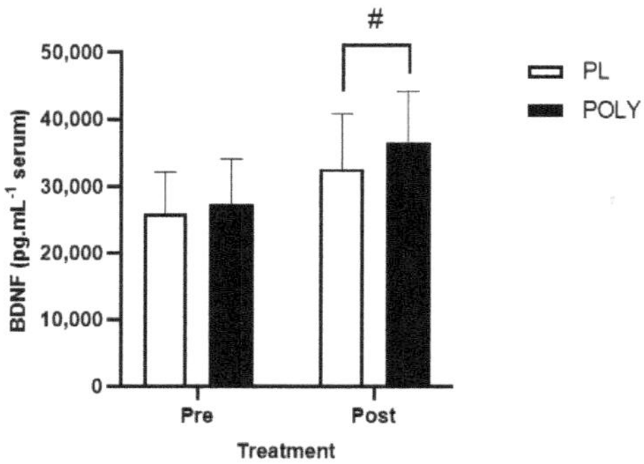

Figure 2. Serum BDNF levels pre- and post-exercise in ozone following 7 days of supplementation of either PL or POLY. Data presented as mean ± SD. # $p = 0.019$ # denotes a treatment effect.

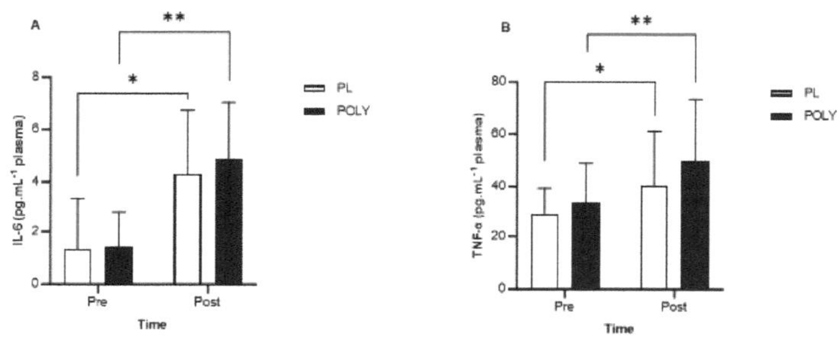

Figure 3. (**A**) Plasma IL-6 (pg/mL) pre- and post-exercise. * $p = 0.001$, ** $p = 0.019$. (**B**) Plasma TNF-α plasma levels (pg/mL) pre- and post-exercise in ozone. * $p = 0.005$, ** $p = 0.016$. Data presented as mean ± SD. * denotes an effect for time.

3.3. Stroop Test

There were no differences in Stroop performance before or after exercise in an ozone-polluted environment (main time effect $p = 0.22$) or between PL and POLY treatments either pre-exercise ($p = 0.83$, d = 0.19), post-preload ($p => 0.99$, d = 0.03) or post the 4 km TT ($p > 0.99$, d = 0.03). The number of errors made was not significantly different in the PL and POLY conditions pre-exercise ($p = 0.82$, d = 0.44), post the preload ($p = 0.97$, d = 0.20), or following the 4 km TT ($p = 0.22$, d = 0.22). Means ± SDs for the Stroop task are shown in Table 1.

Table 1. Stroop test performance before and after exercise in ozone following either PL or POLY supplementation.

	PL			POLY		
	Pre	Post 1	Post 2	Pre	Post 1	Post 2
Stroop speed (s)	13.63 ± 3.07	13.18 ± 3.27	13.48 ± 3.26	14.26 ± 3.65	13.10 ± 3.02	13.58 ± 3.17
Stroop time (s)	27.26 ± 6.14	26.37 ± 6.53	26.96 ± 6.52	28.55 ± 7.33	26.77 ± 7.13	27.66 ± 7.02
Stroop errors	0.20 ± 0.63	0.10 ± 0.32	0.30 ± 0.48	0 ± 0	0.20 ± 6.32	0.20 ± 0.42

Data reported as the mean ± SD from 10 subjects.

3.4. Serial Subtraction Task

A significant main effect for treatment ($p = 0.05$) was observed in the number of responses in the serial subtraction 3's task. However, post hoc analysis showed no treatment differences between PL or POLY either pre- (−0.40, 95% CI −1.93 to 1.13, $p = 0.75$, d = 0.13) or post (−0.80, 95% CI −2.34 to 0.73, $p = 0.35$) exercise in ozone. There was a significant main effect for time in the serial 7's task ($p = 0.03$), but no significant differences were seen with post hoc analysis (Pre: −1.70, 95% CI −4.09 to 0.69, $p = 0.17$, d = 0.45, Post: −1.40, 95% CI −3.79 to 0.99, $p = 0.28$, d = 0.34). There was a significant reduction in errors in the serial 3's task with POLY treatment post-exercise ($p = 0.004$), but no differences in error rate between PL and POLY treatments either pre- ($p > 0.99$, d = 0.00) or post- ($p = 0.12$, d = 0.67) exercising in ozone in the serial 3 task or the serial 7 s (pre: $p = 0.61$, d = 0.27; post: $p = 0.94$, d = 0.08). Means ± SDs for serial subtraction task measures are shown in Table 2.

Table 2. Serial subtraction 3's and 7's task performance before and after exercise in ozone following 7 days of supplementation with PL or POLY.

	PL		POLY	
	Pre	Post	Pre	Post
Serial 3 s	13.80 ± 3.43	14.20 ± 2.20	14.20 ± 2.62	15.00 ± 2.31
Serial 7 s	6.40 ± 3.78	7.70 ± 4.73	8.10 ± 3.84	9.10 ± 3.70
Serial 3 errors	0.40 ± 0.84	0.20 ± 0.42	0.40 ± 0.84	0.0 ± 0.0 *
Serial 7 errors	0.80 ± 0.79	0.90 ± 1.01	0.50 ± 0.71	1.00 ± 1.25

Data reported as the mean ± SD from 10 subjects. Serial = Serial Subtraction Tasks. * $p = 0.004$ pre to post exercise.

4. Discussion

The primary finding of the present study was that serum BDNF levels increased following an acute bout of high-intensity exercise in an ozone-polluted environment. In addition, supplementation with an anthocyanin-rich supplement providing 4.3 mg/kg anthocyanins daily for 7 days resulted in significantly higher BDNF levels post-exercise compared to PL. Plasma IL-6 levels in the present study increased in participants post exercise, including the familiarization trial performed under ambient air, while the levels of TNF-α increased following cycling in ozone. There were no significant improvements in cognitive tasks typically seen following exercise.

Performance in the Stroop test and serial subtraction tasks in the present study did not differ between pre- and post-cycling in ozone in either treatment arm, suggesting a lack of improvement in cognition after exercise in ozone. However, small, nonsignificant effects were observed in the serial subtraction tasks, with a higher number of responses post-exercise and a higher response rate pre-exercise in the POLY group. The acute effects of ozone exposure on cognition are not well established, but adverse effects on cognitive tasks related to short-term memory and attention were consistently observed in a cohort of healthy adults aged 20–50 years after ozone exposure [48]. While cognitive test performance in the present study did not worsen post-exercise, the lack of improvement indicates a potential negative effect of ozone on cognitive domains assessing attention and executive function.

Previous work by Bos et al. [18] found that BDNF increased ~14% after exercise in clean air, but no elevations in BDNF were seen after cycling along a busy road. BDNF levels in the present study increased 29% following exercise in ozone in the PL arm and 35% with polyphenol supplementation and exercise. Evidence suggests a dose–response relationship between acute exercise and BDNF levels [49], with acute high-intensity exercise bouts and graded exercise tests eliciting higher BDNF levels post exercise in healthy subjects. The present study utilized a preload protocol relative to each individual's cycling ability (as measured by peak power output). Cyclists therefore increased their exercise intensity progressively over a 25-min period and then cycled maximally for 4 km. This exercise protocol had higher maximal heart rates and a longer duration (approximately 65 min exposure vs. 20 min) than those in the Bos et al. [18] study. Our findings are in alignment with those of Silveira et al. [50]. While the cyclists in their study were not supplemented, they did show elevations in BDNF after completing a 50 km TT in traffic-related air pollution.

While IL-6 is used to reflect inflammation, it is also now recognized as a myokine, and plasma levels of IL-6 increase during muscular work [51]. In the present study, there was a 3-fold increase in plasma IL-6 levels following exercise regardless of air quality or supplementation, indicating that the increases in IL-6 in this case may be attributed to the exercise protocol independent of ozone exposure. The release of IL-6 stimulates the secretion of the anti-inflammatory IL-10 [52]. In the present study, a significant difference was observed in IL-10 levels post-exercise in ozone with POLY supplementation. Typically, plasma levels of TNF-α do not increase as a result of exercise [53], but elevations in TNF-α have been observed in both bronchoalveolar lavage fluid (BALF) and the cerebral cortex following 6 h of ozone exposure in mice [54]. In the present study, the levels of TNF-α increased following cycling in ozone but not in ambient air. The increase in TNF-α can then be attributed to ozone exposure during exercise, and elevated levels may reflect systemic inflammation and activation of the innate immune system [55]. Ozone exposure can increase the levels of TNF-α, disrupt blood brain barrier permeability, and result in neuroinflammation [56]. In the present study, supplementation with a polyphenol powder providing anthocyanins for 7-days preceding the exercise trials did not attenuate the increase in TNF-α.

Ozone exposure is known to cause oxidative stress, and the disruption to the oxidation–reduction balance leads to progressive damage and causes alterations in the hippocampus at molecular, cellular, and cognitive levels [2,57]. Serum BDNF is known for its role in synaptic plasticity [58], as it regulates the survival and differentiation of neurons and influences the formation of dendrites and dendritic spindles [59]. A systematic review by Gravesteijn, Mensink, and Plat [25] found significant improvement in BDNF in four of 11 studies. However, exercise was not a component in any of these studies. To our knowledge, no other research has explored the effect of a combination of exercise and polyphenol consumption on BDNF levels. The results from the present study show that supplementation of an anthocyanin-rich polyphenol powder combined with exercise elevates BDNF levels after cycling in ozone.

A limitation of the study is the small sample size. Thirteen subjects were initially recruited. Two subjects withdrew due to pronounced symptomatic responses to ozone exposure and another due to work commitments. Furthermore, five of 40 samples were missing for plasma cytokine analysis. We recommend that future studies be conducted to confirm the findings from the present study, and that a larger sample size be recruited. While our subjects performed exercise under conditions of ozone pollution, the effects of polyphenol supplementation combined with exercise in ambient air remains unknown.

5. Conclusions

The results of the present study indicate that exercise combined with polyphenol supplementation increases BDNF levels in healthy cyclists exercising in poor air quality.

Author Contributions: Conceptualization, L.M. and A.B.; methodology, L.M., A.B. and C.P.; validation, L.M.; formal analysis, L.M.; investigation, L.M.; resources, L.M. and A.B.; data curation, L.M.; writing—original draft preparation, L.M.; writing—review and editing, L.M.; A.B. and C.P.; visualization, L.M.; supervision, A.B. and C.P.; project administration, L.M.; funding acquisition, A.B. All authors have read and agreed to the published version of the manuscript.

Funding: Funding for the present work was provided by High Value Nutrition (HVN) Ko Ngā Kai Whai Painga National Science Challenge (HVN 1913 3721400). Lillian Morton was supported by a Callaghan Institute Research Development grant.

Institutional Review Board Statement: The study was conducted according to the guidelines of the Declaration of Helsinki, and approved by the Northern Health and Disability Ethics Committee (21/NTB/68, 19 April 2021), and registered with the Australia New Zealand Clinical Trial Registry (ACTRN12622001198718).

Informed Consent Statement: Witten informed consent was obtained from all subjects involved in the study.

Data Availability Statement: Data are contained within the article.

Acknowledgments: We would like to thank the participants for their involvement in this investigation.

Conflicts of Interest: The authors declare no conflicts of interest. The funders had no role in the design of the study; in the collection, analyses, or interpretation of data; in the writing of the manuscript, or in the decision to publish the results.

References

1. Bromberg, P.A. Mechanisms of the acute effects of inhaled ozone in humans. *Biochim. Biophys. Acta BBA-Gen. Subj.* **2016**, *1860*, 2771–2781. [CrossRef] [PubMed]
2. Bello-Medina, P.C.; Rodríguez-Martínez, E.; Prado-Alcalá, R.A.; Rivas-Arancibia, S. Ozone pollution, oxidative stress, synaptic plasticity, and neurodegeneration. *Neurología* **2022**, *37*, 277–286. [CrossRef] [PubMed]
3. Bosson, J.; Barath, S.; Pourazar, J.; Behndig, A.F.; Sandström, T.; Blomberg, A.; Ädelroth, E. Diesel exhaust exposure enhances the ozone-induced airway inflammation in healthy humans. *Eur. Respir. J.* **2008**, *31*, 1234–1240. [CrossRef]
4. Gackière, F.; Saliba, L.; Baude, A.; Bosler, O.; Strube, C. Ozone inhalation activates stress-responsive regions of the CNS. *J. Neurochem.* **2011**, *117*, 961–972. [CrossRef] [PubMed]
5. Galiè, M.; Covi, V.; Tabaracci, G.; Malatesta, M. The role of Nrf2 in the antioxidant cellular response to medical ozone exposure. *Int. J. Mol. Sci.* **2019**, *20*, 4009. [CrossRef]
6. Nery-Flores, S.D.; Ramírez-Herrera, M.A.; Mendoza-Magaña, M.L.; Romero-Prado, M.M.; Ramírez-Vázquez, J.D.; Bañuelos-Pineda, J.; Espinoza-Gutiérrez, H.A.; Ramírez-Mendoza, A.A.; Tostado, M.C. Dietary curcumin prevented astrocytosis, microgliosis, and apoptosis caused by acute and chronic exposure to ozone. *Molecules* **2019**, *24*, 2839. [CrossRef] [PubMed]
7. Croze, M.L.; Zimmer, L. Ozone atmospheric pollution and Alzheimer's disease: From epidemiological facts to molecular mechanisms. *J. Alzheimer's Dis.* **2018**, *62*, 503–522. [CrossRef]
8. Chen, M.C.; Wang, C.F.; Lai, B.C.; Hsieh, S.W.; Chen, S.C.; Hung, C.H.; Kuo, C.H. Air pollution is associated with poor cognitive function in Taiwanese adults. *Int. J. Environ. Res. Public Health* **2021**, *18*, 316. [CrossRef]
9. Gao, Q.; Zang, E.; Bi, J.; Dubrow, R.; Lowe, S.R.; Chen, H.; Zeng, Y.; Shi, L.; Chen, K. Long-term ozone exposure and cognitive impairment among Chinese older adults: A cohort study. *Environ. Int.* **2022**, *160*, 107072. [CrossRef]
10. Lo, Y.T.; Lu, Y.C.; Chang, Y.H.; Kao, S.; Huang, H.B. Air pollution exposure and cognitive function in Taiwanese older adults: A repeated measurement study. *Int. J. Environ. Res. Public Health* **2019**, *16*, 2976. [CrossRef]
11. Power, M.C.; Adar, S.D.; Yanosky, J.D.; Weuve, J. Exposure to air pollution as a potential contributor to cognitive function, cognitive decline, brain imaging, and dementia: A systematic review of epidemiologic research. *Neurotoxicology* **2016**, *56*, 235–253. [CrossRef] [PubMed]
12. Erickson, M.A.; Jude, J.; Zhao, H.; Rhea, E.M.; Salameh, T.S.; Jester, W.; Pu, S.; Harrowitz, J.; Nguyen, N.; Banks, W.A.; et al. Serum amyloid A: An ozone-induced circulating factor with potentially important functions in the lung-brain axis. *FASEB J.* **2017**, *31*, 3950. [CrossRef] [PubMed]
13. Gaetani, L.; Paoletti, F.P.; Bellomo, G.; Mancini, A.; Simoni, S.; Di Filippo, M.; Parnetti, L. CSF and blood biomarkers in neuroinflammatory and neurodegenerative diseases: Implications for treatment. *Trends Pharmacol. Sci.* **2020**, *41*, 1023–1037. [CrossRef]
14. Terrone, G.; Frigerio, F.; Balosso, S.; Ravizza, T.; Vezzani, A. Inflammation and reactive oxygen species in status epilepticus: Biomarkers and implications for therapy. *Epilepsy Behav.* **2019**, *101*, 106275. [CrossRef] [PubMed]
15. Zhao, T.; Markevych, I.; Romanos, M.; Nowak, D.; Heinrich, J. Ambient ozone exposure and mental health: A systematic review of epidemiological studies. *Environ. Res.* **2018**, *165*, 459–472. [CrossRef] [PubMed]
16. Schuch, F.B.; da Silveira, L.E.; de Zeni, T.C.; da Silva, D.P.; Wollenhaupt-Aguiar, B.; Ferrari, P.; Reischak-Oliveira, Á.; Kapczinski, F. Effects of a single bout of maximal aerobic exercise on BDNF in bipolar disorder: A gender-based response. *Psychiatry Res.* **2015**, *229*, 57–62. [CrossRef]
17. Jiménez-Maldonado, A.; Rentería, I.; García-Suárez, P.C.; Moncada-Jiménez, J.; Freire-Royes, L.F. The impact of high-intensity interval training on brain derived neurotrophic factor in brain: A mini-review. *Front. Neurosci.* **2018**, *12*, 839. [CrossRef]
18. Bos, I.; Jacobs, L.; Nawrot, T.S.; De Geus, B.; Torfs, R.; Panis, L.I.; Degraeuwe, B.; Meeusen, R. No exercise-induced increase in serum BDNF after cycling near a major traffic road. *Neurosci. Lett.* **2011**, *500*, 129–132. [CrossRef]
19. Bos, I.; De Boever, P.; Int Panis, L.; Meeusen, R. Physical activity, air pollution and the brain. *Sports Med.* **2014**, *44*, 1505–1518. [CrossRef]
20. Bos, I.; De Boever, P.; Vanparijs, J.; Pattyn, N.; Panis, L.I.; Meeusen, R. Subclinical effects of aerobic training in urban environment. *Med. Sci. Sports Exerc.* **2013**, *45*, 439–447. [CrossRef]
21. Griffin, É.W.; Mullally, S.; Foley, C.; Warmington, S.A.; O'Mara, S.M.; Kelly, Á.M. Aerobic exercise improves hippocampal function and increases BDNF in the serum of young adult males. *Physiol. Behav.* **2011**, *104*, 934–941. [CrossRef] [PubMed]

22. Miodownik, C.; Maayan, R.; Ratner, Y.; Lerner, V.; Pintov, L.; Mar, M.; Weizman, A.; Ritsner, M.S. Serum levels of brain-derived neurotrophic factor and cortisol to sulfate of dehydroepiandrosterone molar ratio associated with clinical response to L-theanine as augmentation of antipsychotic therapy in schizophrenia and schizoaffective disorder patients. *Clin. Neuropharmacol.* **2011**, *34*, 155–160. [CrossRef] [PubMed]
23. Revi, N.; Rengan, A.K. Impact of dietary polyphenols on neuroinflammation-associated disorders. *Neurol. Sci.* **2021**, *42*, 3101–3119. [CrossRef]
24. Choi, D.Y.; Lee, Y.J.; Hong, J.T.; Lee, H.J. Antioxidant properties of natural polyphenols and their therapeutic potentials for Alzheimer's disease. *Brain Res. Bull.* **2012**, *87*, 144–153. [CrossRef] [PubMed]
25. Gravesteijn, E.; Mensink, R.P.; Plat, J. Effects of nutritional interventions on BDNF concentrations in humans: A systematic review. *Nutr. Neurosci.* **2022**, *25*, 1425–1436. [CrossRef]
26. Hidese, S.; Ogawa, S.; Ota, M.; Ishida, I.; Yasukawa, Z.; Ozeki, M.; Kunugi, H. Effects of L-theanine administration on stress-related symptoms and cognitive functions in healthy adults: A randomized controlled trial. *Nutrients* **2019**, *11*, 2362. [CrossRef]
27. Jiang, T.A. Health benefits of culinary herbs and spices. *J. AOAC Int.* **2019**, *102*, 395–411. [CrossRef] [PubMed]
28. Kawaguchi, K.; Matsumoto, T.; Kumazawa, Y. Effects of antioxidant polyphenols on TNF-alpha-related diseases. *Curr. Top. Med. Chem.* **2011**, *11*, 1767–1779. [CrossRef]
29. Lee, W.H.; Loo, C.Y.; Bebawy, M.; Luk, F.; Mason, R.S.; Rohanizadeh, R. Curcumin and its derivatives: Their application in neuropharmacology and neuroscience in the 21st century. *Curr. Neuropharmacol.* **2013**, *11*, 338–378. [CrossRef]
30. Sangiovanni, E.; Brivio, P.; Dell'Agli, M.; Calabrese, F. Botanicals as modulators of neuroplasticity: Focus on BDNF. *Neural Plast.* **2017**, *2017*, 5965371. [CrossRef]
31. Wang, F.; Zhang, K.; Zhai, M.; Lin, X.; Hu, Y.; Feng, L.; Yang, J.; Yu, H.; Wu, C. Protective effect and mechanism of Lycium barbarum L. polyphenol on cognitive impairment induced by ethanol in mice. *Phytomedicine* **2022**, *100*, 154033. [CrossRef] [PubMed]
32. Zhu, A.; Yuan, C.; Pretty, J.; Ji, J.S. Plant-based dietary patterns and cognitive function: A prospective cohort analysis of elderly individuals in China (2008–2018). *Brain Behav.* **2022**, *12*, e2670. [CrossRef] [PubMed]
33. Ammar, A.; Trabelsi, K.; Boukhris, O.; Bouaziz, B.; Mueller, P.; Glenn, J.M.; Bott, N.T.; Mueller, N.; Chtourou, H.; Driss, T.; et al. Effects of polyphenol-rich interventions on cognition and brain health in healthy young and middle-aged adults: Systematic review and meta-analysis. *J. Clin. Med.* **2020**, *9*, 1598. [CrossRef]
34. Bao, M.J.; Shen, J.; Jia, Y.L.; Li, F.F.; Ma, W.J.; Shen, H.J.; Shen, L.L.; Lin, X.X.; Zhang, L.H.; Dong, X.W.; et al. Apple polyphenol protects against cigarette smoke-induced acute lung injury. *Nutrition* **2013**, *29*, 235–243. [CrossRef] [PubMed]
35. Garcia-Larsen, V.; Thawer, N.; Charles, D.; Cassidy, A.; Van Zele, T.; Thilsing, T.; Ahlström, M.; Haahtela, T.; Keil, T.; Matricardi, P.M.; et al. Dietary intake of flavonoids and ventilatory function in European adults: A GA2LEN study. *Nutrients* **2018**, *10*, 95. [CrossRef]
36. Nyanhanda, T.; Gould, E.M.; McGhie, T.; Shaw, O.M.; Harper, J.L.; Hurst, R.D. Blackcurrant cultivar polyphenolic extracts suppress CCL26 secretion from alveolar epithelial cells. *Food Funct.* **2014**, *5*, 671–677. [CrossRef]
37. Qi, G.; Mi, Y.; Fan, R.; Zhao, B.; Ren, B.; Liu, X. Tea polyphenols ameliorates neural redox imbalance and mitochondrial dysfunction via mechanisms linking the key circadian regular Bmal1. *Food Chem. Toxicol.* **2017**, *110*, 189–199. [CrossRef]
38. Shaw, O.M.; Nyanhanda, T.; McGhie, T.K.; Harper, J.L.; Hurst, R.D. Blackcurrant anthocyanins modulate CCL11 secretion and suppress allergic airway inflammation. *Mol. Nutr. Food Res.* **2017**, *61*, 1600868. [CrossRef]
39. Tabak, C.; Arts, I.C.; Smit, H.A.; Heederik, D.; Kromhout, D. Chronic obstructive pulmonary disease and intake of catechins, flavonols, and flavones: The MORGEN Study. *Am. J. Respir. Crit. Care Med.* **2001**, *164*, 61–64. [CrossRef]
40. Vergara, D.; Ávila, D.; Escobar, E.; Carrasco-Pozo, C.; Sánchez, A.; Gotteland, M. The intake of maqui (*Aristotelia chilensis*) berry extract normalizes H_2O_2 and IL-6 concentrations in exhaled breath condensate from healthy smokers-an explorative study. *Nutr. J.* **2015**, *14*, 1–5. [CrossRef]
41. Preedy, V.R.; Watson, R.R.; Zibadi, S. (Eds.) *Polyphenols in Human Health and Disease*; Academic Press: Cambridge, MA, USA, 2014.
42. Pounis, G.; Arcari, A.; Costanzo, S.; Di Castelnuovo, A.; Bonaccio, M.; Persichillo, M.; Donati, M.B.; de Gaetano, G.; Iacoviello, L. Favorable association of polyphenol-rich diets with lung function: Cross-sectional findings from the Moli-sani study. *Respir. Med.* **2018**, *136*, 48–57. [CrossRef] [PubMed]
43. Morton, L.C.; Paton, C.D.; Merry, T.; Braakhuis, A.J. Effects of 7-day polyphenol powder supplementation on cycling performance and lung function in an ozone-polluted environment. *Eur. J. Appl. Physiol.* **2023**, 1–10. [CrossRef] [PubMed]
44. Marquez, C.M.; Vanaudenaerde, B.; Troosters, T.; Wenderoth, N. High-intensity interval training evokes larger serum BDNF levels compared with intense continuous exercise. *J. Appl. Physiol.* **2015**, *119*, 1363–1373. [CrossRef] [PubMed]
45. Bajaj, J.S.; Heuman, D.M.; Sterling, R.K.; Sanyal, A.J.; Siddiqui, M.; Matherly, S.; Luketic, V.; Stravitz, R.T.; Fuchs, M.; Thacker, L.R.; et al. Validation of EncephalApp, smartphone-based Stroop test, for the diagnosis of covert hepatic encephalopathy. *Clin. Gastroenterol. Hepatol.* **2015**, *13*, 1828–1835. [CrossRef] [PubMed]
46. Bristow, T.; Jih, C.S.; Slabich, A.; Gunn, J. Standardization and adult norms for the sequential subtracting tasks of serial 3's and 7's. *Appl. Neuropsychol. Adult* **2016**, *23*, 372–378. [CrossRef] [PubMed]
47. Cohen, J. *Statistical Power Analysis for the Behavioral Sciences*; Academic Press: Cambridge, MA, USA, 2013.
48. Chen, J.C.; Schwartz, J. Neurobehavioral effects of ambient air pollution on cognitive performance in US adults. *Neurotoxicology* **2009**, *30*, 231–239. [CrossRef] [PubMed]

49. Knaepen, K.; Goekint, M.; Heyman, E.M.; Meeusen, R. Neuroplasticity—Exercise-induced response of peripheral brain-derived neurotrophic factor: A systematic review of experimental studies in human subjects. *Sports Med.* **2010**, *40*, 765–801. [CrossRef]
50. Silveira, A.C.; Hasegawa, J.S.; Cruz, R.; Matsuda, M.; Marquezini, M.V.; Lima-Silva, A.E.; Giles, L.V.; Saldiva, P.; Koehle, M.S.; Bertuzzi, R. Effects of air pollution exposure on inflammatory and endurance performance in recreationally trained cyclists adapted to traffic-related air pollution. *Am. J. Physiol.-Regul. Integr. Comp. Physiol.* **2022**, *322*, R562–R570. [CrossRef]
51. Pedersen, B.K.; Febbraio, M.A. Muscle as an endocrine organ: Focus on muscle-derived interleukin-6. *Physiol. Rev.* **2008**, *88*, 1379–1406. [CrossRef]
52. Steensberg, A.; Fischer, C.P.; Keller, C.; Møller, K.; Pedersen, B.K. IL-6 enhances plasma IL-1ra, IL-10, and cortisol in humans. *Am. J. Physiol.-Endocrinol. Metab.* **2003**, *285*, E433–E437. [CrossRef]
53. Ullum, H.E.; Haahr, P.M.; Diamant, M.A.; Palmo, J.; Halkjaer-Kristensen, J.; Pedersen, B.K. Bicycle exercise enhances plasma IL-6 but does not change IL-1 alpha, IL-1 beta, IL-6, or TNF-alpha pre-mRNA in BMNC. *J. Appl. Physiol.* **1994**, *77*, 93–97. [CrossRef] [PubMed]
54. González-Guevara, E.; Martínez-Lazcano, J.C.; Custodio, V.; Hernández-Cerón, M.; Rubio, C.; Paz, C. Exposure to ozone induces a systemic inflammatory response: Possible source of the neurological alterations induced by this gas. *Inhal. Toxicol.* **2014**, *26*, 485–491. [CrossRef] [PubMed]
55. Dinarello, C.A. Overview of the IL-1 family in innate inflammation and acquired immunity. *Immunol. Rev.* **2018**, *281*, 8–27. [CrossRef] [PubMed]
56. Yan, Z.; Liu, Y.M.; Wu, W.D.; Jiang, Y.; Zhuo, L.B. Combined exposure of heat stress and ozone enhanced cognitive impairment via neuroinflammation and blood brain barrier disruption in male rats. *Sci. Total Environ.* **2023**, *857*, 159599. [CrossRef] [PubMed]
57. Rivas-Arancibia, S.; Guevara-Guzmán, R.; López-Vidal, Y.; Rodríguez-Martínez, E.; Zanardo-Gomes, M.; Angoa-Pérez, M.; Raisman-Vozari, R. Oxidative stress caused by ozone exposure induces loss of brain repair in the hippocampus of adult rats. *Toxicol. Sci.* **2010**, *113*, 187–197. [CrossRef]
58. Bowtell, J.L.; Aboo-Bakkar, Z.; Conway, M.E.; Adlam, A.L.; Fulford, J. Enhanced task-related brain activation and resting perfusion in healthy older adults after chronic blueberry supplementation. *Appl Physiol. Nutr. Metab.* **2017**, *42*, 773–779. [CrossRef]
59. Fang, J.L.; Luo, Y.; Jin, S.H.; Yuan, K.; Guo, Y. Ameliorative effect of anthocyanin on depression mice by increasing monoamine neurotransmitter and up-regulating BDNF expression. *J. Funct. Foods* **2020**, *66*, 103757. [CrossRef]

nutrients

Article

Nutritional Considerations of Irish Performance Dietitians and Nutritionists in Concussion Injury Management

Emma Finnegan, Ed Daly and Lisa Ryan *

Department of Sport, Exercise and Nutrition, Atlantic Technological University (ATU), H91 T8NW Galway, Ireland; emma.finnegan@atu.ie (E.F.); ed.daly@atu.ie (E.D.)
* Correspondence: lisa.ryan@atu.ie

Abstract: Sport-related concussion incidence has increased in many team-based sports, such as rugby, Gaelic (camogie, hurling, football), and hockey. Concussion disrupts athletes' brain function, causing an "energy crisis" that requires energy and nutrient support to restore function and heal. Performance dietitians and nutritionists play a role in supporting athletes' post-injury nutritional demands. This study aimed to investigate Irish performance dietitians' and nutritionists' knowledge and implementation of nutritional strategies to manage and support athletes' recovery following concussion. In-depth, semi-structured interviews were conducted with seventeen (n = 17) Irish performance dietitians and nutritionists recruited from the Sport and Exercise Nutrition register and other sporting body networks across Ireland. Participants practised or had practised with amateur and/or professional athletes within the last ten years. All interviews and their transcripts were thematically analysed to extract relevant insights. These data provided valuable insights revealing performance dietitians and nutritionists: (1) their awareness of concussion events and (2) their use of nutritional supports for concussion management. Furthermore, the research highlighted their implementation of 'novel nutritional protocols' specifically designed to support and manage athletes' concussion recovery. There was a clear contrast between participants who had an awareness and knowledge of the importance of nutrition for brain recovery after sport-related concussion(s) and those who did not. Participants presenting with a practical understanding mentioned re-emphasising certain foods and supplements they were already recommending to athletes in the event of a concussion. Performance dietitians and nutritionists were keeping up to date with nutrition research on concussions, but limited evidence has prevented them from implementing protocols in practice. Meanwhile, participants mentioned trialling/recommending nutritional protocols, such as carbohydrate reloading, reducing omega-6 intake, and acutely supplementing creatine, omega-3 fish oils high in Docosahexaenoic acid, and probiotics to support brain healing. Performance dietitians' and nutritionists' use of nutrition protocols with athletes following concussion was linked to their knowledge and the limited scientific evidence available. Nutrition implementation, therefore, may be overlooked or implemented with uncertainty, which could negatively affect athletes' recovery following sports-related concussions.

Keywords: concussion; mild traumatic brain injury; nutrition; sport; recovery; dietary; supplement; athletes

Citation: Finnegan, E.; Daly, E.; Ryan, L. Nutritional Considerations of Irish Performance Dietitians and Nutritionists in Concussion Injury Management. *Nutrients* **2024**, *16*, 497. https://doi.org/10.3390/nu16040497

Academic Editor: Matthew Barnes

Received: 3 January 2024
Revised: 29 January 2024
Accepted: 1 February 2024
Published: 9 February 2024

1. Introduction

Sport-related concussions (SRCs), also known as mild Traumatic Brain Injuries (mTBIs), are prevalent [1–4], with up to 3.8 million cases reported in the United States annually [5–7]. The term 'mild' does not reflect severity but reflects the absence of structural brain damage. SRC is a type of mTBI with subtle differences. Both (SRC and mTBI) share subjective presentations [8,9] and are often used interchangeably, particularly in the sporting context [2]. Improvements in technology, education, and concussion identification protocols [10] have led to an increase in the reporting of SRC incidents [11,12], though many are still going unreported or undiagnosed [13,14].

SRCs are inevitable in contact and collision sports. Due to their subjective and invisible injury presentation, many frequently go undiagnosed or unreported [2–4,15,16]. In sports, sub-concussive impacts, and repetitive head injuries (RHIs) are concerns due to their long-term effects on athletes' health [17]. In Ireland, many athletes (amateur and professional) engage in collision sports, contact sports, or other activities that will increase their exposure to SRC events [18]. Collision sports, such as rugby union, involve body-to-body collisions as a fundamental element of the game. For contact sports, such as Gaelic football, hurling, camogie, field hockey, and soccer, purposeful body-to-body collisions or outright tackling [19], although not endorsed, are recognised as a natural part of the game [20,21]. Combat sports involve striking (boxing), grappling (wrestling), or a combination (mixed martial arts) [22,23] and involve 'knock out' or a 'technical knockout' for a fight to cease [24]. Additionally, non-field-based activities such as cycling can involve bike collisions and crashing [25]. Concussion does not discriminate based on age, gender, preferred sport/activity, or level (amateur/professional) and impacts individuals of all backgrounds [26–29]. In Ireland, athletes will often play multiple team sports recreationally, at an amateur level (Gaelic, combat, etc.), which typically have limited medical field side support. This situation increases the risk of SRCs going undetected or undiagnosed and athletes' exposure to RHIs [10]. Scullion et al. [30] identified that players and coaches in amateur sports may have limited knowledge and training regarding SRC, in contrast to those in professional or elite team settings [30]. Therefore, providing suitable education, training, and resources to athletes, coaches, and medical professionals would help reduce harmful outcomes and long-term consequences associated with SRC [31].

SRC, according to the "Concussion In Sport Group" (CISG), is provoked by a direct or indirect impact to the head, face, neck, or other body parts, passing an impulsive force to the brain, disrupting its function, and resulting in the rapid onset of transient symptoms [1,9]. Symptoms and signs are subjective, and present immediately or develop over minutes or hours, altering athletes' cognitive and mental state (e.g., confusion, disorientation) [1,9,30,32]. Athletes present with SRC in a variety of ways and do not have to have visible head trauma or a loss of consciousness. SRC, if experienced in isolation and managed properly, should not pose a significant risk to athletes' health. Most individuals should see improvements in their symptoms within 7 to 30 days [3,17,33] and return to their baseline within 3 months [34] following concussion. Recent research has highlighted the potential importance of nutrition in supporting and promoting recovery from brain injury, making it an essential component currently understated for SRC reduction and management [3].

Though an emerging area, in the concussion recovery management literature, nutrition is acknowledged for providing the fuel and nutrients to meet functional healing and repair demands [3,11]. In some instances, athletes have insufficient stores of specific nutrients (such as vitamin D) for neuroprotection and acute healing and recovery support. At present, there are no clear recommendations on strategies and recommended dosing [35,36] post-SRC. Strategies to increase athletes' intake of protein foods would increase amino acid availability and may prevent further tissue breakdown, support healing, and regulate brain metabolism [3,37]. Increasing athletes' consumption of fats, particularly omega-3 fatty acids such as docosahexaenoic acid (DHA) and eicosapentaenoic acid (EPA), through food (fish and algae-based products) and supplements may also support recovery. DHA plays a role in brain development [38] and has been shown to be neuroprotective, having and may aid brain recovery following RHI and concussion [3,39]. Supplementation with a high dose of DHA or a combination of DHA and EPA may help saturate brain cells and promote healing [3], mitigating the long-term adverse effects associated with low brain DHA levels after concussion [40]. No specific DHA recommendations exist for high-risk sub-concussive sports athletes [41]. However, the Food and Drug Administration (FDA) and the European Food Safety Authority (EFSA) recommend consuming at least two servings of fish per week and a maximum of 2–3 g daily via supplement (EPA and DHA) for optimal health [3,42–44]. In addition, the fat-soluble nutrient vitamin D is neuroprotective and promotes healing and neural recovery following a head impact [3]. Athletes with low vitamin D levels have reduced neuroprotection, heightened inflammation, and compromised and prolonged cognitive recovery [3,45]. Supplementing magnesium within 24 h replenishes depleted brain cellular levels, alleviating symptoms and promoting faster recovery [46].

Creatine, an essential amino acid, is crucial in energy production, influencing brain and muscle tissue function and performance, and may play a role in brain injury recovery [47,48]. Without free creatine or phosphocreatine available, energy deprivation occurs during the neurometabolic cascade following the accelerated uptake and use of adenosine triphosphate (ATP). Increasing cellular creatine levels in the hypometabolic period may help restore energy by supporting ATP production from glucose and enhancing oxygen supply to the brain. However, positive effects of creatine have been primarily observed in healthy individuals, animal populations, or cases of severe brain injury. Its effectiveness in addressing concussion-related (RHI or mTBI) issues is uncertain and requires further investigation for preventive and post-SRC protocols.

The field of performance nutrition is dynamic and involves applying evidence-based nutritional strategies to help enhance athletes' training, recovery, and athletic capacities [49]. In the event of an injury, performance dietitians (PDs) and nutritionists (PNs) help athletes in meeting their nutritional needs to support healing and recovery using dietary and supplementation strategies. Given their pivotal role in supporting athletes after injury, this research aimed to understand the nutritional protocols Irish PDs and PNs implement with their athletes post-concussion.

2. Materials and Methods

2.1. Study Design

Braun and Clarke's reflexive thematic analysis (TA) approach was implemented to enable the interpretation of the qualitative data to identify and analyse themes and patterns present throughout the research data [50]. Individual semi-structured interviews were designed, conducted, and reported in line with the COnsolidated Criteria for REporting Qualitative research (COREQ) [51].

Before the study commenced, interview guides were developed by E.F. and piloted with two PNs to test the feasibility of the interview script questions. All participants in this study were performance/sports dietetic and nutrition professionals (female and male) located and practising in Ireland or Northern Ireland and working with professional/elite, semi-professional/sub-elite, or amateur athletes and/or teams aged $\geq$16 years. Professional registrations (the Sport and Exercise Nutrition register (SENr)), sporting bodies, the Irish Rugby Football Union (IRFU), the Gaelic Athletic Association (GAA), Sport Ireland, and sports nutrition networks were used to identify and source PN(s) and/or PD(s) that were currently practising throughout Ireland/had practised within the last ten years. The lead researcher (E.F.) invited suitable candidates to participate in an online one-to-one interview via email.

Data collection began in March 2022 and ceased in August 2022 once data saturation had occurred. The interview format was designed to discern participants' backgrounds, education, and career paths to date; the different types of athletes they worked with; sports; and settings. Section B then proceeded to ask participants about the types of injury their athletes would commonly present with and if, as practitioners, they considered/used nutrition to support athletes' healing and recovery outcomes. The final section sought to identify specific nutrition protocols PD(s)/PN(s) implemented for different types of injury, tissues, and sites to support and facilitate athletes in the recovery and healing process.

2.2. Ethics and Procedure

This study was ethically approved by the Research Sub-Committee of Atlantic Technological University's Academic Council (ATU-RSC_AC_25/11/2021). The lead researcher (E.F.) identified the initial number of participants by distributing a direct invite alongside a participant information sheet detailing the purpose of the study. Before each interview, informal discussions were conducted with participants to discuss the study objectives, protocols, and the confidential management of the resulting data. The lead researcher (E.F.) conducted all interviews using Microsoft Teams, and before each interview, participant consent was recorded. Interviews lasted between 25 and 60 min (Mean ($\overline{x}$) = 41.77 min, Standard Deviation (SD) = 9.9 min) in duration. Interviews were semi-structured, with a topic guide that included a series of ethically approved open-ended questions and supporting questions designed to create discussion on topics relevant to the study. After each interview, each data transcript was collected, and all data related to the study were fully anonymised to protect all professional participants from identification.

2.3. Participants Characteristics

Seventeen (n = 17) PN(s) and/or PD(s), identifying as male (n = 8) and female (n = 9), working with a wide range of professional/elite, semi-professional/sub-elite, or amateur male and female (adult and youth) athletes took part in the interviews. During data collection, participants were practising in the Republic of Ireland and Northern Ireland or had been within the last ten years.

2.4. Sampling and Eligibility Criteria

A purposeful sampling [52,53] methodology was employed to create a sequence of responses across participants. An Irish network of PN(s) and PD(s) was identified, targeted, and contacted, with an invitation to participate in the one-to-one interviews. Professional registrations (SENr), sporting bodies (IRFU, GAA, and Sport Ireland) and sports nutrition networks were used to identify and source PN(s) and/or PD(s) registered to practise throughout Ireland currently (at the time of the study) or within the last ten years. Eligible participants had to be working with adults and youth ($\geq$16 years of age), professional/elite, semi-professional/sub-elite, or amateur athlete(s) and/or teams. E.F. invited suitable candidates to participate in online one-to-one interviews via email. The sampling process was concluded once data saturation was reached.

2.5. Data Collection

Interview questions were used to gather evidence of PD(s)/PN(s) personal experiences with injuries, specifically concussions. They discussed awareness of injury events within their athlete cohorts, their role in prevention and injury management, and how they utilised nutrition to support athletes' return to play (RTP) after concussion.

2.6. Researcher Description

The lead researcher and author (E.F.) identifies as a woman and has been actively involved in sport and nutrition professionally for eight years in consultancy and research settings, working with athletes and performance nutritionists in amateur, semi-professional, and professional sports settings. E.F. is currently a research associate within the Irish Concussion Research Centre (ICRC) engaged in researching strategies for managing, reducing, and educating cohorts about mTBI/concussion, RHI, brain health, and nutrition. Her research focuses on investigating the "Role of Nutrition in Concussion Recovery and Management". During the research process, to increase rigour, E.F. implemented a bracketing method to support their background reflection before data collection commenced to minimise potential bias from personal preconceptions [54].

2.7. Data Analysis

A reflexive TA approach was implemented due to the researcher's role in knowledge production [50]. Reflexive TA would support a richer and more precise reading of the data as it required the researchers to continually question and query any assumptions made during the interpretation and coding of the data [50]. The analysis followed a six-stage approach to identify and construct meaning and patterns from the data [50,55].

2.8. Transcription

Initially, the original audio recordings of each interview were listened to multiple times before being transcribed verbatim by the lead researcher (E.F.). Transcripts were examined for accuracy, cross-checked with original audio recordings, and re-edited as necessary. This familiarisation (Phase 1) with the content of each transcript was continued by E.F., who re-read each transcript on four separate occasions and compiled initial notes per interviewee to support the coding process. This practice enabled E.F. to confirm that questions and responses were linked with each interview audio recording. Transcripts were then read by a second author (L.R.) blinded to the participants and any initial trends generated within the data.

2.9. Coding

Initial codes (Phase 2) were created based on theoretical assumptions, and the research aimed to focus on semantic meanings within interview transcripts. This was carried out by E.F. and reviewed together with L.R. Both researchers independently and systematically coded transcripts and then met to discuss and verify codes and their application to research data. This coding phase created theme semantic blocks (Phase 3) within transcripts, which were then linked to subthemes, and quotations were extracted (Figure S1A) accordingly. The authors reviewed themes (T) in Phase 4 to check and challenge any assumptions. Thematic maps (Figure S1B,C) were developed, and theme linkages were created and reviewed to convey meanings evident throughout the dataset. The initial Ts included (T1) Concussion Awareness—reporting and communication, (T2) Nutritional Support—Awareness, (T3) Knowledge of Nutrition Protocols, (T4) Nutrition Implementation, and (T5) Nutrition Novel Protocols—specific to concussion. Themes were defined and refined (Phase 5) to ensure they individually captured each theme clearly. As a result, theme 1 was renamed, to be more specific, and themes 2, 3, and 4 were joined (Figure 1A,B). The final themes were PDs'/PNs' '(T1) Awareness of Concussion Events' and their use of '(T2) Nutritional Support for Concussion Management', which included 'Novel Nutritional Protocols' to support and manage SRC recovery. For the final stage (Phase 6), an analytic narrative was produced, and this is presented in the Results section (Section 3) in this manuscript.

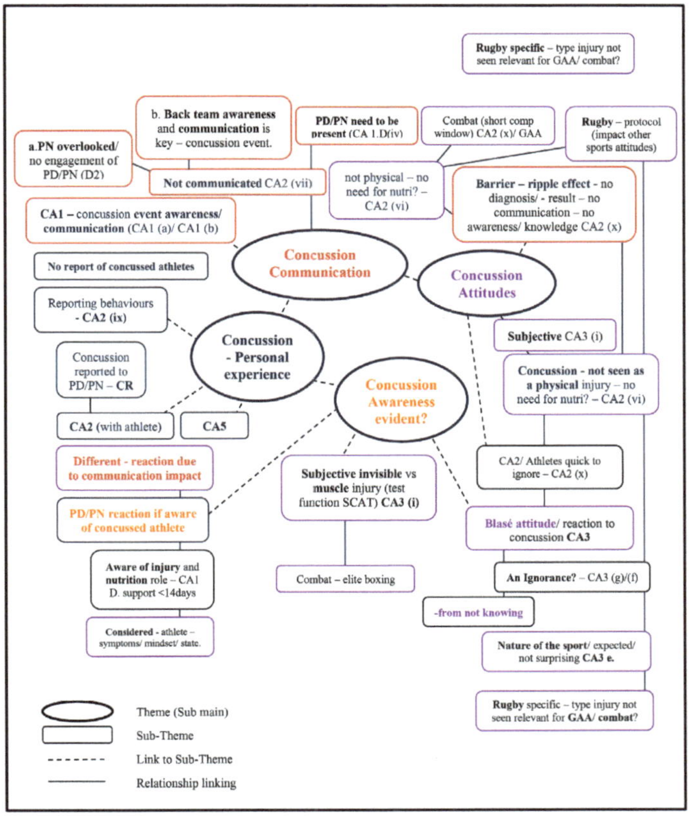

(A)

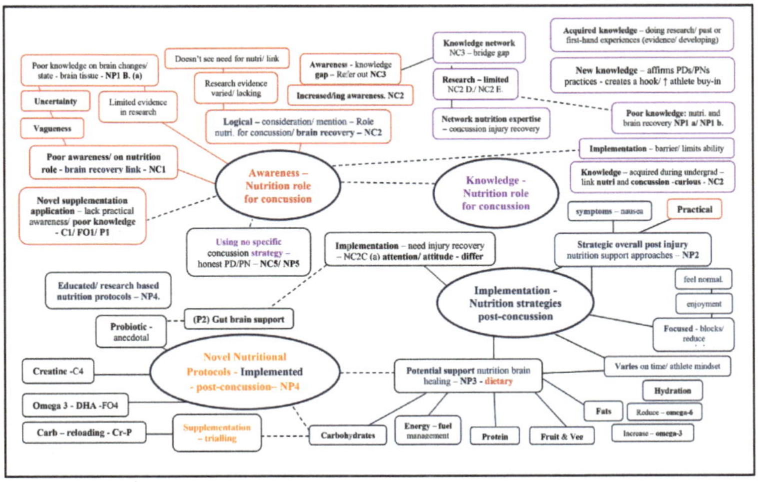

(B)

Figure 1. (**A**) Reflexive Thematic Analysis (Phase 5). Awareness of concussion—thematic map demonstrating four subthemes (s-T). (**B**) Reflexive Thematic Analysis (Phase 5). Nutritional support for concussion management—thematic map demonstrating four subthemes (s-T).

3. Results

The purpose of this study was to develop an understanding of the nutritional protocols implemented by Irish PDs and PNs with their athletes post-concussion. The semi-structured interviews TA identified two main themes (T) with eleven subthemes (s-T). Descriptions of each central theme (T = 2) and its associated subthemes (s-T = 11) are summarised in this section (3.0) with meaningful verbatim quotation evidence to highlight participants' narratives.

3.1. Participant Characteristics

Participants (Table 1) were Irish PDs and PNs working with a wide range of adult and youth (≥16 years) professional/elite, semi-professional/sub-elite, or amateur athletes across the Republic of Ireland and Northern Ireland. At a minimum, participants held Master of Science degrees in sports nutrition and exercise and/or a Doctor of Philosophy (PhD). The PDs and PNs involved in supporting team-based athletes were participating in various Irish native sports, including Gaelic football (https://www.gaa.ie/my-gaa/getting-involved/gaelic-football (accessed on 21 June 2023)), ladies' Gaelic football (LGFA, https://www.gaa.ie/my-gaa/getting-involved/ladies-gaelic-football (accessed on 25 June 2023)), hurling (https://www.gaa.ie/article/hurling (accessed on 25 June 2023)), camogie (https://www.gaa.ie/my-gaa/getting-involved/camogie (accessed on 25 June 2023)) (intercounty, county, and club levels), soccer (Premier League, League of Ireland, and club-level), rugby union, women's hockey (provincial and club-level), and cricket (professional). Individual sports were also represented, such as combat sports, boxing, mixed martial arts, kickboxing, and judo (amateur and professional/elite levels); gymnastics (elite); athletics, running, and cycling (elite, ex-elite, and amateur levels); rowing; endurance events; triathlon (Ironman); and competitive multisport, Olympic lifting, and powerlifting.

3.2. Thematic Results

Two major themes were identified from this research analysis of PDs and PNs: (1) their awareness of concussion events and their use of (2) nutritional supports for concussion management (Figure 2), including 'novel nutritional protocols', to manage SRC.

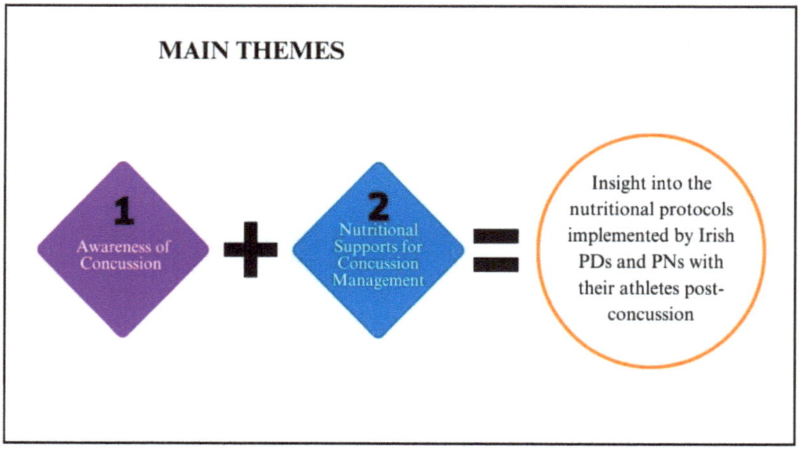

Figure 2. Reflexive thematic analysis. Result: main themes addressing the research question. Note: PD(s): Performance Dietitian(s), PN(s): Performance Nutritionist(s).

These main themes were separated into subthemes, theme 1 and 2 (Tables 2 and 3).

Table 1. Participant profiles and characteristics: PD/PN background, education, roles, employment, and athlete types.

Participants Profile						
	Total Sample (n)			n = 17		
	Gender			Male		Female
	% (n)			59% (10)		51% (7)
Undergraduate degree	BSc Dietetics and nutrition sciences	BSc Human nutrition sciences	BSc Nutrition and sports sciences	BSc Health, sport, and exercise sciences	BA Education with science	Other (BA, BCom, BBS non-science degrees)
% (n)	11.8% (2)	17.6% (3)	5.9% (1)	35.3% (6)	11.8% (2)	17.6% (3)
Post Graduate degree (MSc/PhD)	MSc in Sports Nutrition	Dip Sports Nutrition	MSc Sports and Exercise Nutrition	MSc in Human or/and Nutrition,	MRes in Sport and Exercise Nutrition	Doctor of Philosophy (PhD)
(n)	(4)	(3)	(9)	(2)	(1)	(5) Specialisms included: Energy, Sports, and Exercise Nutrition Bone Health, Exercise Biochemistry, Bioactives in Health and Exercise.
SENr Registered % (n)				Yes 100% (17)		
Previously concussed (history) % (n)			Yes 23.5% (4)		No 76.5% (13)	

PN-ID	Type Athlete/Client	Teams/Organisations	Part/Full-time
PN 1	Elite teams: male senior and U20s Gaelic footballers—county-level.	GAA	Part-time/contract roles
PN 2	Elite teams: male athletes in rugby union—academy and senior squads; male Gaelic footballers—county-level.	IRFU, GAA	Full-time
PN 3	Elite individual athletes (mixed); elite teams: rugby union (senior, academy males/7s, XVs female) and senior (male) Gaelic football and hurling athletes—county and intercounty levels.	Sport Ireland, University scholarships, Athletics Ireland, IRFU, LGFA, GAA	Part-time/contract roles

Table 1. *Cont.*

	Participants Profile		
PN 4	Elite teams: men's hurling and ladies' and men's Gaelic football (male/female) athletes. Individuals: amateur/non-elite-MMA, soccer athletes.	LGFA, GAA	Part-time/contract roles
PN 5	Elite amateur teams: Gaelic football athletes; individual: amateur/non-elite endurance and rugby athletes	GAA	Full-time
PN 6	Individual: retired professional/high-level amateur-endurance (runners, cyclists), kickboxing, high-intensity functional training, powerlifting athletes	N/A	Full-time-self-employed
PN 7	High-level amateur teams: U20 hurlers (county) and senior men's Gaelic footballers (intercounty). Individual: soccer athletes.	GAA	Part-time roles
PN 8	Elite/Professional teams: academy, youth, and senior men's rugby union (current). Women's soccer, senior ladies', and U20s men's Gaelic football and hurling at county and intercounty levels (past). Individual: Triathletes (paralympic squad, past).	IRFU, LGFA, GAA, Women's FC	Full-time
PN 9	Elite: Women's XV and 7s and men's 7s academy and sub-academy rugby union teams. Amateur: junior Gaelic intercounty team athletes.	IRFU, GAA	Full-time
PN 10	Teams: U21s and mixed 1–1 Gaelic footballs. Individual: professional and amateur combat male/female athletes—boxers, MMA, and kickboxing.	GAA	Full-time-self-employed
PN 11	Teams: Elite/high-level women's soccer, hockey, and rugby union squads. Individual: mixed 1–1 athletes.	WFC, women's hockey, IRFU, SN private practice	Part-time/contract roles
PN 12	Elite/high-level amateur teams: U20s and senior Gaelic footballers and hurlers.	GAA	Part-time/contract roles
PN 13	Elite teams: women's hockey, individual junior gymnastic athletes, and endurance athletes (cyclists).	Sport Ireland	Full-time
PN 14	Teams: professional rugby union and high-level amateur Gaelic football athletes. Individual: elite/professional Olympic boxers, rowers, athletics, judo, and cricket athletes.	Sport Ireland	Full-time
PN 15	Teams: senior and U21 Gaelic footballers and hurlers, academy male rugby union athletes. Individual: Gaelic footballers, hurlers, and jockeys.	GAA, IRFU	Part-time roles
PN 16	Team: rugby/soccer/hockey/Gaelic hurling, camogie, football, club, intercounty, ladies, men's athletes. Individual: competitive/high level/weight class athletes/HIFT/multi-sport athletes (boxers, Olympic, power weightlifting/MMA)/endurance athletes.	N/A	Full-time
PN 17	Teams: professional rugby union—male academy/NTS squads (16 years up), high-level amateur intercounty Gaelic football and Camogie athletes. Individual: endurance athletes.	IRFU	Part-time roles

Abbreviation notes: SENr: Sport Exercise Nutrition register; BDA: The British Dietetic Association; PN: Precision Nutrition; ISAK: The International Society for the Advancement of Kinanthropometry; NTOI: Nutritional Therapists of Ireland; IRFU: Irish Rugby Football Union; FC: Football Club; GAA: Gaelic Athletic Association, MMA: Mixed Martial Arts, HIFT: high-intensity functional training, SN: Sports nutrition.

Table 2. Theme 1: Irish performance dietitians and nutritionists' awareness of concussion. Developed themes, subthemes, sample codes, and example quotes.

Theme	Subtheme	Example Quote
1. PD/PN Personal experiences with concussion injuries	Concussion diagnosis reported to PD/PN	. . .your first most common will be, ehmm, connective tissue injuries. So, like your shoulders. . .shoulders, ACLs, ankles syndesmosis, then followed by concussion, and then you have your hamstrings and calves like soft tissues, and then you have your broken bones, and then your kind of back injuries would be. [PN 9]
	Concussions not reported by athletes to PD/PN	. . .you never. . .never even hear of like concussions reported back to you, but God knows, even though it's probably likely you'll never hear back! [PN 12]
	Personal concussion experience	First impact: . . .the first one happened during a hockey match. . . I just stepped back, and the player behind me. . .stepped back, and it was just like totally innocuous. No big deal; we didn't even hit heads that that hard! I played on. . .totally, sort of out of it! I went off, and then I tried to insist on going back on, but then eventually the penny dropped that I wasn't ok and like I couldn't keep my eyes open. . . I felt fine again a few hours later. . . If I'm honest, I didn't change anything about the way I was eating, then. I just. . .sort of slept a bit more. [PN 11] Second impact: . . .next one, then only about four months later, I got a ball right into the face; a hockey ball. I kind of knew then I'm obviously slower. . . I did make the change (nutritionally) at that stage. . .I would be, you know, eating more regularly. . .making sure my protein intake would better across the day. . .the probiotics. . . I was a bit worried. [PN 11] Third impact: . . .the third one. I was playing with my kids in the swimming pool. . .managed to smack my head off the bottom of it. . .then. . .I didn't play hockey for quite a while because I wanted. . .to get a brain scan. . . Three in 18 months is a lot! [PN 11]
2. Concussion injury communication	Back-team communication key-acute injury	. . .I know when there is a decent backroom team that are all together, and I know when. . . they don't really believe in all the different pillars as much as their own pillar. . . If you've got a backroom team that is set up in a very efficient way, it's just then firing off a message to one person who does their part. . . I would work very closely with one set of backroom teams, the doctor and the physio, and the S&C coach. . . Even though they've changed. . . the doctor never has. . . there has always been a kind of a multi-faceted approach. . . Whereas in other situations, it hasn't been as strong, you know, and I think that makes a big difference in terms of catching the acute phase. [PN 4]
	Open Communication	So, making contact. . . as soon as possible, but again. . . if you know the doc is on to them if you know the coach, the manager is on to them. . . if you know the physios are on to them, it is sometimes best to void your time. . . I've gotten a little bit better at identifying when are you helpful and when are you just annoying them you know? [PN 5]

Table 2. *Cont.*

Theme	Subtheme	Example Quote
3. Poor Concussion Reporting-Risk	Lucky or poor communication and reporting?	I'm. . .I'm so I'm so lucky that in just having the conversation with you there now. . . I'm just thinking back like five years, five years working in performance nutrition directly, and I have never had anyone with real. . .real acute injuries like. [PN 10]
	Concussion underdiagnosed or a reality of poor communication?	So, ehhh. . .luckily, we don't really get too many of them; now, like that, I can; I can miss some as well just by not being on site too often. Ehmm. . .again, like I'll go back to my old role of just turning up when, ehhh. . .when the, the rugby season is a little bit over. [PN 4]
4. Concussion Attitudes and Behaviours	Reaction to injury frequency of athletes-nature of sport?	Overall, there's nearly always, have some kind of knock or a niggle or a strain. . . When we're coming out off the back of matches ehmm to be honestly, injuries. . .they're very varied. . . I'm always just always still, even in shock with these guys! Like, how can you cope with it like they're just constantly in a state of basically recovery because they come out so beat and bruised from games. [PN 8]
	Athletes blasé risky attitude–concussion	Oh yeah! I think they are very quick to dismiss. . .injuries, especially when, I suppose, there's no, not that there's no obvious symptoms of it. But you know, they're not carrying their leg, for instance, or, you know? So, I definitely think they will try and mask it. . . I think your senior, more experienced players don't do that as much, but I definitely think your younger players will do what they can to try and get back out. . . [PN 7]
5. Concussion Awareness Evident	Elite-level subjective injury 'carrot' proof protocol	. . .boxers when they're dehydrated, looking at the SCAT test. So, we've actually used that as part of our showing them. . . Showing them that if they're dehydrated, their response to the SCAT is actually a lot less. So, you know, we've. . .put that in place some years ago around, you know, trying to educate them, to show them. . . That if you cut back on your fluids or you dry out too quickly. . .the reason that they may be drying out too quickly is because they're not following a better weight-making process. [PN 14]

Abbreviation notes: PD: performance dietitian, PN: Performance nutritionist, E.F.: interviewer.

Table 3. Theme 2: Nutritional support for concussion management mentioned by Irish performance dietitians and nutritionists. Developed themes, subthemes, sample codes, and example quotes.

Theme	Subtheme	Example Quote
1. Awareness of Nutrition in Concussion Management	Poor awareness	Not too sure, really, just keep up the good habits. But I haven't looked at it… Is there much? Is there much research on concussion and nutrition immediate or…? [PN 1]
	Aware with limited knowledge	Yeah…yeah, I look; I'd be the first admit now I don't… I know "X" and a few lads up in "x" are really interested in this area, and it's it is really interesting! So, I'm kind of keeping an eye on creatine, fish oil supplementation, ehmm, and just to see the effects on recovery… If there's anything there with creatine and fish oils. [PN 5]
2. Knowledge on the role of nutrition in concussion recovery	Acquired knowledge	Yeah, it's; it's an area I'm doing a bit of reading around at moment. But definitely, concussions are not that well-researched. But I think from what I have read, there's a couple things you can do, and creatine, I believe, is important in the…not even the acute phase of, of, of having a concussion, but I think consistently for optimal cognition. [PN 2]
	Personal led knowledge	…what would I implement with somebody else? I, I think, to be honest…the rest and the regular eating are…crucial and then… Whether, whether the extra probiotics or… Do you know whether they make that much of a difference? I don't really know… But the anti-inflammatory, the protein, the carb, I think they would be crucial. Obviously, you know…you know your…your healthy fats as well. But the diet…the diet itself is probably the most important thing. [PN 11]
	Nutrition knowledge network	With regards to concussion, then we have two dietitians. One that actually has worked in rugby and who would I suppose work and are more familiar with the concussion side of things… [PN 13]
	Expertise in nutrition risk	…if you look at concussions, like concussion, is like shortage of energy in the brain at the time of impact, so…you could, like. I'd broadly say it to people, you know…'just to make sure you eat enough during this time, and kind of, you know', were kind of very basic interventions, but nothing, I don't think we ever…got to a stage where we were comfortable giving nutrition advice to someone who was concussed because there was stuff out there on creatine and stuff on there, high dose DHA, but we never…never formalised that to a policy. [PN 9]

Table 3. *Cont.*

Theme	Subtheme	Example Quote
3. Implementation—Nutrition post-concussion	Implementation with uncertainty	Ehmm, so I'm kind of keeping an eye on creatine, fish oil supplementation. . .and just to see the effects on recovery. . .if there's anything there with creatine and fish oils. So, I would be kind of promoting or recommending to just keep those, the dosage on those. . . ehmm, keep including those if the lads have a concussion, and I would be in touch with the lads as well, like. . . . . .focus on the hydration. Keep on top of the omegas and the creatine. I'm not fully sure about the creatine yet, but they're taking it anyway for other reasons and I think there could be? [PN 5]
	Focused energy/symptom management	. . .one of the players who had been concussed had two in four weeks and was, you know, quite nauseous, wasn't able to eat a lot. So, it was more around I suppose having smaller meals, more frequently liquid, a lot of liquid meals and stuff. . . I just didn't really feel like it was settling him, but obviously, we are still, I suppose, were trying to get back to where he needs to be and be ready for when they get the go ahead to go back and train. . . So tried to ensure energy levels were kept up just through kind of liquid-based meals, small little snacks, nothing that was going to cause. . . stomach aggravation. . . So, it was more kind of in that, you know, couple days after. . . after the knock as opposed to long term [PN 7]
	Strategically blocked collaborative athlete support	I try to do it in smaller focuses instead of bombarding them all at once. . . So, let's say they initially we try to break down even with the physios; we'd break down their rehab into, like, phases. . . So, the initial being, their protection phase, for example. . . I try row in with that being with 'this is your initial focus' instead of trying to bombard them with loads. Saying, 'this is what I really want to get out of this block', and then we tried to do it in focus. [PN 8]
	Supplementation–refocus	. . .if they do get a concussion, I kind of re-emphasise that. I'll be like, you know. . . for some, not everyone will take fish oils ehmm, even though they have done. . . So, I'll re-emphasise that you should be taking fish oils, and I'll even tell them to load creatine and during that period. . . [PN 12]
	Dietary fat intake	your brain tissues are very, very reliant on kind of fat as its main fuel source. . . in terms of kind of recovery. . . So, a big, big focus on kind of their healthy omega 3s, and a reduction in obviously their pro-inflammatory omega 6s [PN 6]

Table 3. *Cont.*

Theme	Subtheme	Example Quote
4. Potential barrier	1. athletes' attitudes	I would say that the physical ones. . . they are probably more. . . (shaking head) open to the fact that nutrition can play (emphasised tone) a role immediately. . . Whereas the likes of the concussions, as you said, like it's not visible. . . So maybe a little bit more towards the towards the physical ones. . . [PN 17]
	2. athletes' nutrition adherence	. . .they are obviously fine, but like they. . . Well, see, I don't know if that they are actually taken it! But the guys who have been concussed recently. . . I definitely know one of them 100% was because he was looking for more creatine and everything, you know because he was loading up on it. . . [PN 12]
5. Novel nutrition protocol implementation post-concussion	Acute creatine intake	Again, I've done a little bit of research into it, and there is a small bit around concussion and creatine. [PN 8] Yeah. [E.F.] So, a lot of our athletes would take creatine. But if they haven't or around a concussion, potentially increasing that creatine intake, ehmm. . . In that period of concussion, to help with that energy availability side of things. Ehmm, if the brain can't fully use their glucose efficiently. So, I have trialled that; again, there was a little bit of research around it. But ehmm, aside from that, no there is nothing else. [PN 8]
	Carbohydrate-energy availability	Matthew Frakes is a researcher in Pittsburgh. I think he spoke about the energy availability and that like they compared guys that I don't know-was it like 4 or 500 g of carbs in the 5 days, after concussion versus the guys that had a low carbohydrate diet and the symptoms for the guys that had more carbohydrates were got back to baseline that bit quicker. So, that's kind of something I have been doing; it's like, well, if a guy is in a gradual return to play protocol, then can you eat enough food? [PN 2]

Abbreviation notes: PN: Performance Nutritionist, PD: Performance Dietitian, E.F.: Interviewer.

3.2.1. Irish Performance Dietitians and Nutritionists' Awareness of Concussion

Concussion: Personal Experience

In the context of concussion awareness, participants who cited having prior personal experience diagnosing or reporting concussions exhibited a higher awareness of their impact on athletes. In comparison, those without such experience demonstrated a lower awareness. The participants reporting concussion as common, casual occurrence amongst their athletes showed higher awareness of injury incidence without prompting or hesitation.

> *"I suppose obviously within... within rugby; we have like a lot of the collision-based injuries. So, for example, you know, the likes of concussion come up a lot and kind of ligament... ligament and tendons would be the ones that I see a lot of..."* [PN 17]

In 2014, World Rugby introduced the Head Injury Assessment (HIA) concussion management system into an injury policy [56]. One participant mentioned that head injury such as concussion *"wasn't really like a... like a thing... before HIAs"* [PN 3]. Before this, PDs/PNs involved in rugby were not part of the conversation or made aware of concussion incidence compared to 2022, when HIA was protocol and actively used to assist and improve reporting practices. However, in PDs/PNs working with hockey, soccer, combat, Gaelic football, and some individual athletes, reporting was not evident as they showed no awareness of concussion occurrence as an injury subset. In this instance, PDs/PNs reported that they were fortunate to have no recorded cases of concussion among their athletes:

> *"...I'm so lucky that, in just having the conversation with you there now... I'm just thinking back like five years, five years working in performance nutrition directly, and I have never had anyone with real...real acute injuries like."* [PN 10]

Alternatively, it is possible that they may be unfortunate, and that in reality, under-reporting is going unnoticed. Another participant highlighted the prevalence of injuries among high-level combat athletes and pointed out that *"...you never even hear of like concussions reported back to you, but God knows, even though it's probably likely you'll never hear back!"* [PN 12]. Meanwhile, a PN with a background as a hockey player shared insight into their injury experience, having had *"...three concussions at one point in 18 months"* [PN 11], highlighting differing levels of cognitive decline experienced and their subsequent need for nutrition to fuel their healing and extra rest. However, the PN was unaware of concussion incidences within their own hockey or soccer athletes (see Table 2).

Concussion Communication

The interviews generated patterns linking PDs'/PNs' experiences and awareness of concussion to the level of communication that existed between back-team members and their athletes in the incident of injury. Delving deeper, the data highlighted incidences of poor communication where the PDs/PNs were overlooked and, as result, did not know athletes had sustained an impact or SRC. PDs/PNs admitted feeling the need to be present at training and matches to be aware and in the know regarding SRC events. They felt the onus was on them as practitioners; otherwise, their involvement/awareness of injury events would be easily overlooked, especially if they were not present.

> *"Luckily, we don't really get too many of them now like that I can; I can miss some as well just by not being on site too often..."* [PN 4]

Having an awareness and understanding of an athlete's health and injury status, specifically after concussion, is a multifaceted task that requires collaboration across the entire back team. It is not the sole responsibility of one professional (i.e., doctor or the physio) in isolation to provide support, as highlighted by PN 4:

> *"I know when there is a decent backroom team that are all together, and I know when...they don't really believe in all the different pillars as much as their own pillar... If you've got a backroom team that is set up in a very efficient way, it's just them firing off a message to one person who does their part..."* [PN 4]

PDs/PNs know that differing communication and collaboration levels are present within a sport setting and are aware of their impact on forming *"a decent backroom team"* [PN 4]. A well-coordinated backroom team characterised by shared values, mutual respect, and effective communication collaborating on members' expertise would guarantee the successful implementation of essential measures following an SRC.

While the ideal scenario involves strong collaboration within the back-team setup, it is not always common practice, as expressed by PN 4 sharing the impact of limited collaboration situations where they felt it had not *"... been as strong, you know, and I think that makes a big difference in terms of catching the acute phase"* [PN 4]. In addition, PN 13 commented on the value placed on the PDs'/PNs' discipline and noted that at

> *"... the amateur, intercounty level... nutritionists are nearly shoved to the side 'ahhh we don't need the nutritionist on match day', you know, but like physios they're stade on foot... it's happening at all corners, and that's at the top level"* [PN 13]

This highlighted the potential dangers of scenarios where the back-team setup is not valued, is fragmented, and has poor communication channels. In contrast, when communication channels are open, PDs/PNs have injury awareness. PDs/PNs can effectively prepare and tailor their support and work with back-team members to ensure athletes' best recovery interests are met, emphasising the importance of a cohesive relationship and collaborative approach. Furthermore, providing more insight into the dynamics of the back team, PN 5 stated:

> *"... if you know the doc is on to them if you know the coach, the manager is on to them... if you know the physios are on to them, it sometimes best to void your time... I've gotten a little bit better at identifying when you are helpful and when you are just annoying them, you know?"* [PN 5]

For some participants, their first protocol following a suspected SRC impact is a diagnosis and medical sign-off; they know this is a crucial step before any other back-team member implements support: *"on the day I would be leaving it to the medic, really"* [PN 1]. However, PDs/PNs seemingly underestimate the significance of their role in acute recovery support compared to other back-team members.

> *"I think in that scenario (pause)... I would wait to hear from... some other medical professional before doing anything...*
>
> *Rugby is one of those sports... I think that it's further ahead than a lot of sports certainly in Ireland, where they do have that support on hand."* [PN 16]

Concussion Attitudes

Awareness of concussion incidence amongst PDs/PNs appears to be influenced by a seemingly 'blasé' attitude toward the injury. This may influence an athlete or backroom team member's reaction and subsequent reporting behaviour if a suspected concussive impact occurs. PDs/PNs working with athletes in contact collision-based sports, like rugby, expect injuries due to the nature of the sport and perceive athletes to often be in a heightened recovery state, especially after matches. For example, PN 8 commented:

> *"Overall, there's nearly always have some kind of knock or a niggle or a strain... When we're coming out off the back of matches...*
>
> *They're just constantly in a state of basically recovery because they come out so beat and bruised from games."* [PN 8]

However, could this better awareness be creating a more casual attitude toward concussion, as some participants comment and perceive it as *"just another like... injury"* [PN 8]?

> *"... with guys that are there concussed, which are probably be quite regularly... which is unfortunately the case, your kind of on to them to stay away..."* [PN 2]

Athletes in collision sports may have a casual attitude due to the subjective nature of concussions. For instance, they may believe that they can quickly RTP, as stated in an example of an athlete persona by PN 8: "*. . .ahhh no I'll be fine, I'll be back in a week*" [PN 8]. The frequency of SRC in a collision sport and its subjective presentation (i.e., symptoms) may feed behaviours of poor compliance to recovery support programs. As stated by one PN, speaking specifically about professional rugby athletes,

> "*They don't really care. . . I think it's cause it's such a common injury, like while concussion in GAA might be less common. When it's so common in rugby. . .concussion is just like another. . .another injury*" [PN 8]

Athletes tend to disregard subjective and invisible injuries, especially when they are eager to RTP. As noted by PN 7, athletes can be "*. . .very quick to dismiss. . .injuries, especially when, I suppose, there's no, not that there's no obvious symptoms of it. . .you know, they're not carrying their leg*" [PN 7] due to physical symptoms such as limping or bruising. This behaviour is commonly observed among younger rugby and Gaelic athletes, who may be more inclined to take risks to get back on the field, as mentioned both by PN 7 and PN 8.

Concussion Awareness Evidence

In elite-level combat sports, where concussions are frequently reported, some PDs/PNs proactively implement objective tests and diagnostic protocols to help athletes better understand the impact of SRC on their brains. One such protocol involved using the 'Sport Concussion Assessment Tool 5 (SCAT5)' [57,58] to assess brain function and provide athletes with objective evidence (subjective) of injury and concussion. In addition, PN 14 explains that SCAT5 results help demonstrate the significance of proper hydration to an athlete on their brain function and may support concussion prevention, given that "*if they're dehydrated, their response to the SCAT5 is actually a lot less*" [PN 14].

Several participants showed awareness and knowledge of the acute metabolic and physiological changes that occur in the brain tissue following a concussion, which reduces energy availability, mentioning the following statements:

> "*But like, even if you look at concussions, like concussions, like a shortage of energy in the brain at the time of impact*" [PN 9] (referring to increasing energy/caloric intake).

Additionally, in the period following the concussion,

> "*to help with that energy availability side of things. . . Ehmm, if the brain can't fully use their glucose efficiently" [PN 8] (referring to implementing creatine supplementation).*

These statements reflect PDs'/PNs' genuine understanding and knowledge of the manifestation of concussion as an injury and the associated metabolic and functional changes in the brain tissues' physiology.

3.2.2. Theme 2: Nutritional Support for Concussion Management

Awareness of Using Nutrition in Concussion Management

Participants' consideration of nutritional strategies to support their athletes with SRC was linked closely to their awareness and understanding of nutrition for its role in healing the brain tissue during recovery. This was evidently reflected through PDs'/PNs' implementation of nutritional support protocols for athletes with SRC.

However, participants had mixed levels of awareness and knowledge; some presented uncertainty around SRC as an injury and its subsequent need for nutrition, impacting their knowledge of strategies to support and manage recovery. PDs'/PNs' lack of awareness and nutrition knowledge was a concern as they were not well informed about its role following SRC. As a result, they did not see or consider the benefits of using nutritional support to promote brain tissue healing, which could pose a risk to their athletes.

> "*Not too sure, really, just keep up the good habits. But I haven't looked at it. . . Is there much? Is there much research on concussion and nutrition immediate or. . .?*" [PN 1]

A link was identified between participants who were unaware of concussion incidence within their team setup and/or athletes. These participants did not consider and were unaware of any physiological and metabolic changes that happen in the brain after impact, providing vague responses revealing a limited understanding. In addition, they had poor knowledge of the significance of adjusting athletes' nutritional intake (for perceived 'invisible injury') to meet altered requirements to facilitate healing and recovery post-SRC. For example, PN 15 commented,

> *"I think it's a really good way of putting it in terms of like an invisible injury. You don't, you don't necessarily think that there's a, there's a change required. I guess they're not wrong in saying that there probably isn't from a nutrient point of view."* [PN 15]

A number of PDs/PNs were aware of concussion events and the role of nutrition in brain health as they actively kept up to date with scientific research. However, informed participants were not confident or certain on nutrition protocols and considered strategies based on their acquired knowledge influenced by limited scientific evidence.

> *"I know there is a little bit on creatine and omega-3 fish oils as well. Ehmm, so again, not a whole lot we can do."* [PN 7]

Participants who demonstrated a more certain type of knowledge actively kept informed by scientific research related to concussions/brain injuries and the role of nutrition in brain health and function. However, they were unsure of protocols as they, too, were influenced and limited by *"no real hard and fast evidence on it"* [PN 9].

> *"Yeah, it's, it's an area I'm doing a bit of reading around at moment. But definitely, concussions are not that well-researched. But I think from what I have read there's a couple things you can do and creatine, I believe is important in the... not even the acute phase of, of, of having a concussion, but I think consistently for optimal cognition."* [PN 2]

PDs'/PNs' personal experiences with concussion and head injuries provided them with experiential knowledge on the importance of a nutritious dietary intake and regular eating habits for brain recovery. This experience led them to logically consider implementing nutrition strategies to support their athletes' recovery following SRC prospectively.

> *"So, what would I implement with somebody else? I think to be honest...the rest and the regular eating are, are crucial and then...the extra probiotics or, ehmm you know, whether they make that much of a difference. I don't really know. But the anti-inflammatory, the protein, the carb, I think they would be crucial. Obviously, you know...your healthy fats as well. But the diet...the diet itself is probably the most important thing."* [PN 11]

Some participants who lacked knowledge of potential SRC management protocols were not negatively limited as they had access to a network of expert nutritionists. This network helped bridge their knowledge gap and supported them implement necessary nutrition protocols with their athletes in the event of an acute injury.

> *"With regards to concussion, then we have two dietitians. One that actually has worked in rugby and who would I suppose work and are more familiar with the concussion side of things..."* [PN 13]

This evidence presents an opportunity for PD/PN professionals who can often work independently to have an open network to share expertise and support the expansion of nutrition knowledge. The PDs/PNs who mentioned being able to refer to a niche network of nutrition experts with experience in SRC, as a result, had the support they needed to implement safe nutritional protocols to manage their athletes' recovery. Interestingly, PN 9, despite having extensive knowledge on concussion and the sequel metabolic brain changes that occur, mentioned only implementing nutritional strategies at an individual level with athletes, unlike with other protocols formulated into their injury (rugby) management guidelines and policy. Experts expressed hesitancy and discomfort in recommending nutritional protocols following a concussive impact (invisible brain injury). This reluctance stemmed from the variability in research, such as the lack of human-specific studies and numerous unanswered questions and knowledge gaps.

PN 9 highlighted these concerns:

> *"But like, even if you look at concussions, like concussions, like shortage of energy in the brain at the time of impact. . .you could, like, I'd broadly say it to people, you know. . .'just to make sure you eat enough during this time, and kind of, you know', were kind of very basic interventions. But nothing, I don't think we ever. . .got to a stage where we were comfortable giving nutrition advice to someone who was concussed because there was stuff out there on creatine and stuff on the high dose DHA, but. . .we never formalised that to a policy."* [PN 9]

This led the nutrition focus to remain on physical or visible type injuries, which may cause other sports (outside of rugby) to follow suit and, as a result, neglect nutrition as a strategy (or PDs/PNs role) for brain healing following SRC due to the subjective and non-physical presentation of the injuries (creating a potential implementation barrier).

Implementation—Nutrition Post-Concussion

Participants who did mention attempts to implement or actively trial specific nutritional strategies to facilitate athlete recovery following SRC did so with an element of uncertainty. Following a known SRC, some PDs/PNs took a comprehensive approach aiming to minimise athletes' mental load and any potential challenges faced by athletes during their injury recovery. They addressed athletes' nutrition requirements, overseeing fuel selection (i.e., carbohydrates and fats), quality (i.e., protein), and nutrient variety (i.e., micronutrients) and implementing specific supplements for optimal performance and to facilitate SRC recovery.

In the event of injury, an athlete's focus needs to shift from performing at their very best to healing and recovery to support their return to sport (RTS) [1]. During this period, the athlete's mood may fluctuate between motivated and capable to depleted, depressed, and unmotivated, which may impact their nutritional habits. For example, suppose athletes' habits fall by the wayside. In that case, their level of engagement with the PD/PN may become disjointed, which may/will impact the level of nutrition support they receive, and subsequently their recovery will suffer.

> *". . .if the player isn't overly motivated, they'll get blanket ehmm. . .they get blanket attention. The motivated player will get more attention. The educated player will snap back into their habits. . ."* [PN 1]

Some PDs/PNs were mindful of this shift and took practical steps to implement nutrition strategies specific to their athlete's needs that would minimise their mental load. These strategies focused on ensuring athletes ate enough food to fuel and nourish brain tissue healing and support them in feeling better overall.

> *"So tried to ensure energy levels were kept up just through kind of liquid-based meals, small little snacks, nothing that was going to cause. . .stomach aggravation. . . So, it was more kind of in that, you know, couple days after. . .after the knock as opposed to long term"* [PN 7]

Strategies to facilitate acute energy requirements post-SRC need to be tailored and consider the varying (subjective) symptoms experienced by athletes, such as being *"quite nauseous"* and unable *"to eat a lot"* (i.e., nausea), through implementing *"smaller meals, more frequently, liquid"* [PN 7] to help simplify and support adherence. PNs/PDs focus on and manage athletes' dietary changes to nourish and support brain tissue healing by encouraging and supporting athletes' intake of *"anti-inflammatory foods. . .your fruits, fruit and veg, fish"* [PN 11] and promoting their intake of poly-unsaturated dietary fats via omega-3 rich foods and supplements. Dietary fat plays a significant role in providing fuel and nutrient support for the brain. However, following injury, specific types become exceedingly important, and it is advised to limit the consumption of *"pro-inflammatory omega-6s"* [PN 6] foods to prevent an imbalance of omega 3s to 6s. Proactive PDs/PNs are strategic and align nutrition support with their athletes' mindset and recovery goals at the forefront whilst syncing with other back-team members: "*. . .initially we try to break down even with the physios; we'd break down their rehab into, like, phases*" [PN 8]. Participants know their role in injury support and that when implementing nutrition, their concussed athlete needs clear "*. . .smaller focuses instead of bombarding them all at once*" [PN 8]. This approach aims to keep the athlete accountable and focused during SRC recovery, making the process less daunting and challenging.

> "*So, the initial being, their protection phase, for example. . . I try row in with that being with 'this is your initial focus' instead of trying to bombard them with loads. Saying, 'this is what I really want to get out of this block', and then we tried to do it in focus.*" [PN 8]

Furthermore, PDs/PNs provide flexible availability with open channels of communication for athletes to seek and receive support during SRC recovery through casual check-ins, "*corridor conversations*" [PN 5], WhatsApp messaging, and planned one-to-one sit-down meetings around training schedules, either "*early from a training session, or you meet them there beforehand*" [PN 5]. Open channels and connecting with athletes in casual environments are highly beneficial. They provide opportunities to establish trust and build rapport as some athletes may not be very forthcoming. For athletes who may not have as much access to in-person support, PDs/PNs provide "*Zoom conversations, sharing resources on the screen*" [PN 5], communication, and support that work around lifestyles and outside stressors that factor into athletes' SRC recovery trajectory.

Potential Barriers

Athletes' attitudes on SRC as an injury and their value on the importance of nutrition and its role in their RTP strongly dictate buy-in and protocol implementation. Athletes tend to place a higher value on more physical injuries. They are more "*. . .open to the fact that nutrition can play a role immediately*" [PN 17], creating an adherence motive, compared to the invisible presentation of head injuries and concussions. In assisting athletes' SRC recovery outcomes, PDs/PNs prescribe daily supplements that are brain-supportive and tick all their nutritional gap boxes. However, the reality is they are unable to control behaviours, as one participant admitted, "*Well, see, I don't know if that actually taken it!*" [PN 12]. Meanwhile, PN 5 stated empathetic know-how in the event of injury that "*most, or some of their*" athletes' "*good habits to go out the window*" [PN 5], commenting that in such incidences, "*. . .ideally you want to be on to those lads*" to remind athletes to "*keep on top of the. . .omegas and the creatine*" [PN 5]. Participants stressed the need to remind athletes of the basics that they should be adhering to habitually and taking, for example, fish oils. However, PDs/PNs are cognisant that adherence is subjective and "*not everyone will take fish oils*" [PN 12]. Unlike measurable supplement adherence evidence,

> "*. . .the guys who have been concussed recently. . . I definitely know one of them 100% was because he was looking for more creatine and everything, you know, because he was loading up on it*" [PN 12]

Novel Nutritional Protocol Implementation Post-Concussion

PDs and PNs mentioned exploring, considering, and trialling several novel nutrition protocols that may support the recovery of athletes who have suffered SRC. Numerous participants mentioned that their athletes had already been prescribed creatine for muscle mass and performance (i.e., strength) properties. For example, in rugby:

> "*. . .a lot of our athletes would take creatine. But if they haven't or around a concussion, potentially increasing that creatine intake*" [PN 8]

Creatine is considered in combat sports when there is a "known concussion in boxing. . ." [PN 15] to potentially help "where the boxer has to be pulled out, we have actually put in creatine to try and see if that can help in terms of the recovery from that" [PN 15]. One participant (n = 1/17) recommended a protocol implementing creatine supplementation with concussed Gaelic athletes. It entailed a loading phase, shifting athletes' everyday prescribed performance dose from "5 g a day" to "20 g a day" [PN 12] following the SRC event (see Figure 3).

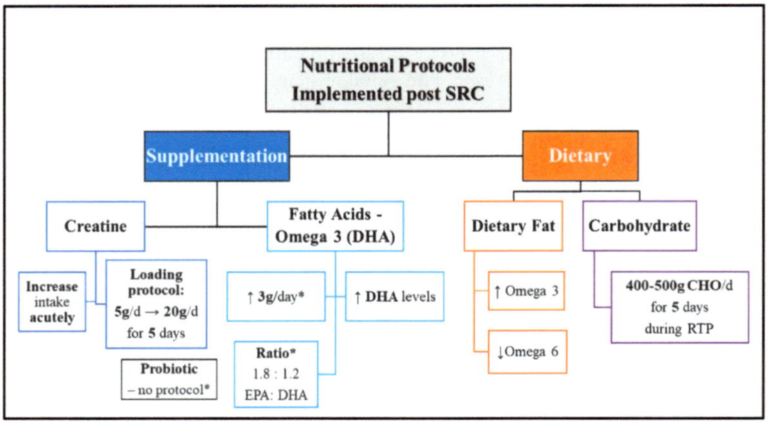

Figure 3. Novel nutritional protocols implemented post-SRC by PD/PN participants. Abbreviations—DHA: Docosahexaenoic acid, EPA: Eicosapentaenoic acid, CHO: Carbohydrate; RTP: Return to Play/Practice. Symbols: ↓: Reduce, ↑: Increase, g: grams, d: day, *: note.

> *"I'll even tell them to load creatine and during that period. . .the week after a concussion, instead of just taking 5 g a day, I'll get them to load like 20 g a day of creatine just for that little period. . .then the rest is kind of lead. . .by the physio"* [PN 12]

Participants cited using omega-3 fish oil supplementation with their athletes; some had no clear rationale, and others prescribed it for brain health, *"cognition"* [PN 2], and recovery properties. Following SRC, it was cited that athlete's intake of *"healthy omega-3s"* [PN 6] should be increased and their *"omega-6s"* [PN 6] reduced. One PN (n = 1/17) recommended omega-3 supplementation following SRC and shared the protocol they implemented with Gaelic athletes. It included using a daily 3 g dose of an omega-3 fish oil to achieve a target ratio of 1.8 to 1.2, EPA:DHA, aiming to get athletes' *"DHA levels up a little bit more"* [PN 12] (see Figure 3).

> *"Ehmm, 3 about 3 g of. . .so that's about 1.8 g. I think it's like 1.8 to. . .the ratio was like 1.8 to 1.2, EPA:DHA. . .with the concussion. I'm trying to get the DHA levels up a little bit more."* [PN 12]

The next protocol cited by one (n = 1/17) participant involved acute carbohydrate loading, which had been discovered from research findings indicating potential effectiveness in increasing energy availability in the brain after SRC, which may shorten symptom duration [59,60]. The protocol involved concussed collision-based sports (American football) athletes consuming 400–500 g of carbohydrates daily for 5 days during their RTP to meet post-SRC caloric requirements. The PN mentioned that they were trialling this protocol in their rugby setting by simply ensuring that athletes who had been concussed consumed enough carbohydrate-rich foods acutely following SRC.

> *". . .like 4 or 500 g of carbs in the 5 days, after concussion versus the guys that had a low carbohydrate diet and the symptoms for the guys that had more carbohydrates were got back to baseline that bit quicker.*
>
> *So, that is kind of something I have been doing; it's like, well, if a guy is in a gradual return to play protocol, then can you eat enough food? Specifically, carbohydrates. . .in that 5-day period. So that's one new area. . ."* [PN 2]

PN 2 stressed the importance of ensuring athletes consume enough carbohydrate-rich foods post-SRC when implementing the protocol on a trial basis to potentially increase energy availability in the brain tissue and support overall recovery (see Figure 3).

The final nutritional protocol includes the use of a probiotic supplement; this was considered by one participant (n = 1/17) and came to fruition after PN 11 shared anecdotal experience after personally sustaining three concussions within 18 months. PN 11 highlighted how fuelling at regular intervals was essential to support their brain recovery and recommended that athletes supplement their food with a probiotic to help the gut–brain connection following concussion (see Figure 3).

> "*. . .I would recommend a probiotic as well for a little while anyway. . . I know it's not maybe an area that's not that well researched yet, but the link between the gut and the head* (holding head)." [PN 11]

4. Discussion

The primary aim of the research was to understand the nutritional protocols implemented by Irish PDs and PNs with their athletes post-concussion to identify whether nutrition is being used to manage and support recovery following SRC diagnosis.

The interviews revealed that the levels of implementing nutrition practices among Irish PDs and PNs to support recovery following acute SRC diagnosis vary a lot. In the study, practitioners' prior exposure to SRC greatly influenced their current knowledge, consideration, and use of nutrition as a support protocol in concussion management. A number of external factors heavily influenced participants' awareness of concussion; these included other team members' (athletes and back-team support) attitudes and behaviours around communicating, reporting, and recognising SRC, as well as acknowledging (the perceived 'invisible injury') concussion as an actual injury. PDs/PNs habitually implemented a range of nutritional strategies with their athletes. Some participants mentioned trialling or recommending nutritional protocols based on their personal experiences—either having personally sustained or having supported athletes with SRCs. These included carb-reloading by increasing carbohydrate-rich foods, reducing the consumption of omega-6 rich foods, promoting the intake of omega-3 fatty acids, and acutely supplementing omega-3s high in DHA and creatine and adding in a probiotic to support brain healing after a concussion.

4.1. Nutrition Protocols Being Implemented Irish PDs/PNs

Some participants did not have any knowledge of the role of nutrition in supporting an athlete's recovery following a head impact and concussion diagnosis. PDs/PNs stated feeling unsure and ill-equipped and did not clearly understand their potential role as practitioners or how to implement nutrition in supporting concussion recovery. Many, in this instance, recommend nutrition strategies that adopted a comprehensive approach embodying athletes' individual needs post-SRC without truly knowing or understanding the purpose behind them. Meanwhile, the strategies that PDs/PNs mentioned included being proactive, reaching out to athletes, and evaluating specific nutritional requirements following SRC to fuel and support their brain healing and recovery. Participants emphasised the importance of supporting athletes' physical and mental health by ensuring nutrition support was tailored and did not strain their mental energy. Overall, PDs/PNs took a proactive and comprehensive approach when applying nutrition to help manage concussion recovery, resetting athletes' habits and refocusing support to facilitate brain healing. Meanwhile, a range of acute nutritional strategies specific to support SRC were mentioned by PDs/PNs; these included supplementing with creatine monohydrate, consuming omega-3 fish oils rich in DHA, incorporating a probiotic, and replenishing carbohydrates through dietary means.

Creatine monohydrate supplementation was actively cited by participants (n = 11/17) and used to promote athletes' strength and performance to be further incorporated and implemented in the event of a concussion. Using creatine acutely following an impact to saturate the brain has the potential to replenish levels by 3–10%, thereby restoring energy homeostasis and potentially blunting symptoms experienced by athletes [48,61,62]. The brain synthesises creatine endogenously; therefore, exogenous supplementation with the purpose of repleting levels may differ for individuals due to dietary preferences and age (> in older adults) [47,63]. Nonmeat or seafood eaters such as pescatarians, vegans, and vegetarians have a lower dietary intake of creatine and skeletal muscle stores, making them more responsive to supplementation than meat eaters (omnivores) [64]. Furthermore, during a period of neurometabolic stress, like after a concussive impact [47,63], brain tissue shows slower responsiveness and ability to replenish creatine levels [47,64] compared to muscle cells. Therefore, loading creatine to saturate brain cells may prove effective following SRC. However, it is crucial to determine a specific dosage tailored for injured brain tissue [47,62,65].

In a non-injured state, a creatine dose of 5 g (g) (approximately 0.3 g/kg body weight) four times daily (totalling approximately 20 g/day) over 5–7 days is suggested [66]. However, brain tissue may require higher doses (>20 g/day) for a more extended period to accumulate adequate levels [47]. Therefore, utilising creatine as a strategy like those employed for brain disease states, involving high doses administered over extended periods (e.g., 0.3–0.8 g/kg/day), may be more effective post-SRC [65].

Several participants mentioned prescribing 5 g of creatine daily to their athletes for muscle mass and performance (i.e., strength) properties. However, this strategy may not be sufficient following SRC and should be tailored to athletes' creatine requirements (i.e., are they currently taking/not taking the supplement?) at the time of their impact. In combat sports, athletes must make weight to compete; this often includes cutting strategies that should be strategically planned and managed by PDs/PNs. Creatine promotes intramuscular water retention; therefore, to reduce weight (water), some athletes undergo a supplementation washout. Theoretically, these weight-cutting practices may make athletes more susceptible to concussion, especially if cuts are managed closely by a PD/PN. Dehydrated athletes who fail to rehydrate sufficiently post-weigh-in will be more susceptible to concussion, having reduced cognitive function and brain protection [67,68].

Further, in the absence of a PD/PN, athletes become more vulnerable as they may not receive creatine supplementation when a known concussion occurs. One participant [PN 12] (n = 1/17) recommended a creatine protocol involving a loading phase, which is being implemented with Gaelic athletes following SRC. The protocol included acutely increasing athletes' daily creatine monohydrate dose from "5 g a day" to "20 g a day" [PN 12] following SRC (see Figure 3).

Presently, the optimal protocol for creatine supplementation in the context of SRC requires further investigation. While interval doses of 5 g, totalling 20 g daily for a 5 to 7-day period, are considered safe, these recommendations primarily support muscle tissue strength and performance capacities and may not be as effective in enhancing SRC recovery [48,69].

4.1.1. Omega-3–Docosahexaenoic Acid (DHA)

Omega-3 fish oil supplementation was actively implemented by participants with athletes to support brain health, cognitive function [PN 2], healing, and tissue recovery [3,38]. Participants cited a general need to increase athletes' intake of omega-3-type fatty acids using foods and supplements post-SRC without stating clear rationales or protocols. PN 6 clearly specified ensuring that athletes reduce their intake of foods high in omega-6 type fatty acids due to their pro-inflammatory properties, which may hinder brain recovery if prolonged [36].

In practice, athletes' omega-3 intake is generally poor, and this is partly due to 'Westernised' dietary intakes being more abundant in convenience and processed foods rich in omega-6 fats (i.e., processed meats, fried and greasy foods, and vegetable oils). Consequently, athletes risk having pro-inflammatory brain environments deficient in DHA, with limited neuroprotection and worse adverse effects (i.e., symptomology, oxidative stress, inflammation), impacting their healing and recovery following concussion or RHIs [3,40].

One participant [PN 12] (n = 1/17) recommended an omega-3 supplementation strategy post-SRC that was implemented with Gaelic athletes. The aim was for athletes to consume a daily dose of 3 g of omega-3 to achieve a target ratio of 1.8 to 1.2 of EPA:DHA, aiming to increase brain DHA levels following a concussive impact (see Figure 3).

> *"Ehmm, 3 about 3 g of, so that's about 1.8 g. I think it's like 1.8 to. . .the ratio was like 1.8 to 1.2, EPA:DHA. . .with the concussion. I'm trying to get the DHA levels up a little bit more. . ."* [PN 12]

However, further investigation (by E.F.) into the specific supplement and brand mentioned identified that the dosing cited (*1 cap = 500 mg EPA, 250 mg DHA/1000 mg omega-3 (PN 12 mentioned a 3 g dose, which equates to 3000 mg omega-3 = 1500 mg EPA and 750 mg DHA and 750 mg omega-3 filler–ratio 2:1:1)) may not constitute a realistic SRC recovery protocol.

Further research is needed, but current evidence supports PNs' use of omega-3s, suggesting that high-dose DHA, either alone or combined with EPA, may optimise recovery and provide a protective nutritional foundation for the brain tissue after SRC. Several protocols are currently being tested to rebuild brain tissue and aid recovery following SRC. Dr Lewis recommends a three-step protocol utilising a high-quality 1000 mg omega-3 fish oil (EPA + DHA). The protocol involves (1) saturating the brain cells with a 9000 mg dose for 7 days, followed by (2) a 6000 mg dose for an additional 7 days, and (3) a maintenance dose of 3000 mg daily after that (protocol link: https://atlantictu-my.sharepoint.com/:b:/g/personal/emma_finnegan_atu_ie/EWWfBeX5lttCtsWGfSz2faMBH--eSJv2oNySP5afNaIWuw?e=SFfYpw (accessed on 25 June 2023), [69]). Falk [70] trialled a combined omega-3 protocol using a tiered dose of 6000 mg for 4 weeks and 1200 mg for 8 weeks (1000 mg (500 mg DHA and 100 mg EPA) capsule) and found it helped settle post-SRC symptoms (92.8%) [3,71]. Additionally, Miller [39] identified that a dose of 2000 mg/day of DHA is well tolerated by concussed athletes and quickly alleviates their symptoms [3,39]. Meanwhile, Heileson [40] further found that a dose of 2000 mg DHA in athletes in precompetitive and competitive seasons was effective at reducing head trauma biomarkers (serum Nf-L) associated with RHI.

4.1.2. Carbohydrates

Acutely reloading carbohydrates post-concussion was mentioned by one participant [PN 2] (n = 1/17); this protocol is based on research suggesting that it may increase brain tissue energy availability effectively [59]. Carbohydrates are a preferred brain fuel source; therefore, consuming them will ensure a supply of glucose is available to enhance brain function and performance. In the case of SRC, the rationale is to provide glucose support to the brain, which may help alleviate symptoms related to energy availability discrepancies by delivering substrate to make ATP and fuel recovery. The protocol involved concussed athletes consuming a dose of 400–500 g of carbohydrate (via corn starch, using a 26 g dose) at controlled time points (a) within 30–60 min following diagnosis, then hourly (over 4 h), and then (b) twice daily for 5 days during their RTP [59]. PN 12 mentioned implementing aspects of Frakes' [59] protocol in a rugby setting by ensuring athletes ate enough carbohydrate-rich foods acutely post-SRC. At present, the literature on the impact of acute carbohydrate administration for fuelling the acute hypermetabolic period following SRC is mixed and very limited [39]. Despite this, it is important to consider the quality of carbohydrate foods consumed as processed and refined types can have a less favourable impact on healing and recovery from concussion.

4.1.3. Probiotics

One participant [PN 11] (n = 1/17) highlighted the significance of incorporating a probiotic supplement after SRC following personal experience (see Figure 3), having sustained three consecutive impacts within 18 months. PN [11] shared that including a probiotic in their recovery plan, along with maintaining regular eating intervals, had helped support their gut function. SRC is a neurological injury that can result in symptoms like vomiting, which are triggered by the mismatched signals between the brain's vagal nerves and the stomach. This mismatch leads to an inflammatory response that disrupts gut function, affecting food transit, metabolism, and nutrient absorption. Consequently, it can disrupt the gut microbiome's balance, leading to dysbiosis and prolonging inflammation and recovery [72,73]. Pilot findings have confirmed that the changes that occur in an athlete's gut microbiome following SRC do negatively influence performance and prolong inflammation [74].

Therefore, restoring the microbiome environment of an injured athlete may positively interrupt the gut response, mitigate symptoms, and ease neurological deficits following SRC. Therefore, probiotics have the potential to positively alter the gut microbiome and support communication between the gut and the brain. This may help reduce athletes' symptoms and inflammation and improve their digestion. As a result, nutrient absorption and energy availability to the brain may be facilitated, as reported anecdotally by PN [11] (see Figure 3), to support SRC healing and recovery.

4.2. *Impact of Back-Team Collaboration and Communication*

4.2.1. Communication, Collaboration, and SRC Reporting

Effective communication and collaboration amongst backroom team practitioners and athletes are key mediators in establishing effective recovery strategies after injury diagnosis [17,75], especially after SRC. PDs/PNs know that differing levels of communication exist as part of working in a team and recognise that a *"decent backroom team"* [PN 5] needs internal collaboration to formulate and deliver suitable protocols to manage SRC recovery. Participants highlighted the importance of having a well-coordinated, athlete-centric backroom team defined by shared values, professional respect, and effective communication. This cohesive backroom teamwork ensures the prompt and effective implementation of protocols and support for athletes when sidelined due to injury. Open channels of communication promote collaboration and enable the sharing of insights from multiple perspectives to make informed athlete-centred decisions, such as athletes' RTP strategies. On the other hand, when communication breaks down, it can lead to increased misunderstandings and a risk of one-sided decision making [17,75]. The limited recognition of PDs'/PNs' role by other team members in the event of injury has led to incidents where participants experienced closed communication channels, impacting their awareness of their athlete's history with SRC. Instead, each backroom practitioner should understand and endorse a multifaceted approach when supporting athletes, with clarity on their role and one another's contribution within that following SRC diagnosis. Otherwise, a lack of awareness and respect among backroom practitioners and misaligned values may compromise the quality of care provided to injured athletes [75,76]. PDs'/PNs' awareness of SRC incidences is shaped by the culture and reporting practices within their sports setup. This was evident by the limited awareness amongst participants regarding athletes' SRC experiences, highlighting the crucial role of collaboration and open communication channels. Interestingly, those involved in rugby or elite-level sports exhibited greater awareness of SRC than those in Gaelic, hockey, combat, or amateur-level sports. Additionally, symptoms of SRC are not externally visible and are solely experienced by athletes, which increases the risk of underreporting, injury masking, and underestimating its severity due to insufficient knowledge. Nonetheless, practitioners on the sideline rely heavily on athletes' self-reporting of symptoms [77,78]. Poor communication among backroom team practitioners, combined with these factors, may be the underlying cause of PDs'/PNs' limited understanding of their role and responsibilities in facilitating athletes' SRC recovery.

4.2.2. Roles and Perceived Responsibility

The attitudes of athletes and backroom team practitioners toward concussion, along with the subjective nature of the injury, contribute to underreporting and shape the perceptions of PDs/PNs regarding their role, influencing recovery outcomes. PDs/PNs involvement in a team or individual athlete support setting goes beyond a tick-the-box exercise and is a vital component of the team and athletes' backroom support. Their role extends not only to situations where there is a perceived need or when an athlete's performance is a priority but also when physical and invisible injuries occur. Athletes require individual support for tissue healing and rehabilitation. This cannot happen if a PD's/PN's role is not valued but seen as a nonchalant tick-the-positive nutrition box exercise or a lower priority and sometimes cancelled to save funds. Coaches, physios, medics, and athletes should be aware that the role of the PD/PN goes beyond superficial support and requires involvement during all aspects of communication around athletes' acute health, performance, and injury outcomes. All members have an active duty of care with a common goal to support and prevent a breakdown in all pillars of health on the athlete's and teams' path to their goals and recovery.

4.3. Limitations

The findings of this research reflect a particular period, and it is important to acknowledge that performance and injury nutrition are rapidly evolving fields. Therefore, the factors highlighted in this study may not remain applicable in the future. Despite the relatively small Irish cohort of PDs/PNs (n = 17), this study has provided valuable insights into areas that require consideration by sport performance dietitians, nutritionists, coaches, and other team professionals in the context of managing SRC. The research has identified current best-practice nutritional strategies and potential protocols to implement and support athletes' SRC recovery, acknowledging the clear gaps in research and their impact on PD/PN decisions and their implementation of SRC management protocols with athletes. It is important to note that PDs/PNs often have limited or no concussion education. Participants demonstrated varying levels of knowledge regarding concussion as an injury and the potential role of nutrition as a management strategy. The sporting environment within the team and professional practitioner setup significantly influenced participants' awareness, diagnosis, and management of athletes' SRC. Moreover, specific attitudes and norms related to sporting culture were observed across different sports, levels, and team environments. In addition, the availability of support resources for athletes was strongly influenced by the level of sport at play (elite vs. amateur) and the teams' gender (female vs. male), which impacted PDs'/PNs' awareness and the level of support provided to athletes following SRC.

4.4. Future Recommendations

1. Further research that is robust and can be safely implemented to support and manage concussion recovery in a sporting context is needed. Irish PDs/PNs have cited using creatine, omega-3 fatty acids, probiotics, and carbohydrate reloading strategies. The availability of human-based evidence is limited, highlighting the necessity for additional investigation and research in this area.
2. Concussion and head injury education and training should be mandatory for all healthcare practitioners supporting athletes, including nutrition experts (PDs and PNs), psychologists, and physical therapists (physio, rehabilitation, and athletic) working with or as part of the back team. According to the latest concussion management protocols, a diagnosis should ideally be conducted by medical healthcare professionals such as a doctor or physiotherapist [1], which is not feasible for many sports settings (i.e., amateur, underage, and female). To address this limitation, we recommended that all healthcare practitioners in the multidisciplinary care team receive comprehensive training on brain injuries and concussions.
3. Open and transparent communication among all back-team members, actively involving PDs/PNs in player analysis, performance, and injury discussions, is needed. This collaborative approach will help mitigate the risk of missing acute injury management and the subsequent risk of poor recovery outcomes for athletes.

4. Regular monitoring of athletes' hydration and mental capacity status should be implemented during pre-match hydration test protocols to identify and prevent cognitive decline and, as a result, help reduce the risk of an impact occurring during gameplay. PDs/PNs can use the CRT6 and SCAT6 tools to educate athletes about the effects of their hydration and its impact on brain function. They can use it as evidence to address suboptimal nutrition, assess performance, and measure the recovery of athletes with SRC. By conducting regular evaluations and the monitoring of athletes, PDs/PNs can enhance nutrition protocols for concussion recovery and support athletes, ultimately helping them prevent injury and achieve optimal recovery and RTP outcomes.

5. Conclusions

PDs'/PNs' use of nutrition protocols with athletes following acute SRC diagnosis was linked to their knowledge and the scientific evidence available. Nutrition implementation, as a result, may be overlooked or implemented with uncertainty due to limited evidence, which could negatively affect the potential for optimal SRC recovery outcomes. From PD/PN practices, it is evident that there is a need for research to uncover safe and practical nutritional protocols that they can use to mitigate the effects of SRC and support athletes' recovery and return to play.

Supplementary Materials: The following supporting information can be downloaded at: https://www.mdpi.com/article/10.3390/nu16040497/s1, Figure S1: (**A**): Reflexive Thematic Analysis Planning (Phase 3). Generating initial themes. Note: T: Theme, PD(s): Performance Dietitian(s), PN(s): Performance Nutritionist(s), C: Creatine, FO: Fish Oil, Cr-P: Carbohydrate reloading protocol, Diff: different. (**B**): Reflexive Thematic Analysis (Phase 4). Generating themes on nutritional support for concussion management. Note: PD(s): Performance Dietitian(s), PN(s): Performance Nutritionist(s), CA: Concussion Awareness, CR: Concussion Report, CI: Concussion Injury, SRC: Sport-related concussion, MMA: Mixed Martial Arts. (**C**): Reflexive Thematic Analysis (Phase 4). Generating themes on nutritional support for concussion management. Note: PD(s): Performance Dietitian(s), PN(s): Performance Nutritionist(s), C: Creatine, FO: Fish Oil, Cr-P: Carbohydrate reloading protocol. Table S1. Thematic Analysis (Phase 2). Initial code generation based on theoretical assumptions and research aims (semantic approach).

Author Contributions: E.F., L.R. and E.D. were involved in conceptualising and designing the study. E.F. contributed to data acquisition, analysis, and manuscript writing. L.R. and E.D. contributed to data analysis and manuscript writing. All authors, E.F., L.R. and E.D., reviewed and edited previous drafts of the manuscript. Additionally, all authors participated in discussions, provided feedback, and approved the manuscript before submission. All authors have read and agreed to the published version of the manuscript.

Funding: This research received no external funding.

Institutional Review Board Statement: This study received ethical approval the Research Sub-Committee of Atlantic Technological University's Academic Council (ATU-RSC_AC_25/11/2021).

Informed Consent Statement: Informed consent was obtained from all subjects involved in the study. Each participant completed informed consent forms prior to attending virtual interviews on Microsoft Teams.

Data Availability Statement: The original data, unfortunately, are unavailable to protect participant confidentiality. However, the data presented in the study article are included in the Supplementary Materials. Further inquiries can be directed to the corresponding author.

Acknowledgments: The authors would like to extend their gratitude to the performance dietitians and nutritionists who generously gave their time to contribute to this research project.

Conflicts of Interest: The authors declare that the research was conducted in the absence of any commercial or financial relationships that could be construed as potential conflicts of interest.

References

1. Patricios, J.S.; Schneider, K.J.; Dvorak, J.; Ahmed, O.H.; Blauwet, C.; Cantu, R.C.; Davis, G.A.; Echemendia, R.J.; Makdissi, M.; McNamee, M.; et al. Consensus statement on concussion in sport: The 6th international conference on concussion in sport–Amsterdam, October 2022. *Br. J. Sports Med.* **2023**, *57*, 695–711. [CrossRef]
2. Hallock, H.; Mantwill, M.; Vajkoczy, P.; Wolfarth, B.; Reinsberger, C.; Lampit, A.; Finke, C. Sport-related concussion: A cognitive perspective. *Neurol. Clin. Pract.* **2023**, *13*, e200123. [CrossRef]
3. Finnegan, E.; Daly, E.; Pearce, A.J.; Ryan, L. Nutritional interventions to support acute mTBI recovery. *Front. Nutr.* **2022**, *9*, 977728. [CrossRef]
4. Van Pelt, K.L.; Puetz, T.; Swallow, J.; Lapointe, A.P.; Broglio, S.P. Data-driven risk classification of concussion rates: A systematic review and meta-analysis. *Sports Med.* **2021**, *51*, 1227–1244. [CrossRef]
5. Harmon, K.G.; Drezner, J.A.; Gammons, M.; Guskiewicz, K.M.; Halstead, M.; Herring, S.A.; Kutcher, J.S.; Pana, A.; Putukian, M.; Roberts, W.O. American medical society for sports medicine position statement: Concussion in sport. *Br. J. Sports Med.* **2013**, *47*, 15–26. [CrossRef]
6. Daneshvar, D.H.; Nowinski, C.J.; McKee, A.C.; Cantu, R.C. The epidemiology of sport-related concussion. *Clin. Sports Med.* **2011**, *30*, 1–17. [CrossRef] [PubMed]
7. Langlois, J.A.; Rutland-Brown, W.; Wald, M.M. The epidemiology and impact of traumatic brain injury: A brief overview. *J. Head Trauma Rehabil.* **2006**, *21*, 375–378. [CrossRef] [PubMed]
8. Schneider, K.J.; Patricios, J.; Echemendia, R.J.; Makdissi, M.; Davis, G.A.; Ahmed, O.H.; Blauwet, C.; Dvorak, J.; Engebretsen, L. Concussion in sport: The consensus process continues. *Br. J. Sports Med.* **2022**, *56*, 1059–1060. [CrossRef] [PubMed]
9. McCrory, P.; Meeuwisse, W.; Dvorak, J.; Aubry, M.; Bailes, J.; Broglio, S.; Cantu, R.C.; Cassidy, D.; Echemendia, R.J.; Castellani, R.J.; et al. Consensus statement on concussion in sport—The 5th international conference on concussion in sport held in Berlin, October 2016. *Br. J. Sports Med.* **2017**, *51*, 838–847. [CrossRef]
10. Daly, E.; Pearce, A.J.; Finnegan, E.; Cooney, C.; McDonagh, M.; Scully, G.; McCann, M.; Doherty, R.; White, A.; Phelan, S.; et al. An assessment of current concussion identification and diagnosis methods in sports settings: A systematic review. *BMC Sports Sci. Med. Rehabil.* **2022**, *14*, 125. [CrossRef] [PubMed]
11. Walrand, S.; Gaulmin, R.; Aubin, R.; Sapin, V.; Coste, A.; Abbot, M. Nutritional factors in sport-related concussion. *Neurochirurgie* **2021**, *67*, 255–258. [CrossRef]
12. Lust, C.A.C.; Mountjoy, M.; Robinson, L.E.; Oliver, J.M.; Ma, D.W. Sports-related concussions and subconcussive impacts in athletes: Incidence, diagnosis, and the emerging role of EPA and DHA. *Appl. Physiol. Nutr. Metab.* **2020**, *45*, 886–892. [CrossRef]
13. Beidler, E.; Wallace, J.; Alghwiri, A.A.; O'Connor, S. Collegiate athletes' concussion awareness, understanding, and -reporting behaviors in different countries with varying concussion publicity. *J. Athl. Train.* **2021**, *56*, 77–84. [CrossRef]
14. O'Connor, S.; Geaney, D.; Beidler, E. Non-disclosure in Irish collegiate student-athletes: Do concussion history, knowledge, pressure to play and gender impact concussion reporting? *Phys. Sportsmed.* **2020**, *48*, 186–193. [CrossRef]
15. Leahy, R.; Farrington, S.; Whyte, E.; O'Connor, S. Concussion reporting, knowledge and attitudes in Irish amateur Gaelic games athletes. *Phys. Ther. Sport* **2019**, *43*, 236–243. [CrossRef]
16. Nolan, K.E.; Caccese, J.B.; Kontos, A.P.; Buckley, T.A.; Garcia, G.P.; Port, N.; Broglio, S.P.; McAllister, T.W.; McCrea, M.; Pasquina, P.F.; et al. Primary and Secondary risk factors associated with concussion symptom clusters in collegiate athletes: Results from the NCAA-DoD grand alliance CARE consortium. *Orthop. J. Sports Med.* **2023**, *11*, 23259671231163581. [CrossRef]
17. Ryan, L.; Daly, E.; Blackett, A.D. Sport-related concussion disclosure in women's rugby—A social identity approach. *Front. Sports Act. Living* **2023**, *5*, 1058305. [CrossRef]
18. Piedade, S.R.; Hutchinson, M.R.; Ferreira, D.M.; Cristante, A.F.; Maffulli, N. The management of concussion in sport is not standardized. A systematic review. *J. Saf. Res.* **2021**, *76*, 262–268. [CrossRef] [PubMed]
19. Rotundo, M.; Sokol-Randell, D.; Bleakley, C.M.; Donnelly, P.; Tierney, G. Characteristics of potential concussive events in elite hurling: A video-analysis study. *Ir. J. Med. Sci.* **2023**, *17*, 3175–3185. [CrossRef] [PubMed]
20. Walshe, A.; Daly, E.; Ryan, L. Epidemiology of sport-related concussion rates in female contact/collision sport: A systematic review. *BMJ Open Sport Exerc. Med.* **2022**, *8*, e001346. [CrossRef] [PubMed]
21. Meehan, W.P.; Taylor, A.M.; Berkner, P.; Sandstrom, N.J.; Peluso, M.W.; Kurtz, M.M.; Pascual-Leone, A.; Mannix, R. Division III collision sports are not associated with neurobehavioral quality of life. *J. Neurotrauma* **2016**, *33*, 254–259. [CrossRef] [PubMed]
22. Turnagöl, H.H.; Koşar, N.; Güzel, Y.; Aktitiz, S.; Atakan, M.M. Nutritional considerations for injury prevention and recovery in combat sports. *Nutrients* **2021**, *14*, 53. [CrossRef] [PubMed]
23. Lemme, N.J.; Johnston, B.; DeFroda, S.F.; Owens, B.D.; Kriz, P.K. Incidence of combat sport-related mild traumatic brain injuries presenting to the emergency department from 2012 to 2016. *Clin. J. Sport Med.* **2020**, *30*, 585–590. [CrossRef] [PubMed]
24. Neidecker, J.; Sethi, N.K.; Taylor, R.; Monsell, R.; Muzzi, D.; Spizler, B.; Lovelace, L.; Ayoub, E.; Weinstein, R.; Estwanik, J.; et al. Concussion management in combat sports: Consensus statement from the association of ringside physicians. *Br. J. Sports Med.* **2019**, *53*, 328–333. [CrossRef] [PubMed]
25. Heron, N.; Jones, N.; Cardwell, C.; Gomes, C. 'If in doubt, sit them out': How long to return to elite cycling competition following a sports-related concussion (SRC)? *Int. J. Environ. Res. Public Health* **2023**, *20*, 5449. [CrossRef]

26. Lumba-Brown, A.; Yeates, K.O.; Sarmiento, K.; Breiding, M.J.; Haegerich, T.M.; Gioia, G.A.; Turner, M.; Benzel, E.C.; Suskauer, S.J.; Giza, C.C.; et al. Diagnosis and management of mild traumatic brain injury in children: A systematic review. *JAMA Pediatr.* **2018**, *172*, e182847. [CrossRef]
27. Marchand, N.E.; Jensen, M.K. The role of dietary and lifestyle factors in maintaining cognitive health. *Am. J. Lifestyle Med.* **2018**, *12*, 268–285. [CrossRef] [PubMed]
28. Verboon, L.N.; Patel, H.C.; Greenhalgh, A.D. The immune system's role in the consequences of mild traumatic brain injury (concussion). *Front. Immunol.* **2021**, *12*, 620698. [CrossRef]
29. Shukla, D.; Devi, B.I. Mild traumatic brain injuries in adults. *J. Neurosci. Rural. Pract.* **2010**, *1*, 82–88. [CrossRef]
30. Scullion, E.; Heron, N. A scoping review of concussion guidelines in amateur sports in the United Kingdom. *Int. J. Environ. Res. Public Health* **2022**, *19*, 1072. [CrossRef]
31. Conaghan, C.; Daly, E.; Ryan, L. An accessible concussion education tool that improves athlete, coach and parent knowledge and attitudes. *Austin. Sports Med.* **2022**, *7*, 1049.
32. Halstead, M.E.; Walter, K.D.; Moffatt, K.; Council on Sports Medicine and Fitness. Sport-Related Concussion in Children and Adolescents. *Pediatrics* **2018**, *142*, e20183074. [CrossRef]
33. Iverson, G.L.; Gardner, A.J.; Terry, D.P.; Ponsford, J.L.; Sills, A.K.; Broshek, D.K.; Solomon, G.S. Predictors of clinical recovery from concussion: A systematic review. *Br. J. Sports Med.* **2017**, *51*, 941–948. [CrossRef]
34. Kim, S.; Han, S.C.; Gallan, A.J.; Hayes, J.P.; Fakhran, S.; Delic, J.; Alhilali, L.; Jagannathan, J.; McDevitt, J.; Krynetskiy, E.; et al. Neurometabolic indicators of mitochondrial dysfunction in repetitive mild traumatic brain injury. *Concussion* **2017**, *2*, CNC45. [CrossRef] [PubMed]
35. Flueck, J.L.; Parnell, J.A. Protein considerations for athletes with a spinal cord injury. *Front. Nutr.* **2021**, *8*, 142441. [CrossRef] [PubMed]
36. Smith-Ryan, A.E.; Hirsch, K.R.; Saylor, H.E.; Gould, L.M.; Blue, M.N.M. Nutritional considerations and strategies to facilitate injury recovery and rehabilitation. *J. Athl. Train.* **2020**, *55*, 918–930. [CrossRef] [PubMed]
37. Abdullah, M.I.; Ahmad, A.; Wafa, S.W.W.S.S.T.; Latif, A.Z.A.; Yusoff, N.A.M.; Jasmiad, M.K.; Udin, N.; Karim, K.A. Determination of calorie and protein intake among acute and sub-acute traumatic brain injury patients. *Chin. J. Traumatol.* **2020**, *23*, 290–294. [CrossRef] [PubMed]
38. Dighriri, I.M.; Alsubaie, A.M.; Hakami, F.M.; Hamithi, D.M.; Alshekh, M.M.; Khobrani, F.A.; Dalak, F.E.; Hakami, A.A.; Alsueaadi, E.H.; Alsaawi, L.S.; et al. Effects of omega-3 polyunsaturated fatty acids on brain functions: A systematic review. *Cureus* **2022**, *14*, e30091. [CrossRef] [PubMed]
39. Miller, S.M.; Zynda, A.J.; Sabatino, M.J.; Jo, C.; Ellis, H.B.; Dimeff, R.J. A pilot randomized controlled trial of docosahexaenoic acid for the treatment of sport-related concussion in adolescents. *Clin. Pediatr.* **2022**, *61*, 785–794. [CrossRef] [PubMed]
40. Heileson, J.L.; Anzalone, A.J.; Carbuhn, A.F.; Askow, A.T.; Stone, J.D.; Turner, S.M.; Hillyer, L.M.; Ma, D.W.L.; Luedke, J.A.; Jagim, A.R.; et al. The effect of omega-3 fatty acids on a biomarker of head trauma in NCAA football athletes: A multi-site, non-randomized study. *J. Int. Soc. Sports Nutr.* **2021**, *18*, 65. [CrossRef]
41. Thielecke, F.; Blannin, A. Omega-3 fatty acids for sport performance—Are they equally beneficial for athletes and amateurs? A narrative review. *Nutrients* **2020**, *12*, 3712. [CrossRef]
42. Armstrong, A.; Anzalone, A.J.; Pethick, W.; Murray, H.; Dahlquist, D.T.; Askow, A.T.; Heileson, J.L.; Hillyer, L.M.; Ma, D.W.L.; Oliver, J.M. An evaluation of omega-3 status and intake in Canadian elite rugby 7s players. *Nutrients* **2021**, *13*, 3777. [CrossRef] [PubMed]
43. Ritz, P.P.; Rogers, M.B.; Zabinsky, J.S.; Hedrick, V.E.; Rockwell, J.A.; Rimer, E.G.; Kostelnik, S.B.; Hulver, M.W.; Rockwell, M.S. Dietary and biological assessment of the omega-3 status of collegiate athletes: A cross-sectional analysis. *PLoS ONE* **2020**, *15*, e0228834. [CrossRef] [PubMed]
44. EFSA Panel on Dietetic Products, Nutrition and Allergies (NDA). Scientific Opinion on the Tolerable Upper Intake Level of eicosapentaenoic acid (EPA), docosahexaenoic acid (DHA) and docosapentaenoic acid (DPA). *EFSA J.* **2012**, *10*, 2815.
45. Lawrence, D.W.; Sharma, B. A review of the neuroprotective role of vitamin D in traumatic brain injury with implications for supplementation post-concussion. *Brain Inj.* **2016**, *30*, 960–968. [CrossRef]
46. Standiford, L.; O'Daniel, M.; Hysell, M.; Trigger, C. A randomized cohort study of the efficacy of PO magnesium in the treatment of acute concussions in adolescents. *Am. J. Emerg. Med.* **2020**, *44*, 419–422. [CrossRef]
47. Prokopidis, K.; Giannos, P.; Triantafyllidis, K.K.; Kechagias, K.S.; Forbes, S.C.; Candow, D.G. Effects of creatine supplementation on memory in healthy individuals: A systematic review and meta-analysis of randomized controlled trials. *Nutr. Rev.* **2023**, *81*, 416–427. [CrossRef]
48. Forbes, S.C.; Cordingley, D.M.; Cornish, S.M.; Gualano, B.; Roschel, H.; Ostojic, S.M.; Rawson, E.S.; Roy, B.D.; Prokopidis, K.; Giannos, P.; et al. Effects of creatine supplementation on brain function and health. *Nutrients* **2022**, *14*, 921. [CrossRef]
49. Beck, K.L.; Thomson, J.S.; Swift, R.J.; von Hurst, P.R. Role of nutrition in performance enhancement and postexercise recovery. *Open Access J. Sports Med.* **2015**, *6*, 259–267. [CrossRef]
50. Braun, V.; Clarke, V. Reflecting on reflexive thematic analysis. *Qual. Res. Sport Exerc. Health* **2019**, *11*, 589–597. [CrossRef]
51. Tong, A.; Sainsbury, P.; Craig, J. Consolidated criteria for reporting qualitative research (COREQ): A 32-item checklist for interviews and focus groups. *Int. J. Qual. Health Care* **2007**, *19*, 349–357. [CrossRef]

52. Draper, A.; Swift, J.A. Qualitative research in nutrition and dietetics: Data collection issues. *J. Hum. Nutr. Diet.* **2011**, *24*, 3–12. [CrossRef]
53. Valerio, M.A.; Rodriguez, N.; Winkler, P.; Lopez, J.; Dennison, M.; Liang, Y.; Turner, B.J. Comparing two sampling methods to engage hard-to-reach communities in research priority setting. *BMC Med. Res. Methodol.* **2016**, *16*, 146. [CrossRef]
54. Tufford, L.; Newman, P. Bracketing in qualitative research. *Qual. Soc. Work.* **2010**, *11*, 80–96. [CrossRef]
55. Braun, V.; Clarke, V. Using thematic analysis in psychology. *Qual. Res. Psychol.* **2006**, *3*, 77–101. [CrossRef]
56. Fuller, G.W.; Kemp, S.; Decq, P. The International Rugby Board (IRB) pitch side concussion assessment trial: A pilot test accuracy study. *Br. J. Sports Med.* **2015**, *49*, 529–535. [CrossRef]
57. Sport concussion assessment tool—5th edition. *Br. J. Sports Med.* **2017**, *51*, 851–858. [CrossRef]
58. Echemendia, R.J.; Meeuwisse, W.; McCrory, P.; Davis, G.A.; Putukian, M.; Leddy, J.; Makdissi, M.; Sullivan, S.J.; Broglio, S.P.; Raftery, M.; et al. The Sport Concussion Assessment Tool 5th Edition (SCAT5). *Br. J. Sports Med.* **2017**, *51*, 848–850. [CrossRef] [PubMed]
59. Frakes, M.R. The Impact of Dietary Intake on Concussion Recovery in Division I NCAA Athletes. Ph.D. Thesis, University of Mississippi, Mississippi, MS, USA, 2020. Available online: https://egrove.olemiss.edu/etd/1870 (accessed on 22 June 2023).
60. Frakes, M.; Valliant, M.W.; Crowther, M.; Michel, J.; Callaway, K.; Morgan, B.; Franks, C.; Beyke, A. Collegiate athletes that consumed adequate energy post-concussion reported fewer days of concussion-related symptoms. *Med. Sci. Sports Exerc.* **2019**, *51*, 864–865. [CrossRef]
61. Vagnozzi, R.; Signoretti, S.; Floris, R.; Marziali, S.; Manara, M.; Amorini, A.M.; Belli, A.; Di Pietro, V.; D'Urso, S.; Pastore, F.S.; et al. Decrease in n-acetylaspartate following concussion may be coupled to decrease in creatine. *J. Head Trauma Rehabil.* **2013**, *28*, 284–292. [CrossRef] [PubMed]
62. Ashbaugh, A.; McGrew, C. The role of nutritional supplements in sports concussion treatment. *Curr. Sports Med. Rep.* **2016**, *15*, 16–19. [CrossRef] [PubMed]
63. Solis, M.Y.; Artioli, G.G.; Otaduy, M.C.G.; Leite, C.D.C.; Arruda, W.; Veiga, R.R.; Gualano, B. Effect of age, diet, and tissue type on PCr response to creatine supplementation. *J. Appl. Physiol.* **2017**, *123*, 407–414. [CrossRef] [PubMed]
64. Kaviani, M.; Shaw, K.; Chilibeck, P.D. Benefits of creatine supplementation for vegetarians compared to omnivorous athletes: A systematic review. *Int. J. Environ. Res. Public Health* **2020**, *17*, 3041. [CrossRef] [PubMed]
65. Giza, C.C.; Hovda, D.A. The new neurometabolic cascade of concussion. *Neurosurgery* **2014**, *75* (Suppl. S4), S24–S33. [CrossRef] [PubMed]
66. Kreider, R.B.; Kalman, D.S.; Antonio, J.; Ziegenfuss, T.N.; Wildman, R.; Collins, R.; Candow, D.G.; Kleiner, S.M.; Almada, A.L.; Lopez, H.L. International Society of Sports Nutrition position stand: Safety and efficacy of creatine supplementation in exercise, sport, and medicine. *J. Int. Soc. Sports Nutr.* **2017**, *14*, 18. [CrossRef]
67. Januszko, P.; Lange, E. Nutrition, supplementation and weight reduction in combat sports: A review. *AIMS Public Health* **2021**, *8*, 485–498. [CrossRef]
68. Rici, T.; Forbes, S.C.; Candow, D.G. Creatine supplementation: Practical strategies and considerations for mixed martial arts. *J. Exerc. Nutr.* **2020**, *3*, s2. Available online: https://www.journalofexerciseandnutrition.com/index.php/JEN/article/view/58 (accessed on 28 June 2023).
69. Turner, C.E.; Byblow, W.D.; Gant, N. Creatine Supplementation enhances corticomotor excitability and cognitive performance during oxygen deprivation. *J. Neurosci.* **2015**, *35*, 1773–1780. [CrossRef]
70. The Omega-3 Protocol for Brain Health—Brain Health Education and Research Institute [Internet]. Available online: http://www.brainhealtheducation.org/resources/brain-injury-protocol/ (accessed on 21 June 2023).
71. Falk, H.; Korley, F. A pilot study of omega-3 polyunsaturated fatty acid treatment in mild acute TBI (Optima-TBI pilot). *J. Neurotrauma.* **2018**, *35*, A144. [CrossRef]
72. Baracaldo-Santamaría, D.; Ariza-Salamanca, D.F.; Corrales-Hernández, M.G.; Pachón-Londoño, M.J.; Hernandez-Duarte, I.; Calderon-Ospina, C.A. Revisiting excitotoxicity in traumatic brain injury: From bench to bedside. *Pharmaceutics* **2022**, *14*, 152. [CrossRef]
73. Brenner, L.A.; Forster, J.E.; Stearns-Yoder, K.A.; Stamper, C.E.; Hoisington, A.J.; Brostow, D.P.; Mealer, M.; Wortzel, H.S.; Postolache, T.T.; Lowry, C.A. Evaluation of an Immunomodulatory Probiotic Intervention for Veterans with Co-occurring Mild Traumatic Brain injury and posttraumatic stress disorder: A pilot study. *Front. Neurol.* **2020**, *11*, 1015. [CrossRef]
74. Soriano, S.; Curry, K.; Sadrameli, S.S.; Wang, Q.; Nute, M.; Reeves, E.; Kabir, R.; Wiese, J.; Criswell, A.; Schodrof, S.; et al. Alterations to the gut microbiome after sport-related concussion in a collegiate football players cohort: A pilot study. *Brain, Behav. Immun. Health* **2022**, *21*, 100438. [CrossRef]
75. Ekstrand, J.; Lundqvist, D.; Davison, M.; D'Hooghe, M.; Pensgaard, A.M. Communication quality between the medical team and the head coach/manager is associated with injury burden and player availability in elite football clubs. *Br. J. Sports Med.* **2019**, *53*, 304–308. [CrossRef]
76. Ghrairi, M.; Loney, T.; Pruna, R.; Malliaropoulos, N.; Valle, X. Effect of poor cooperation between coaching and medical staff on muscle re-injury in professional football over 15 seasons. *Open Access J. Sports Med.* **2019**, *10*, 107–113. [CrossRef] [PubMed]

77. Corman, S.R.; Adame, B.J.; Tsai, J.-Y.; Ruston, S.W.; Beaumont, J.S.; Kamrath, J.K.; Liu, Y.; Posteher, K.A.; Tremblay, R.; van Raalte, L.J. Socioecological influences on concussion reporting by NCAA Division 1 athletes in high-risk sports. *PLoS ONE* **2019**, *14*, e0215424. [CrossRef] [PubMed]
78. Knollman-Porter, K.; Thaxton, S.; Hughes, M.R.; Constantinidou, F. Management and recovery patterns following sport-related mild traumatic brain injury in male and female college athletes. *Top. Lang. Disord.* **2019**, *39*, 257–275. [CrossRef]

nutrients

Article

The Mediating Effect of Coping Strategies and Emotion Regulation in the Relationship between Impulsivity, Metacognition, and Eating Disorders

Ana Estévez [1,*], Janire Momeñe [1], Laura Macía [1], Iciar Iruarrizaga [2], Leticia Olave [2] and Gema Aonso-Diego [1]

1 Department of Psychology, Faculty of Health Sciences, University of Deusto, Avda. de las Universidades 24, 48007 Bilbao, Spain; janiremomene@deusto.es (J.M.); laura.macia@deusto.es (L.M.); gema.aonso@deusto.es (G.A.-D.)
2 Department of Experimental Psychology, Cognitive Psychology and Speech & Language Therapy, Faculty of Psychology, Complutense University of Madrid, 28040 Madrid, Spain; iciariru@psi.ucm.es (I.I.); leticiaolave@ucm.es (L.O.)
* Correspondence: aestevez@deusto.es

Abstract: Background. Risk factors for eating disorders are multifaceted and complex, so it is crucial to elucidate the role of executive functions, including impulsivity and metacognition, and coping strategies in the severity of eating behaviors. The study aims were threefold: (1) to analyze gender differences in impulsivity, metacognition, coping strategies, emotion regulation, and eating disorders; (2) to examine the correlation between the study variables; and (3) to test the mediating role of coping and emotion-regulation strategies in the relationship between metacognition, impulsivity, and eating disorders. Methods. A total of 1076 participants (M_{age} = 21.78, SD = 5.10; 77.7% women) completed a set of questionnaires. Two mediation analyses were conducted to test the mediating role of coping strategies, including emotion regulation, in the relationship between executive functions (i.e., impulsivity and metacognition) and eating disorders. Results. Women displayed higher coping strategies, specifically emotional expression, wishful thinking, and social support, whereas men presented greater social withdrawal. Mediational analyses showed a significant association between impulsivity, metacognition, and eating disorders, whose relationship was partially mediated by coping strategies and mainly by emotion regulation. Conclusion. Interventions based on coping strategies and emotion regulation could be a feasible and effective option to deal with eating disorders among the young population.

Keywords: eating disorders; gender differences; impulsivity; coping strategies; metacognition

Citation: Estévez, A.; Momeñe, J.; Macía, L.; Iruarrizaga, I.; Olave, L.; Aonso-Diego, G. The Mediating Effect of Coping Strategies and Emotion Regulation in the Relationship between Impulsivity, Metacognition, and Eating Disorders. *Nutrients* **2024**, *16*, 1884. https://doi.org/10.3390/nu16121884

Academic Editor: Sébastien Guillaume

Received: 21 May 2024
Revised: 10 June 2024
Accepted: 12 June 2024
Published: 14 June 2024

1. Introduction

Eating disorders constitute a spectrum of psychiatric conditions characterized by disturbances in eating behaviors, attitudes toward food, body weight, and shape. These disorders significantly impact individuals' physical and mental health (e.g., depression, anxiety) [1], including suicide [2], and notably, the mortality rate for eating disorders is strikingly high [3–5]. Among the most prevalent eating disorders are anorexia nervosa, bulimia nervosa, and binge eating disorder, each presenting distinct clinical features and diagnostic criteria [6].

The etiology of eating disorders is multifaceted, influenced by a complex interplay of genetic, biological [7], psychological (e.g., stressful life events) [8,9], and sociocultural factors (e.g., cultural norms) [10]. Two variables that have received the most attention are those related to executive function, specifically lack of control or impulsivity, and metacognitive strategies.

Impulsivity, broadly defined as a predisposition towards rapid, unplanned reactions to internal or external stimuli without consideration of potential consequences, has been deeply studied within the realm of eating disorders, showing a different profile of impulsivity for each diagnosis [11,12]. Previous evidence suggests a strong relationship between impulsivity and different eating disorders (i.e., anorexia nervosa, bulimia nervosa, and binge eating disorder) [13–17], as well as the risk of developing an eating disorder [18]. Impulsivity manifests in binge eating episodes, purging behaviors, or excessive exercise, which are undertaken without forethought or control [19,20].

On the other hand, metacognition, the process of thinking about one's own thinking, beliefs, and cognitive processes, has emerged as a critical factor in understanding eating behaviors and the development and maintenance of eating disorders. This variable has been related to a large number of psychological disorders [21,22], addictive behaviors [23,24], as well as eating disorders and problematic eating behaviors [25–29], both in anorexia and bulimia [30–32] and binge eating [33].

Despite the large number of studies confirming the association between impulsivity and metacognitive strategies with eating disorders, the causal mechanism remains unclear. Some studies have pointed to the importance of coping strategies, including emotion regulation, in explaining this relationship [34–37].

Coping and emotion regulation strategies have been widely studied in relation to eating disorders [38–42]. Nonetheless, to our knowledge, no previous studies have analyzed the mediating role of coping strategies and emotion regulation in the relationship between metacognition or impulsivity and eating disorders. However, it has been studied in other psychological variables, such as anxiety [43,44], attachment [45], excessive worry [46], posttraumatic symptoms [47], Internet addiction [48], and overall mental health [49], which show elevate comorbidity with eating disorders [1,50].

Based on the Self-Regulatory Executive Function model (S-REF) [51–54], metacognitive beliefs activate a combination of coping strategies. In other words, whereas metacognition refers to the awareness and understanding of one's own cognitive processes, including thoughts, beliefs, and strategies, coping strategies encompass the behavioral, cognitive, and emotional efforts employed to manage stressors and adapt to adverse circumstances. Positive metacognitive beliefs (e.g., self-efficacy and perceived control over stressors) promote the utilization of proactive coping strategies (e.g., problem-solving, seeking social support, or positive reappraisal). Conversely, negative metacognitive beliefs, such as catastrophic thinking, may predispose individuals to employ maladaptive coping strategies (e.g., avoidance, rumination, social withdrawal), which exacerbate emotional distress and increase vulnerability to engaging in binge eating, purging, or restrictive eating behaviors, as well as maintaining eating disorders over time.

In this line, impulsivity often undermines the effectiveness of coping efforts by leading individuals to employ maladaptive or reactive strategies in response to stressors [55–58]. Impulsive individuals may resort to impulsive coping mechanisms, such as avoidance or dysfunctional emotion regulation, as a solution to alleviate distress in the short term.

Despite the amount of research on this issue, no study has tested the mediating role of coping strategies and emotion regulation in the relationship between metacognition or impulsivity and eating disorders. Furthermore, previous studies focusing on these variables (i.e., metacognition, impulsivity, coping strategies, and emotion regulation) were conducted with a clinical population [14,25,30,33], and mostly among the adolescent population [26,27,59]. Also, to our knowledge, no previous study has been conducted among the Spanish population in which eating-related characteristics could differ from other countries [60]. Understanding the role of metacognitive beliefs and impulsivity in shaping eating behaviors has important implications for the development of targeted interventions for eating disorders.

Given this background, the study aims were threefold: (1) to analyze gender differences in the study variables (i.e., eating disorders, impulsivity, metacognition, emotion regulation, and some coping strategies); (2) to examine the correlation between the study variables; and (3) to test the mediating role of coping and emotion-regulation strategies in the relationship between metacognition, impulsivity, and eating disorders.

2. Material and Methods

2.1. Participants and Procedure

The study sample included 1076 participants (M_{age} = 21.78, SD = 5.10, aged between 18 and 61 years). Most participants were women (77.7%, n = 836), 21.7% (n = 233) were men, and the remaining seven participants (0.70%) were trans men. The majority were students (78.6%, n = 845) and single (93.1%, n = 1000). Finally, 34.57% (n = 372) of the participants had received psychological treatment at some point in their lives, of which 5.10% (n = 19) were for eating disorders.

The recruitment was conducted through two channels: online and face-to-face. For online recruitment, surveys were conducted through a SurveyMonkey platform. For the face-to-face channel, participants were recruited at the Complutense University of Madrid. Participants filled out the questionnaires in the classroom during teaching hours through pencil and paper or an online survey in the university classrooms. The only exclusion criterion was being under 18 years of age.

All participants provided written informed consent before study participation, indicating that they had read the study information and agreed to participate voluntarily. The study adhered to the ethical principles of the Declaration of Helsinki and was approved by the university ethics committee (ref. ETK-38/23-24). Participants were assured of the confidentiality and anonymity of their responses, as well as their voluntary participation. The participants did not receive any kind of compensation.

2.2. Instruments

All participants completed a battery in which sociodemographic data (i.e., age, gender, working status, and marital status) were collected. Additionally, participants completed four questionnaires concerning eating disorders, metacognition, impulsivity, coping strategies, and emotion regulation.

2.2.1. Eating Disorders

The Eating Disorder Inventory (EDI-2) [61], validated in Spain by Muro-Sans et al. (2006) [62], is a widely used self-report questionnaire designed to assess various aspects of disordered eating behaviors and attitudes. This inventory included a total of 91 items divided into 11 scales that evaluate central aspects of eating disorders, that is, drive for thinness, bulimia, body dissatisfaction, ineffectiveness, perfectionism, interpersonal distrust, interoceptive awareness, maturity fears, asceticism, impulse regulation, and social insecurity. All items are rated using a Likert-type scale, where individuals rate the extent to which each statement applies to them, ranging from 0 ("never") to 5 ("always"). The internal consistency measured by Cronbach's α of the total scale was 0.95.

2.2.2. Metacognitive Strategies

Metacognitive strategies were assessed with the homonymous subscale of the Inventory of Cognitive Activity in Anxiety Disorders, subscale for obsessive-compulsive disorder (*Inventario de Actividad Cognitiva en Trastornos de Ansiedad—Trastorno Obsesivo-Compulsivo*; IACTA-TOC) [63]. The total inventory consists of 21 items, including the metacognition subscale, which comprises 7 items rated on a Likert-type scale (ranging from 0 "almost never" to 4 "almost always"). The subscale assessed the frequency of certain thoughts in individuals (e.g., "I place great importance on the thoughts that occupy my mind", "at times, I may mistake my thoughts for reality", "I am vigilant and attentive to situations related to my thoughts"). In our sample, Cronbach's alpha was 0.88 for the metacognition subscale.

2.2.3. Impulsivity

The Barratt Impulsiveness Scale (BIS-11) [64], adapted to Spanish by Oquendo et al. (2001) [65], is a self-report questionnaire assessing several aspects of impulsivity. The BIS-11 is a 30-item questionnaire, rated on a 4-point Likert-type scale, ranging from 1 (never/rarely) to 4 (almost always/always). Items are grouped into three subscales: attentional impulsiveness, motor impulsiveness, and non-planning impulsiveness. In the present study, Cronbach's alpha was 0.76 for the global scale.

2.2.4. Coping Strategies

The Coping Strategies Inventory (CSI) [66], validated in Spanish by Cano-García et al. (2007) [67], is a self-report measure designed to assess coping strategies employed by individuals to manage stress and adversity. The CSI includes 40 items grouped into eight factors: problem-solving, cognitive restructuring, social support, emotional expression, problem avoidance, wishful thinking, social withdrawal, and self-criticism. Among the eight factors, there are four with positive valence, that is, higher scores indicate adaptive coping strategies (i.e., problem-solving, emotional expression, social support, and cognitive restructuring), whereas the four remaining factors have a negative valence, namely, higher scores indicate maladaptive coping strategies (i.e., self-criticism, wishful thinking, problem avoidance, and social withdrawal). All items are rated on a five-point Likert-type scale ranging from 0 (not at all) to 4 (completely). The internal consistency in the present study ranged from 0.69 in the social withdrawal subscale to 0.88 in the self-criticism subscale.

2.2.5. Emotion Regulation

The Difficulties in Emotion Regulation Scale (DERS) [68], adapted to Spanish by Hervás and Jódar (2008) [69], was used to assess difficulties in the awareness, understanding, or modulation of emotion. The Spanish validation comprises a total of 28 items rated on a Likert-type scale (1 = almost never, 5 = almost always) assessing five emotion-regulation deficits: (1) non-acceptance of emotions; (2) daily interference ('difficulties engaging in goal-directed behavior' in the original subscale); (3) emotional inattention ('lack of emotional awareness' in the original subscale); (4) emotional confusion ('lack of emotional clarity' in the original subscale); and (5) lack of emotional control ('limited access to emotion regulation strategies' and 'impulse control difficulties' in the original subscales). In the present study, the scale has shown adequate psychometric properties ($\alpha = 0.93$).

2.3. Data Analysis

Descriptive statistics and frequencies were computed to summarize the sociodemographic characteristics and the study variables. Independent samples *t*-tests were conducted to examine gender differences in the study variables. Effect sizes were calculated using Cohen's *d* [70]. Pearson correlation coefficients were computed to assess the relationships between study variables.

Two mediation analyses were performed to test the mediating role of emotion regulation and coping strategies in the relationship between impulsivity and metacognition and eating disorders. Therefore, we considered coping strategies (i.e., problem-solving, cognitive restructuring, social support, emotional expression, problem avoidance, wishful thinking, social withdrawal, and self-criticism) and emotion regulation as mediation variables. Given the high correlation between the subscales of emotion regulation and the total score (ranging between 0.723 and 0.878) and between the subscale of impulsivity and the total score (ranging between 0.728 and 0.788), we deemed the total score in these questionnaires.

This analysis was conducted with Process 4 for SPSS Statistics 28 [71], using 5000 bootstrapping samples. All analyses were performed using the SPSS package, and the confidence levels were set at 95%.

3. Results

The study found significant gender differences in age, body mass index (BMI), weight, and height (all *p*-values ≤ 0.001), with women being younger and having lower BMI, weight, and height. Additionally, more men were married and employed. Conversely, there were no gender differences in the study variables, including eating disorders, impulsivity, metacognition, emotion regulation, and some coping strategies. However, there were gender differences in emotional expression, wishful thinking, social support, and social withdrawal, where women scored higher (see Table 1).

Table 1. Descriptive statistics of the sociodemographic characteristics and the study variables.

	Total Sample (N = 1076)	Male (n = 233)	Female (n = 834)	p-Value	Effect Size
	M (SD)	M (SD)	M (SD)		
Age	21.78 (5.10)	25.19 (6.91)	20.84 (4.00)	<0.001	0.768
Weight (kg)	61.98 (11.78)	73.24 (10.50)	58.84 (10.12)	<0.001	1.396
High (m)	1.66 (0.09)	1.77 (0.07)	1.63 (0.06)	<0.001	2.145
BMI	22.25 (3.24)	23.25 (2.78)	21.97 (3.32)	<0.001	0.419
BMI categories				<0.001	0.142
Underweight (<18.5) [a]	89 (8.44%)	5 (2.16%)	84 (10.19%)		
Normal weight (18.5–24.9) [a]	792 (75.07%)	176 (75.19%)	616 (74.76%)		
Overweight (25–29.9) [a]	145 (13.74%)	45 (19.48%)	100 (12.14%)		
Obesity (>30) [a]	29 (2.75%)	5 (2.16%)	24 (2.91%)		
Marital status [a]				<0.001	0.152
Single	993 (93.06%)	209 (89.70%)	784 (94.00%)		
Married	21 (1.97%)	14 (6.01%)	7 (0.84%)		
Other	53 (4.97%)	10 (4.29%)	43 (5.16%)		
Working status [a]				<0.001	0.350
Student	839 (78.56%)	120 (51.50%)	719 (86.11%)		
Worker	218 (20.41%)	106 (45.49%)	112 (13.41%)		
Other	11 (1.03%)	7 (3.00%)	4 (0.48%)		
Eating disorder	157.88 (55.36)	154.71 (51.05)	158.65 (56.65)	0.355	0.073
Impulsivity	66.72 (9.41)	67.25 (9.28)	66.52 (9.39)	0.307	0.078
Metacognition	9.61 (6.30)	10.21 (6.26)	9.43 (6.29)	0.092	0.124
Coping strategies					
Problem-solving	12.44 (4.57)	12.61 (4.49)	12.41 (4.58)	0.560	0.044
Self-criticism	7.14 (5.25)	7.59 (5.09)	7.04 (5.29)	0.160	0.106
Emotional expression	10.94 (4.81)	10.00 (4.66)	11.23 (4.80)	0.001	0.260
Wishful thinking	13.03 (5.23)	12.23 (5.31)	13.27 (5.20)	0.007	0.198
Social support	14.04 (5.09)	13.07 (4.92)	14.31 (5.11)	0.001	0.247
Cognitive restructuring	10.83 (4.74)	11.06 (4.90)	10.78 (4.68)	0.414	0.058
Problem avoidance	6.98 (4.10)	7.27 (4.08)	6.89 (4.09)	0.200	0.093
Social withdrawal	5.98 (4.23)	6.48 (4.24)	5.82 (4.21)	0.037	0.156
Emotion regulation	63.16 (19.28)	61.53 (16.97)	63.59 (19.85)	0.120	0.112

Note: [a] frequency (percentage). M = mean; SD = standard deviation; BMI = body mass index.

Bivariate correlation analyses revealed a strong relationship among the study variables. The only non-significant relationships found were between specific coping strategies and eating disorders ($r = 0.06$), impulsivity ($r \leq -0.055$), metacognition ($r \leq 0.042$), and emotion regulation ($r = 0.059$) (see Table 2).

Table 2. Correlations of the study variables.

	1	2	3	4	5	6	7	8	9	10	11
1. Eating disorder											
2. Impulsivity	0.347 **										
3. Metacognition	0.595 **	0.255 **									
4. Problem-solving	−0.291 **	−0.169 **	−0.167 **								
5. Self-criticism	0.426 **	0.164 **	0.396 **	−0.076 *							
6. Emotional expression	−0.163 **	−0.059	0.028	0.389 **	0.043						
7. Wishful thinking	0.328 **	0.079 *	0.299 **	−0.014	0.378 **	0.129 **					
8. Social support	−0.284 **	−0.091 **	−0.159 **	0.356 **	−0.153 **	0.437 **	0.055				
9. Cognitive restructuring	−0.241 **	−0.055	−0.115 **	0.451 **	−0.025	0.254 **	−0.088 **	0.382 **			
10. Problem avoidance	0.060	0.105 **	0.042	−0.056	0.077 *	−0.066 *	0.103 **	0.017	0.358 **		
11. Social withdrawal	0.436 **	0.136 **	0.337 **	−0.237 **	0.407 **	−0.252 **	0.278 **	−0.394 **	−0.139 **	0.254 **	
12. Emotion regulation	0.714 **	0.393 **	0.595 **	−0.259 **	0.417 **	−0.068 *	0.323 **	−0.197 **	−0.190 **	0.059	0.391 **

Note: * $p \leq 0.05$; ** $p \leq 0.01$.

The mediation analyses showed that impulsivity and metacognition have significant indirect effects on eating disorders through the mediator variables (i.e., coping strategies and emotion regulation). Both mediation models achieved similar results with a significant direct effect of impulsivity and metacognition on eating disorders, emotion regulation, and coping strategies (except for cognitive restructuring and problem avoidance). Additionally, all indirect effects through emotion regulation and coping strategies were statistically significant, except for the pathway mediated by problem-solving, emotional expression, cognitive restructuring, and problem avoidance. Overall, these results demonstrated the intricate connections between impulsivity, metacognition, and eating disorders, whose relationship was partially mediated by emotion regulation and coping strategies, as evidenced by the statistically significant direct and total effects (see Tables 3 and 4). The two mediating models are displayed in Figures 1 and 2, respectively.

Table 3. Standardized direct and indirect effects of impulsivity on eating disorders.

	β	*p*-Value	LLCI	ULCI
Direct effects				
Impulsivity → Eating disorders	0.075	0.002	0.169	0.714
Impulsivity → Emotion regulation	0.402	<0.001	0.688	0.925
Impulsivity → Problem-solving	−0.163	<0.001	−0.107	−0.047
Impulsivity → Self-criticism	0.169	<0.001	0.058	0.128
Impulsivity → Emotion expression	−0.077	0.020	−0.069	−0.006
Impulsivity → Wishful thinking	0.087	0.008	0.012	0.083
Impulsivity → Social support	−0.109	0.001	−0.093	−0.024
Impulsivity → Cognitive restructuring	−0.067	0.042	−0.064	−0.001
Impulsivity → Social withdrawal	0.131	<0.001	0.030	0.086
Impulsivity → Problem avoidance	0.099	0.003	0.015	0.071
Emotional regulation → Eating disorders	0.535	<0.001	1.405	1.719
Problem-solving → Eating disorders	−0.048	0.075	−1.258	0.06
Self-criticism → Eating disorders	0.111	<0.001	0.636	1.741
Emotional expression → Eating disorders	−0.043	0.100	−1.116	0.098
Wishful thinking → Eating disorders	0.080	0.001	0.333	1.376
Social support → Eating disorders	−0.070	0.011	−1.347	−0.173
Cognitive restructuring → Eating disorders	−0.024	0.419	−0.964	0.401
Social withdrawal → Eating disorders	0.104	<0.001	0.656	2.112
Problem avoidance → Eating disorders	−0.010	0.686	−0.814	0.536
Indirect effects				
Emotion regulation	0.215		1.036	1.499
Problem-solving	0.008		−0.005	0.107
Self-criticism	0.019		0.048	0.185
Emotional expression	0.003		−0.003	0.053
Wishful thinking	0.007		0.007	0.089
Social support	0.008		0.007	0.095
Cognitive restructuring	0.002		−0.013	0.043
Social withdrawal	0.014		0.025	0.152
Problem avoidance	−0.001		−0.039	0.025
Total effects (Impulsivity → mediating variables → Eating disorders)	0.349	0.001	1.691	2.400

Note: LLCI = lower-limit confidence intervals; ULCI = upper-limit confidence interval.

Table 4. Standardized direct and indirect effects of metacognition on eating disorders.

	β	*p*-Value	LLCI	ULCI
Direct effects				
Impulsivity → Eating disorders	0.233	<0.001	1.606	2.539
Metacognition → Emotion regulation	0.596	<0.001	1.679	1.996
Metacognition → Problem-solving	−0.181	<0.001	−0.175	−0.085
Metacognition → Self-criticism	0.410	<0.001	0.292	0.389
Metacognition → Emotion expression	0.015	0.656	−0.037	0.059
Metacognition → Wishful thinking	0.287	<0.001	0.188	0.291
Metacognition → Social support	−0.179	<0.001	−0.195	−0.093
Metacognition → Cognitive restructuring	−0.134	<0.001	−0.147	−0.052
Metacognition → Social withdrawal	0.339	<0.001	0.187	0.268
Metacognition → Problem avoidance	0.019	0.565	−0.030	0.055
Emotional regulation → Eating disorders	0.453	<0.001	1.149	1.464
Problem-solving → Eating disorders	−0.038	0.149	−1.099	0.167
Self-criticism → Eating disorders	0.084	0.001	0.365	1.435
Emotional expression → Eating disorders	−0.072	0.005	−1.44	−0.264
Wishful thinking → Eating disorders	0.066	0.006	0.2	1.206
Social support → Eating disorders	−0.057	0.03	−1.196	−0.062
Cognitive restructuring → Eating disorders	−0.036	0.198	−1.086	0.225
Social withdrawal → Eating disorders	0.071	0.009	0.238	1.632
Problem avoidance → Eating disorders	0.009	0.715	−0.527	0.767
Indirect effects				
Emotion regulation	0.27		2.01	2.799
Problem-solving	0.007		−0.027	0.155
Self-criticism	0.035		0.117	0.515
Emotional expression	−0.001		−0.059	0.037
Wishful thinking	0.019		0.052	0.295
Social support	0.01		0.007	0.187
Cognitive restructuring	0.005		−0.024	0.123
Social withdrawal	0.024		0.032	0.4
Problem avoidance	0		−0.016	0.022
Total effects (Metacognition → mediating variables → Eating disorders)	0.602	<0.001	4.892	5.801

Note: LLCI = lower-limit confidence intervals; ULCI = upper-limit confidence interval.

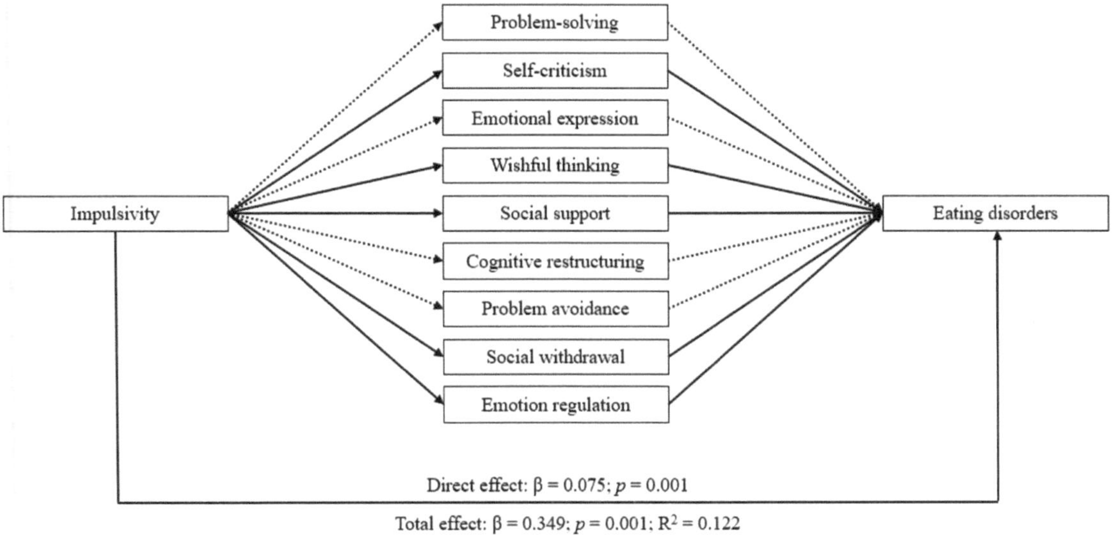

Figure 1. The mediating role of coping strategies and emotion regulation in the relationship between impulsivity and eating disorders. Note: Solid lines indicate significant indirect effects at a 95% confidence interval. Dashed lines indicate non-significant indirect effects at a 95% confidence interval.

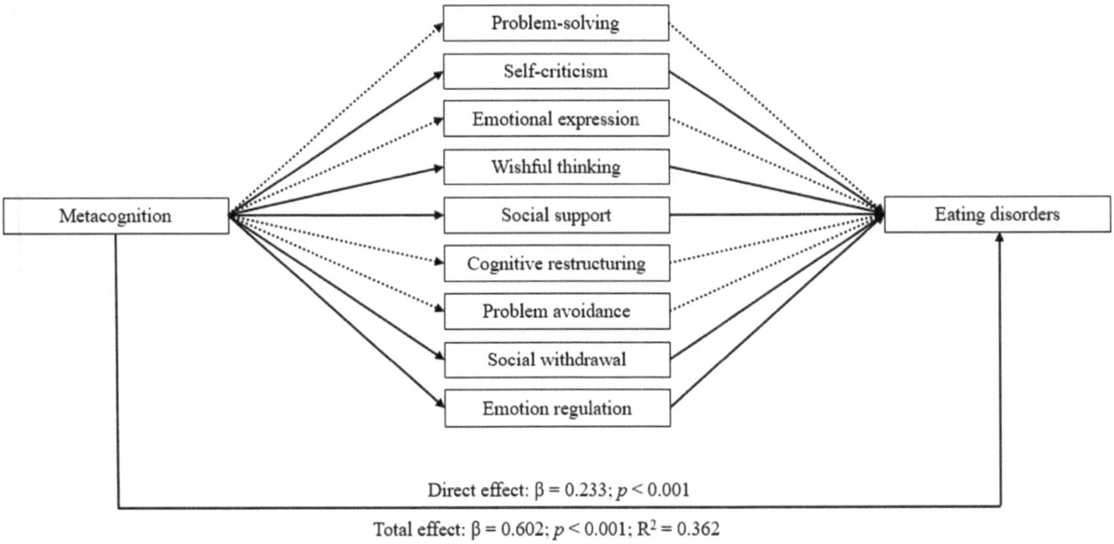

Figure 2. The mediating role of coping strategies and emotion regulation in the relationship between metacognition and eating disorders. Note: Solid lines indicate significant indirect effects at a 95% confidence interval. Dashed lines indicate non-significant indirect effects at a 95% confidence interval.

4. Discussion

The current study aimed to test the mediating role of coping strategies, including emotion regulation, in the relationship between impulsivity and metacognition, and eating disorders. Two results are underlined: (1) Women displayed higher coping strategies, specifically emotional expression, wishful thinking, and social support, whereas men presented greater social withdrawal; and (2) there was a significant association between impulsivity, metacognition, and eating disorders, whose relationship was partially mediated by coping strategies and mainly by emotion regulation.

The results did not find gender differences in eating disorder severity, impulsivity levels, metacognition, or emotion regulation, although differences between men and women were found in some coping strategies. In contrast to the present findings, previous studies have consistently indicated that women exhibit a higher prevalence of eating disorders and greater severity, both in the general population [72,73] and in young adults [74]; higher emotion regulation [75]; and higher scores on some coping strategies [76], although other studies suggest that men score higher on other coping strategies (e.g., avoidance, distraction, and social diversion) [77].

On the other hand, there was a high correlation between coping strategies, especially emotion regulation, and the severity of eating disorders. Emotion regulation has been widely studied as a transdiagnostic construct and also its relationship with several psychological disorders [78–81], including eating disorders [82–85]. Likewise, a strong relationship was also observed between executive functions, specifically impulsivity and metacognition, with eating disorders, coping strategies, and emotion regulation. Theories such as that proposed by Sharp et al. (2013) [86] indicate that women with eating disorders may articulate their mental states extensively and in detail, demonstrating a cognitive understanding of affectivity but with minimal connection to experiential or affective core [87]. In this regard, cognitive strategies characterized by excessive rumination, for instance, tend to focus on issues such as weight, food, and body image, potentially serving as a cognitive-emotional avoidance strategy, thus perpetuating the maintenance of the eating problem [88–91], as they impede cognitive and emotional insight [92].

Finally, the results regarding the mediation analysis yielded similar outcomes for impulsivity and metacognition as independent variables. In both models, coping strategies and emotion regulation partially mediated the relationship between impulsivity and metacognition and eating disorders, except for the pathway mediated by problem-solving, emotional expression, cognitive restructuring, and problem avoidance. This relationship has been demonstrated in other psychological disorders (e.g., anxiety, addictive disorder, mental health) [43,44,48,49], but, to our knowledge, it had not been confirmed in relation to eating disorders until now.

This finding leads to significant clinical implications for the young adult population, as interventions targeting effective coping strategies for dealing with emotional distress may prevent youth from disordered eating. First, it is worth mentioning that therapists' vulnerabilities, biases, and difficulties must be taken into account in addressing eating disorders [93]. Also, several studies have shown the effectiveness of treatments focused on emotion regulation, metacognition, and coping strategies. The systematic review by Sloan et al. (2017) [94] found emotion regulation to be an effective transdiagnostic intervention for eating disorders and other psychological disorders (e.g., anxiety, depression, personality disorders, substance use). Balzan et al. (2023) [95] showed promising results of a metacognition-based intervention in adolescents with anorexia nervosa. Other studies have also examined the effect of coping-based intervention on mental health with excellent results [96,97], although to our knowledge, no studies have conducted coping-based intervention targeted at eating disorders.

When drawing conclusions from the study, it is important to consider certain limitations. Firstly, this is a cross-sectional study, thus causal relationships between variables cannot be established. Moreover, the sample is predominantly composed of women. Hence, future studies should strive to balance gender representation. Although the age range is broad, the sample predominantly comprises young student populations, thus limiting the generalizability of the results to a broader population. Additionally, data collection relied on self-reports, potentially introducing biases such as social desirability. Lastly, given that the sample consisted of the general population rather than clinical populations, caution must be exercised in extrapolating the findings to individuals with eating disorders.

5. Conclusions

In conclusion, understanding eating disorders is paramount for early detection, intervention, and successful treatment outcomes. These findings showed that coping and emotion regulation strategies partially mediated the relationship between executive functions (i.e., impulsivity and metacognition) and eating disorders. Therefore, by elucidating the intricate interplay of executive functions and coping strategies contributing to these disorders, clinicians and researchers can advance our knowledge and develop therapeutic strategies to reduce the impact of eating disorders on individuals and society.

Author Contributions: Conceptualization, G.A.-D., L.M., J.M. and A.E.; Methodology, G.A.-D.; Software, G.A.-D.; Validation, L.M.; Formal Analysis, G.A.-D.; Investigation, G.A.-D.; Resources, Data Curation, I.I. and L.O.; Writing—Original Draft Preparation, G.A.-D.; Writing—Review and Editing, L.M., A.E., I.I., J.M. and L.O.; Visualization, L.M., A.E., I.I., J.M. and L.O.; Supervision, L.M., A.E., I.I., J.M. and L.O.; Project Administration, A.E.; Funding Acquisition, A.E. All authors have read and agreed to the published version of the manuscript.

Funding: This research was funded by the Directorate General for the Regulation of Gambling (ref.: SUBV23/00001) and by a Postdoctoral grant from Ministry of Science (MCIN/AEI/10.13039/501100011033) and from European Union NextGenerationEU/PRTR (ref.: JDC2022-048311-I).

Institutional Review Board Statement: The study was conducted in accordance with the Declaration of Helsinki and approved by the ethics committee of University of Deusto (ref. ETK-38/23-24, approval date: 19 December 2023).

Informed Consent Statement: Informed consent was obtained from all subjects involved in the study. Written informed consent has been obtained from the participants to publish this paper.

Data Availability Statement: The data presented in this study are available on request from the corresponding author. The data are not publicly available because they include confidential information of the participants.

Conflicts of Interest: The authors declare no conflicts of interest.

References

1. Hambleton, A.; Pepin, G.; Le, A.; Maloney, D.; Aouad, P.; Barakat, S.; Boakes, R.; Brennan, L.; Bryant, E.; Byrne, S.; et al. Psychiatric and Medical Comorbidities of Eating Disorders: Findings from a Rapid Review of the Literature. *J. Eat. Disord.* **2022**, *10*, 132. [CrossRef]
2. Amiri, S.; Khan, M.A.B. Prevalence of Non-Suicidal Self-Injury, Suicidal Ideation, Suicide Attempts, Suicide Mortality in Eating Disorders: A Systematic Review and Meta-Analysis. *Eat. Disord.* **2023**, *31*, 487–525. [CrossRef] [PubMed]
3. Jagielska, G.; Kacperska, I. Outcome, Comorbidity and Prognosis in Anorexia Nervosa. *Psychiatr. Pol.* **2017**, *51*, 205–218. [CrossRef] [PubMed]
4. Van Eeden, A.E.; Van Hoeken, D.; Hoek, H.W. Incidence, Prevalence and Mortality of Anorexia Nervosa and Bulimia Nervosa. *Curr. Opin. Psychiatry* **2021**, *34*, 515–524. [CrossRef]
5. Van Hoeken, D.; Hoek, H.W. Review of the Burden of Eating Disorders: Mortality, Disability, Costs, Quality of Life, and Family Burden. *Curr. Opin. Psychiatry* **2020**, *33*, 521–527. [CrossRef] [PubMed]
6. American Psychiatric Association. *Diagnosis and Statistical Manual of Mental Disorders—Fifth Edition Text Revision. DSM-5-TR*; American Psychiatric Association: Washington, DC, USA, 2023.
7. Himmerich, H.; Bentley, J.; Kan, C.; Treasure, J. Genetic Risk Factors for Eating Disorders: An Update and Insights into Pathophysiology. *Ther. Adv. Psychopharmacol.* **2019**, *9*, 1–20. [CrossRef] [PubMed]
8. Kober, H.; Boswell, R.G. Potential Psychological & Neural Mechanisms in Binge Eating Disorder: Implications for Treatment. *Clin. Psychol. Rev.* **2018**, *60*, 32–44. [CrossRef]
9. Alfoukha, M.M.; Hamdan-Mansour, A.M.; Banihani, M.A. Social and Psychological Factors Related to Risk of Eating Disorders Among High School Girls. *J. Sch. Nurs.* **2017**, *35*, 169–177. [CrossRef]
10. Weissman, R.S. The Role of Sociocultural Factors in the Etiology of Eating Disorders. *Psychiatr. Clin. N. Am.* **2019**, *42*, 121–144. [CrossRef]
11. Ciberti, A.; Cavalletti, M.; Palagini, L.; Mariani, M.G.; Dell'osso, L.; Mauri, M.; Maglio, A.; Mucci, F.; Marazziti, D.; Miniati, M. Decision-Making, Impulsiveness and Temperamental Traits in Eating Disorders. *Clin. Neuropsychiatry* **2020**, *17*, 199–208. [CrossRef]
12. Slof-Op't Landt, M.C.T.; Claes, L.; van Furth, E.F. Classifying Eating Disorders Based on "Healthy" and "Unhealthy" Perfectionism and Impulsivity. *Int. J. Eat. Disord.* **2016**, *49*, 673–680. [CrossRef] [PubMed]

13. Boswell, R.G.; Grilo, C.M. General Impulsivity in Binge-Eating Disorder. *CNS Spectr.* **2021**, *26*, 538–544. [CrossRef] [PubMed]
14. Goodwin, A.L.; Butler, G.K.L.; Nikčević, A.V. Impulsivity Dimensions and Their Associations with Disinhibited and Actual Eating Behaviour. *Eat. Behav.* **2023**, *49*, 101752. [CrossRef] [PubMed]
15. Carr, M.M.; Wiedemann, A.A.; Macdonald-Gagnon, G.; Potenza, M.N. Impulsivity and Compulsivity in Binge Eating Disorder: A Systematic Review of Behavioral Studies. *Prog. Neuro-Psychopharmacol. Biol. Psychiatry* **2021**, *110*, 110318. [CrossRef] [PubMed]
16. Shaker, N.M.; Azzam, L.A.B.; Zahran, R.M.; Hashem, R.E. Frequency of Binge Eating Behavior in Patients with Borderline Personality Disorder and Its Relation to Emotional Regulation and Impulsivity. *Eat. Weight Disord.* **2022**, *27*, 2497–2506. [CrossRef]
17. Soidla, K.; Akkermann, K. Perfectionism and Impulsivity Based Risk Profiles in Eating Disorders. *Int. J. Eat. Disord.* **2020**, *53*, 1108–1119. [CrossRef] [PubMed]
18. Bénard, M.; Bellisle, F.; Kesse-Guyot, E.; Julia, C.; Andreeva, V.A.; Etilé, F.; Reach, G.; Dechelotte, P.; Tavolacci, M.P.; Hercberg, S.; et al. Impulsivity Is Associated with Food Intake, Snacking, and Eating Disorders in a General Population. *Am. J. Clin. Nutr.* **2019**, *109*, 117–126. [CrossRef]
19. Testa, G.; Granero, R.; Misiolek, A.; Vintró-Alcaraz, C.; Mallorqui-Bagué, N.; Lozano-Madrid, M.; Heras, M.V.D.L.; Sánchez, I.; Jiménez-Murcia, S.; Fernández-Aranda, F. Impact of Impulsivity and Therapy Response in Eating Disorders from a Neurophysiological, Personality and Cognitive Perspective. *Nutrients* **2022**, *14*, 5011. [CrossRef]
20. Lozano-Madrid, M.; Granero, R.; Lucas, I.; Sánchez, I.; Sánchez-González, J.; Gómez-Peña, M.; Moragas, L.; Mallorquí-Bagué, N.; Tapia, J.; Jiménez-Murcia, S.; et al. Impulsivity and Compulsivity in Gambling Disorder and Bulimic Spectrum Eating Disorders: Analysis of Neuropsychological Profiles and Sex Differences. *Eur. Psychiatry* **2023**, *66*, e91. [CrossRef]
21. Turiaco, F.; Bruno, A.; Mento, C.; Cedro, C.; Pandolfo, G.; Muscatello, M.R.A. Impulsivity and Metacognition in a Psychiatric Population. *Clin. Neuropsychiatry* **2022**, *19*, 97–102. [CrossRef]
22. Sun, X.; Zhu, C.; So, S.H.W. Dysfunctional Metacognition across Psychopathologies: A Meta-Analytic Review. *Eur. Psychiatry* **2017**, *45*, 139–153. [CrossRef] [PubMed]
23. Hamonniere, T.; Varescon, I. Metacognitive Beliefs in Addictive Behaviours: A Systematic Review. *Addict. Behav.* **2018**, *85*, 51–63. [CrossRef] [PubMed]
24. Jauregui, P.; Urbiola, I.; Estevez, A. Metacognition in Pathological Gambling and Its Relationship with Anxious and Depressive Symptomatology. *J. Gambl. Stud.* **2016**, *32*, 675–688. [CrossRef]
25. Palmieri, S.; Mansueto, G.; Ruggiero, G.M.; Caselli, G.; Sassaroli, S.; Spada, M.M. Metacognitive Beliefs across Eating Disorders and Eating Behaviours: A Systematic Review. *Clin. Psychol. Psychother.* **2021**, *28*, 1254–1265. [CrossRef]
26. Laghi, F.; Bianchi, D.; Pompili, S.; Lonigro, A.; Baiocco, R. Metacognition, Emotional Functioning and Binge Eating in Adolescence: The Moderation Role of Need to Control Thoughts. *Eat. Weight. Disord. Stud. Anorex. Bulim. Obes.* **2018**, *23*, 861–869. [CrossRef] [PubMed]
27. Limbers, C.A.; Greenwood, E.; Shea, K.; Fergus, T.A. Metacognitive Beliefs and Emotional Eating in Adolescents. *Eat. Weight Disord.* **2021**, *26*, 2281–2286. [CrossRef] [PubMed]
28. Olstad, S.; Solem, S.; Hjemdal, O.; Hagen, R. Metacognition in Eating Disorders: Comparison of Women with Eating Disorders, Self-Reported History of Eating Disorders or Psychiatric Problems, and Healthy Controls. *Eat. Behav.* **2015**, *16*, 17–22. [CrossRef]
29. Gerges, S.; Azzi, V.; Bianchi, D.; Laghi, F.; Pompili, S.; Malaeb, D.; Obeid, S.; Soufia, M.; Hallit, S. Exploring the Relationship between Dysfunctional Metacognitive Processes and Orthorexia Nervosa: The Moderating Role of Emotion Regulation Strategies. *BMC Psychiatry* **2023**, *23*, 674. [CrossRef]
30. Davenport, E.; Rushford, N.; Soon, S.; Mcdermott, C. Dysfunctional Metacognition and Drive for Thinness in Typical and Atypical Anorexia Nervosa. *J. Eat. Disord.* **2015**, *3*, 1–9. [CrossRef]
31. Georgantopoulos, G.; Konstantakopoulos, G.; Michopoulos, I.; Dikeos, D.; Gonidakis, F. The Relationship between Metacognitive Beliefs and Symptoms in Eating Disorders. *Psychiatriki* **2020**, *31*, 225–235. [CrossRef]
32. Sapuppo, W.; Ruggiero, G.M.; Caselli, G.; Sassaroli, S. The Body of Cognitive and Metacognitive Variables in Eating Disorders: Need of Control, Negative Beliefs about Worry Uncontrollability and Danger, Perfectionism, Self-Esteem and Worry. *Isr. J. Psychiatry* **2018**, *55*, 55–65. [PubMed]
33. Aloi, M.; Rania, M.; Carbone, E.A.; Caroleo, M.; Calabrò, G.; Zaffino, P.; Nicolò, G.; Carcione, A.; Lo Coco, G.; Cosentino, C.; et al. Metacognition and Emotion Regulation as Treatment Targets in Binge Eating Disorder: A Network Analysis Study. *J. Eat. Disord.* **2021**, *9*, 1–9. [CrossRef]
34. Ruscitti, C.; Rufino, K.; Goodwin, N.; Wagner, R. Difficulties in Emotion Regulation in Patients with Eating Disorders. *Borderline Personal. Disord. Emot. Dysregulation* **2016**, *3*, 3. [CrossRef] [PubMed]
35. Mallorquí-Bagué, N.; Testa, G.; Lozano-Madrid, M.; Vintró-Alcaraz, C.; Sánchez, I.; Riesco, N.; Granero, R.; Perales, J.C.; Navas, J.F.; Megías-Robles, A.; et al. Emotional and Non-emotional Facets of Impulsivity in Eating Disorders: From Anorexia Nervosa to Bulimic Spectrum Disorders. *Eur. Eat. Disord. Rev.* **2020**, *28*, 410–422. [CrossRef] [PubMed]
36. Luca, M. Maladaptive Rumination as a Transdiagnostic Mediator of Vulnerability and Outcome in Psychopathology. *J. Clin. Med.* **2019**, *8*, 314. [CrossRef]
37. Tecuta, L.; Gardini, V.; Digiuseppe, R.; Tomba, E. Do Metacognitions Mediate the Relationship between Irrational Beliefs, Eating Disorder Symptoms and Cognitive Reappraisal? *Psychother. Res.* **2021**, *31*, 483–492. [CrossRef]
38. Dingemans, A.; Danner, U.; Parks, M. Emotion Regulation in Binge Eating Disorder: A Review. *Nutrients* **2017**, *9*, 1274. [CrossRef] [PubMed]

39. Meule, A.; Richard, A.; Schnepper, R.; Reichenberger, J.; Georgii, C.; Naab, S.; Voderholzer, U.; Blechert, J. Emotion Regulation and Emotional Eating in Anorexia Nervosa and Bulimia Nervosa. *Eat. Disord.* **2019**, *29*, 175–191. [CrossRef] [PubMed]
40. Mikhail, M.E.; Kring, A.M. Emotion Regulation Strategy Use and Eating Disorder Symptoms in Daily Life. *Eat. Behav.* **2019**, *34*, 101315. [CrossRef]
41. Dworschak, C.; Polack, R.G.; Winschel, J.; Joormann, J.; Kober, H. Emotion Regulation and Disordered Eating Behaviour in Youths: Two Daily-Diary Studies. *Eur. Eat. Disord. Rev. J. Eat. Disord. Assoc.* **2023**, *31*, 655–669. [CrossRef]
42. Tragantzopoulou, P.; Giannouli, V. Unveiling Anxiety Factors in Orthorexia Nervosa: A Qualitative Exploration of Fears and Coping Strategies. *Healthcare* **2024**, *12*, 925. [CrossRef]
43. Gargabi, Z.H.; Nouri, R.; Moradi, A.; Sarami, G. Evaluation of Coping Styles, Metacognition and Their Relationship with Test Anxiety. *J. Mazand. Univ. Med. Sci.* **2014**, *24*, 144–155.
44. Yousefi, M.; Barzegar, M.; Kouroshnia, M.; Khayyer, M. Investigating The Mediating Role of Cognitive Emotion Regulation Strategies in The Relationship Between Meta-Cognitive Beliefs and Learning Anxiety. *Iran. Evol. Educ. Psychol. J.* **2021**, *3*, 256–267. [CrossRef]
45. Mohammadkhani, S.; Hasani, J.; Akbari, M.; Panah, N.Y. Mediating Role of Emotion Regulation in the Relationship of Metacognitive Beliefs and Attachment Styles with Risky Behaviors in Children of Iran-Iraq War Veterans with Psychiatric Disorders. *Iran. J. Psychiatry Clin. Psychol.* **2019**, *25*, 396–411. [CrossRef]
46. Ceren Yıldırım, J.; Bahtiyar, B. The Association between Metacognitions and Worry: The Mediator Role of Experiential Avoidance Strategies. *J. Psychol.* **2022**, *156*, 552–567. [CrossRef]
47. Mazloom, M.; Yaghubi, H.; Mohammadkhani, S. Post-Traumatic Stress Symptom, Metacognition, Emotional Schema and Emotion Regulation: A Structural Equation Model. *Personal. Individ. Differ.* **2016**, *88*, 94–98. [CrossRef]
48. Li, Q.; Dai, W.; Zhong, Y.; Wang, L.; Dai, B.; Liu, X. The Mediating Role of Coping Styles on Impulsivity, Behavioral Inhibition/Approach System, and Internet Addiction in Adolescents From a Gender Perspective. *Front. Psychol.* **2019**, *10*, 2402. [CrossRef] [PubMed]
49. Bacadini França, A.; Samra, R.; Magalhães Vitorino, L.; Waltz Schelini, P. The Relationship Between Mental Health, Metacognition, and Emotion Regulation in Older People. *Clin. Gerontol.* **2024**, *47*, 298–306. [CrossRef]
50. Udo, T.; Grilo, C.M. Psychiatric and Medical Correlates of DSM-5 Eating Disorders in a Nationally Representative Sample of Adults in the United States. *Int. J. Eat. Disord.* **2019**, *52*, 42–50. [CrossRef] [PubMed]
51. Wells, A.; Matthews, G. Modelling Cognition in Emotional Disorder: The S-REF Model. *Behav. Res. Ther.* **1996**, *34*, 881–888. [CrossRef] [PubMed]
52. Sharma, V.; Sagar, R.; Kaloiya, G.; Mehta, M. The Scope of Metacognitive Therapy in the Treatment of Psychiatric Disorders. *Cureus* **2022**, *14*, e23424. [CrossRef]
53. Kraft, B.; Jonassen, R.; Stiles, T.C.; Landrø, N.I. Dysfunctional Metacognitive Beliefs Are Associated with Decreased Executive Control. *Front. Psychol.* **2017**, *8*, 259977. [CrossRef]
54. Wells, A. Breaking the Cybernetic Code: Understanding and Treating the Human Metacognitive Control System to Enhance Mental Health. *Front. Psychol.* **2019**, *10*, 2621. [CrossRef] [PubMed]
55. Miller, A.E.; Racine, S.E. Emotion Regulation Difficulties as Common and Unique Predictors of Impulsive Behaviors in University Students. *J. Am. Coll. Health* **2022**, *70*, 1387–1395. [CrossRef]
56. Lazuras, L.; Ypsilanti, A.; Powell, P.; Overton, P. The Roles of Impulsivity, Self-Regulation, and Emotion Regulation in the Experience of Self-Disgust. *Motiv. Emot.* **2019**, *43*, 145–158. [CrossRef]
57. Altan-Atalay, A.; Zeytun, D. The Association of Negative Urgency with Psychological Distress: Moderating Role of Proactive Coping Strategies. *J. Psychol.* **2020**, *154*, 487–498. [CrossRef] [PubMed]
58. Maier, M.J.; Schiel, J.E.; Rosenbaum, D.; Hautzinger, M.; Fallgatter, A.J.; Ehlis, A.C. To Regulate or Not to Regulate: Emotion Regulation in Participants With Low and High Impulsivity. *Front. Behav. Neurosci.* **2021**, *15*, 645052. [CrossRef]
59. Laghi, F.; Pompili, S.; Bianchi, D.; Lonigro, A.; Baiocco, R. Dysfunctional Metacognition Processes as Risk Factors for Drunkorexia during Adolescence. *J. Addict. Dis.* **2020**, *38*, 291–300. [CrossRef]
60. Strodl, E.; Markey, C.; Aimé, A.; Rodgers, R.F.; Dion, J.; Coco, G.L.; Gullo, S.; McCabe, M.; Mellor, D.; Granero-Gallegos, A.; et al. A Cross-Country Examination of Emotional Eating, Restrained Eating and Intuitive Eating: Measurement Invariance across Eight Countries. *Body Image* **2020**, *35*, 245–254. [CrossRef]
61. Garner, D.M. *Eating Disorder Inventory—2*; Psychological Assessment Resources: Lake Magdalene, FL, USA, 1991.
62. Muro-Sans, P.; Amador-Campos, J.A.; Peró-Cebollero, M. Factor Structure of Eating Disorders Inventory-2 in a Spanish Sample. *Eat. Weight Disord. Stud. Anorex. Bulim. Obes.* **2006**, *11*, e42–e52. [CrossRef]
63. Leal-Carcedo, L. *Validación del Inventrio de Actividad Cognitiva en Los Trastornos de Nasiedad, Subescala Para el Trastorno Obsesivo-Compulsivo (IACTA-TOC)*; Universidad Complutense de Madrid: Madrid, Spain, 2012.
64. Barratt, E.S. Impulsiveness and Anxiety: Information Processing and Electroencephalograph Topography. *J. Res. Pers.* **1987**, *21*, 453–463. [CrossRef]
65. Oquendo, M.A.; Baca-García, E.; Graver, R.; Morales, M.; Montalvan, V.; Mann, J.J. Spanish Adaptation of the Barratt Impulsiveness Scale (BIS-11). *Eur. J. Psychiatry* **2001**, *15*, 147–155.
66. Tobin, D.L.; Holroyd, K.A.; Reynolds, R.V.; Wigal, J.K. The Hierarchical Factor Structure of the Coping Strategies Inventory. *Cognit. Ther. Res.* **1989**, *13*, 343–361. [CrossRef]

67. Cano-García, F.J.; Rodríguez-Franco, L.; García-Martínez, J. Adaptación Española Del Inventario de Estrategias de Afrontamiento. *Actas Españolas Psiquiatr.* **2007**, *35*, 29–39.
68. Gratz, K.L.; Roemer, L. Multidimensional Assessment of Emotion Regulation and Dysregulation: Development, Factor Structure, and Initial Validation of the Difficulties in Emotion Regulation Scale. *J. Psychopathol. Behav. Assess.* **2004**, *26*, 41–54. [CrossRef]
69. Hervás, G.; Jódar, R. Adaptación Al Castellano de La Escala de Dificultades En La Regulación Emocional. *Clínica Salud* **2008**, *19*, 139–156.
70. Cohen, J. *Statistical Power Analysis for the Behavioral Sciences*; Hillsdate: Hillsdale, MI, USA, 1988.
71. Hayes, A.F. *An Introduction to Mediation, Moderation, and Conditional Process Analysis: A Regression-Based Approach*; Guilford Press: New York, NY, USA, 2013.
72. Lindvall-Dahlgren, C.; Wisting, L.; Rø, Ø. Feeding and Eating Disorders in the DSM-5 Era: A Systematic Review of Prevalence Rates in Non-Clinical Male and Female Samples. *J. Eat. Disord.* **2017**, *5*, 56. [CrossRef]
73. Qian, J.; Wu, Y.; Liu, F.; Zhu, Y.; Jin, H.; Zhang, H.; Wan, Y.; Li, C.; Yu, D. An Update on the Prevalence of Eating Disorders in the General Population: A Systematic Review and Meta-Analysis. *Eat. Weight Disord.* **2022**, *27*, 415–428. [CrossRef] [PubMed]
74. Cheah, W.L.; Shin, E.C.V.; Hazmi, H. Examining Gender Difference in Disordered Eating Behaviour and Its Associated Factors among College and University Students in Sarawak. *Nutr. Health*, 2022; *Advance online publication*. [CrossRef]
75. Nolen-Hoeksema, S. Emotion Regulation and Psychopathology: The Role of Gender. *Annu. Rev. Clin. Psychol.* **2012**, *8*, 161–187. [CrossRef]
76. Graves, B.S.; Hall, M.E.; Dias-Karch, C.; Haischer, M.H.; Apter, C. Gender Differences in Perceived Stress and Coping among College Students. *PLoS ONE* **2021**, *16*, e0255634. [CrossRef] [PubMed]
77. Cabras, C.; Mondo, M. Coping Strategies, Optimism, and Life Satisfaction among First-Year University Students in Italy: Gender and Age Differences. *Int. J. Educ. Res.* **2018**, *75*, 643–654. [CrossRef]
78. Sakiris, N.; Berle, D. A Systematic Review and Meta-Analysis of the Unified Protocol as a Transdiagnostic Emotion Regulation Based Intervention. *Clin. Psychol. Rev.* **2019**, *72*, 101751. [CrossRef]
79. Cludius, B.; Mennin, D.; Ehring, T. Emotion Regulation as a Transdiagnostic Process. *Emotion* **2020**, *20*, 37–42. [CrossRef] [PubMed]
80. Hu, T.; Zhang, D.; Wang, J.; Mistry, R.; Ran, G.; Wang, X. Relation between Emotion Regulation and Mental Health: A Meta-Analysis Review. *Psychol. Rep.* **2014**, *114*, 341–362. [CrossRef] [PubMed]
81. Igra, L.; Shilon, S.; Kivity, Y.; Atzil-Slonim, D.; Lavi-Rotenberg, A.; Hasson-Ohayon, I. Examining the Associations between Difficulties in Emotion Regulation and Symptomatic Outcome Measures among Individuals with Different Mental Disorders. *Front. Psychol.* **2023**, *14*, 944457. [CrossRef] [PubMed]
82. Mallorquí-Bagué, N.; Vintró-Alcaraz, C.; Sánchez, I.; Riesco, N.; Agüera, Z.; Granero, R.; Jiménez-Múrcia, S.; Menchón, J.M.; Treasure, J.; Fernández-Aranda, F. Emotion Regulation as a Transdiagnostic Feature Among Eating Disorders: Cross-Sectional and Longitudinal Approach. *Eur. Eat. Disord. Rev.* **2018**, *26*, 53–61. [CrossRef] [PubMed]
83. Prefit, A.B.; Cândea, D.M.; Szentagotai-Tătar, A. Emotion Regulation across Eating Pathology: A Meta-Analysis. *Appetite* **2019**, *143*, 104438. [CrossRef] [PubMed]
84. Leppanen, J.; Brown, D.; McLinden, H.; Williams, S.; Tchanturia, K. The Role of Emotion Regulation in Eating Disorders: A Network Meta-Analysis Approach. *Front. Psychiatry* **2022**, *13*, 793094. [CrossRef]
85. Brockmeyer, T.; Skunde, M.; Wu, M.; Bresslein, E.; Rudofsky, G.; Herzog, W.; Friederich, H.C. Difficulties in Emotion Regulation across the Spectrum of Eating Disorders. *Compr. Psychiatry* **2014**, *55*, 565–571. [CrossRef]
86. Sharp, C.; Ha, C.; Carbone, C.; Kim, S.; Perry, K.; Williams, L.; Fonagy, P. Hypermentalizing in Adolescent Inpatients: Treatment Effects and Association With Borderline Traits. *J. Personal. Disord.* **2013**, *27*, 3–18. [CrossRef] [PubMed]
87. Blatt, S.J.; Auerbach, J.S.; Behrends, R.S. Changes in the Representation of Self and Significant Others in the Treatment Process: Links between Representation, Internalization, and Mentalization. In *Mind to Mind: Infant Research, Neuroscience, and Psychoanalysis*; Jurist, E.L., Slade, A., Bergner, S., Eds.; Other Press: New York, NY, USA, 2008; pp. 225–263.
88. Rawal, A.; Park, R.J.; Williams, J.M.G. Rumination, Experiential Avoidance, and Dysfunctional Thinking in Eating Disorders. *Behav. Res. Ther.* **2010**, *48*, 851–859. [CrossRef]
89. Cowdrey, F.A.; Park, R.J. The Role of Experiential Avoidance, Rumination and Mindfulness in Eating Disorders. *Eat. Behav.* **2012**, *13*, 100–105. [CrossRef] [PubMed]
90. Litwin, R.; Goldbacher, E.M.; Cardaciotto, L.A.; Gambrel, L.E. Negative Emotions and Emotional Eating: The Mediating Role of Experiential Avoidance. *Eat. Weight Disord.* **2017**, *22*, 97–104. [CrossRef] [PubMed]
91. Espel-Huynh, H.M.; Muratore, A.F.; Virzi, N.; Brooks, G.; Zandberg, L.J. Mediating Role of Experiential Avoidance in the Relationship between Anxiety Sensitivity and Eating Disorder Psychopathology: A Clinical Replication. *Eat. Behav.* **2019**, *34*, 101308. [CrossRef] [PubMed]
92. Park, R.J.; Dunn, B.D.; Barnard, P.J. Schematic Models and Modes of Mind in Anorexia Nervosa I: A Novel Process Account. *Int. J. Cogn. Ther.* **2011**, *4*, 415–437. [CrossRef]
93. Tragantzopoulou, P.; Giannouli, V. "You Feel That You Are Stepping into a Different World": Vulnerability and Biases in the Treatment of Anorexia Nervosa. *Eur. J. Psychother. Couns.* **2023**, *25*, 351–368. [CrossRef]

94. Sloan, E.; Hall, K.; Moulding, R.; Bryce, S.; Mildred, H.; Staiger, P.K. Emotion Regulation as a Transdiagnostic Treatment Construct across Anxiety, Depression, Substance, Eating and Borderline Personality Disorders: A Systematic Review. *Clin. Psychol. Rev.* **2017**, *57*, 141–163. [CrossRef] [PubMed]
95. Balzan, R.P.; Gilder, M.; Thompson, M.; Wade, T.D. A Randomized Controlled Feasibility Trial of Metacognitive Training with Adolescents Receiving Treatment for Anorexia Nervosa. *Int. J. Eat. Disord.* **2023**, *56*, 1820–1825. [CrossRef]
96. Tharaldsen, K.B.; Bru, E. Evaluating the Mindfulness-Based Coping Program: An Effectiveness Study Using a Mixed Model Approach. *Ment. Illn.* **2012**, *4*, 43–51. [CrossRef]
97. Herrero, R.; Mira, A.; Cormo, G.; Etchemendy, E.; Baños, R.; García-Palacios, A.; Ebert, D.D.; Franke, M.; Berger, T.; Schaub, M.P.; et al. An Internet Based Intervention for Improving Resilience and Coping Strategies in University Students: Study Protocol for a Randomized Controlled Trial. *Internet Interv.* **2019**, *16*, 43–51. [CrossRef] [PubMed]

nutrients

MDPI

Article

Effects of Acute Guarana (*Paullinia cupana*) Ingestion on Mental Performance and Vagal Modulation Compared to a Low Dose of Caffeine

Tyler N. Talik [1], Eduardo Macedo Penna [2], Brian P. Hack [1], Alec Harp [1] and Mindy Millard-Stafford [1,*]

[1] School of Biological Sciences, Georgia Institute of Technology, Atlanta, GA 30318, USA; tylertpro1@gmail.com (T.N.T.); bhack@gatech.edu (B.P.H.); aharp6@gatech.edu (A.H.)
[2] Physical Education Faculty, Federal University of Pará, Castanhal 68746-630, PA, Brazil; eduardomp@ufpa.br
* Correspondence: mindy.millardstafford@ap.gatech.edu

Abstract: Guarana (GUA), a Brazilian seed extract, contains caffeine and other bioactive compounds that may have psychoactive effects. To assess the acute effects of GUA compared to a low dose of caffeine (CAF) on cognitive and mood parameters, twenty participants completed a double-blind, crossover experiment where they ingested capsules containing the following: (1) 100 mg CAF, (2) 500 mg GUA containing 130 mg caffeine, or (3) placebo (PLA). Cognitive tests (Simon and 2N-Back Task) were performed at the baseline (pre-ingestion) and 60 min after ingestion. The response time for the cognitive tests and heart rate variability were unaffected ($p > 0.05$) by treatment, although 2N-Back was overall faster ($p = 0.001$) across time. The accuracy in the 2N-Back Task showed a significant interaction effect ($p = 0.029$) due to higher post-ingestion versus pre-ingestion levels ($p = 0.033$), but only with the PLA. The supplements also had no effect on cognitive measures following physical fatigue ($n = 11$). There was an interaction effect on perceived mental energy, where the pre-ingestion of GUA had lower mental pep ratings compared to post-ingestion ($p = 0.006$) and post-exercise ($p = 0.018$) levels. Neither the acute ingestion of GUA nor low dose of CAF influenced cognitive performance or provided consistent benefit on mood or mental workload through vagal modulation. Additional investigations are beneficial to determining the lowest effective dose for CAF or GUA to influence mood and/or cognitive performance.

Keywords: cognition; mood; fatigue; perception; emotion; HRV; vagus nerve

Citation: Talik, T.N.; Penna, E.M.; Hack, B.P.; Harp, A.; Millard-Stafford, M. Effects of Acute Guarana (*Paullinia cupana*) Ingestion on Mental Performance and Vagal Modulation Compared to a Low Dose of Caffeine. *Nutrients* **2024**, *16*, 1892. https://doi.org/10.3390/nu16121892

Academic Editors: Roser Granero and Gemma Guillazo-Blanch

Received: 22 May 2024
Revised: 6 June 2024
Accepted: 12 June 2024
Published: 15 June 2024

1. Introduction

Mental performance is characterized by the effectiveness of an individual's cognitive function to accomplish tasks [1]. Mood, feelings, and emotions may also influence mental performance [2], specifically mental fatigue which is a cause of impaired attention and reduced accuracy [3,4]. To combat mental fatigue and enhance cognitive functions, strategies such as exercise and nutritional aids have been suggested [5,6]. Among these, caffeine stands out as the most popular and extensively used stimulant, with over 90% of adults in the United States consuming it regularly [7]. Acute caffeine ingestion significantly improves various cognitive and mood-related variables, including response time, attention, and mental fatigue [8]. The beneficial effects of caffeine are primarily attributed to its role as an adenosine receptor antagonist in the brain [9], blocking adenosine from binding to the receptors and activating them [10], thereby inducing the sympathetic physiological responses of wakefulness, alertness, and arousal [10]. Furthermore, this activation may also lead to physiological changes such as increased blood pressure and heightened muscular activity [11,12].

Factors such as daily consumption habits, age, gender, body size, medical conditions, and genetics [13] all influence individual mood and cognitive responses to caffeine doses [14]. Habitual caffeine consumers often experience more significant cognitive improvements, especially in spatial memory and rapid visual information processing, than non-habitual drinkers [15]. Moreover, the effective caffeine dosage for acute cognitive benefits is debated but also generally observed at 200 mg or higher [16], although smaller doses (below 3 mg per kilogram of body weight) may enhance performance in attention-related tasks [17]. While black coffee is the most common source of caffeine, Guarana, an Amazonian rainforest plant, has emerged with potential cognitive and mood benefits [18]. Guarana seed extracts, depending on the source and processing, have a caffeine content of 5% to 10% [18,19], 0.9% to 2.4% higher than coffee beans [20]. A few studies have indicated that the low natural dose of caffeine, commonly found in Guarana, can separately enhance memory, vigilance, alertness, and information processing speed [21,22]. Whether the effect of Guarana is due solely to its caffeine content for cognitive effects remains unclear.

Guarana also contains bioactive compounds (e.g., flavonoids, methylxanthines, and proanthocyanidins), which may exert certain effects [23,24]. However, few studies have systematically controlled the impact of caffeine versus matched caffeine levels in Guarana. Faster response times (RT) in a Go/No-go Task were found with Guarana (GUA) compared to caffeine (CAF) [25]; but in another study, no differences were found between GUA and CAF for RT during a Simon Task [26]. Furthermore, a meta-analysis of eight placebo-controlled studies indicated that GUA slightly improves RT in cognitive tests without affecting performance accuracy [27]. Moreover, other individual studies have revealed the potential of GUA to enhance alertness, secondary memory accuracy, and working memory, as measured by different cognitive and mood assessments [28,29]. However, not all studies consistently support the effect of Guarana, when compared to the placebo, on cognitive function, underscoring the need for further investigation into its specific effects and the role that its caffeine content may play.

The knowledge about the effects of Guarana to counter fatigue has wide applications, including enhancing athletic performance. Mental fatigue has been shown to reduce endurance, sprint, and jump performance in athletes [30,31]. Caffeine has been recognized to improve various exercise performance metrics [32]. In comparison, limited research has compared Guarana's effect on cognitive performance and mood to that of caffeine, especially in situations eliciting mental or physical fatigue. Investigations of Guarana have mainly focused on working memory and response inhibition after exhaustive cycling [33] or running [34] with unmatched doses of CAF, leaving a knowledge gap in the benefits of GUA over CAF following physical and/or mental fatigue. Whether the caffeine level naturally found in GUA is primarily responsible for the benefits and if a low dose of caffeine (either in GUA or caffeine by itself) improves mental performance remains unclear.

Therefore, we had the following two questions: (1) Does a low dose of caffeine elicit mental performance benefits? And (2) if so, would Guarana perform similarly when the caffeine dose available in the supplement is similarly matched? The acute effects of GUA ingestion on mood (Brunel Mood Scale), cognitive performance (2N-Back and Simon Tasks), motivation/mental energy (Motivation and Energy Visual Analog Scales), and mental fatigue (NASA Task Load) were compared to a low dose of CAF and a placebo. In addition, the effect of GUA following physical fatigue and the role of sympathetic activation as a mechanism for these effects was analyzed. We hypothesized that GUA would improve both mood and performance on cognitive tasks without added mental fatigue compared to the placebo control but elicit similar effects to a low dosage of CAF.

2. Materials and Methods

2.1. Experimental Design

The study utilized a double-blind, placebo-controlled crossover with a Latin square block design for treatment assignments. Participants visited the laboratory four times (once for preliminary testing/familiarization with procedures followed by three experimental trials), each separated by at least one week, occurring at the same hour of day within each participant. A schematic of the test protocol is shown (Figure 1).

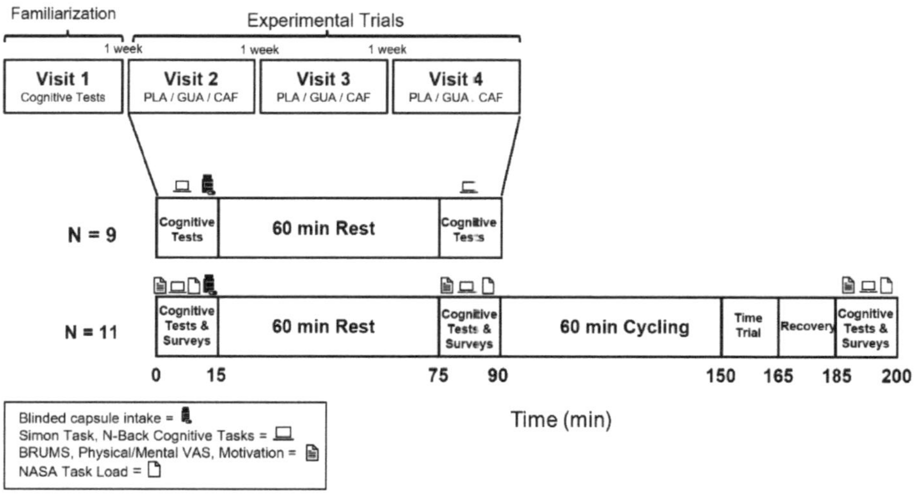

Figure 1. Schematic of the test protocol. CAF = Caffeine; GUA = Guarana; PLA = Placebo. BRUMS, VAS, NASA are survey instruments described in methods.

2.2. Participants

Twenty participants (healthy adult volunteers) were recruited at two locations, one in Brazil and the other in the United States. The selection of participants was a convenient sampling of willing volunteers (non-compensated) available to the research group. All provided written consent as approved by the local Institutional Review Boards. All procedures were conducted according to the Declaration of Helsinki. Participants were requested to avoid any caffeine consumption and vigorous training 24 h before the experimental sessions. The participants' physical characteristics (17 men, 3 women) were as follows: age = 22.5 ± 4.2 y, height = 1.79 ± 0.07 m, body mass = 70.3 ± 11.1 kg). Eleven athlete participants were recruited to perform the cognitive testing protocol, followed by a cycling exercise to elicit physical fatigue. For the exercise subgroup, average caffeine intake was estimated to be 131 ± 78 mg/day. Habitual intake ranged from none (two participants) to ~250 mg (two participants listed two to three cups of coffee per day).

2.3. Interventions

2.3.1. Preliminary Testing and Familiarization

Participants were informed about all the procedures during the first laboratory visit and familiarized with the Simon and 2N-back cognitive tasks. In addition to brief written instructions provided by the task program, verbal instructions for both tasks were given by researchers to participants. Participants were then given as many attempts as needed to learn the tasks with practice versions of each task that included computerized feedback on accuracy. Familiarization with each cognitive test was complete when the participants indicated that they felt comfortable after performing the experimental versions of the Simon and 2N-Back Tasks. Mood and fatigue surveys were verbally explained by researchers and practiced once by only the exercise subgroup.

In the exercise subgroup, a ramp test was performed to measure endurance capacity on an electronically braked cycle ergometer (Lode Excalibur, Groningen, The Netherlands) to set workloads at moderate intensity during the experimental sessions as described previously [35].

2.3.2. Supplement Administration

The CAF, GUA, and PLA treatments were administered orally in a capsule form with 50 mL of tap water, while the participants were blindfolded. Since the capsules were selected and coded by a team member not involved in the data collection, the researchers were blinded. The exercise subgroup was asked after each experimental session about which substance they thought had been ingested, but none were able to correctly identify any capsule.

The same absolute low dose of CAF and GUA dose was administered (not adjusted relative to participants' body mass). The CAF capsules contained 100 mg caffeine anhydrous, while the GUA capsules contained 500 mg GUA (with 100 mg caffeine listed on the label), purchased from the same manufacturer (Nutricost, Vineyard, UT, USA). Following the conclusion of the experiment, independent verification (North American Lab, National Sanitation Foundation [NSF], Ann Arbor, MI, USA) of CAF content was obtained. The NSF found that GUA had higher caffeine content (130 mg) compared with the label (100 mg). Based on the participants' body mass (BM), the caffeine dosage averaged 1.45 ± 0.24 (1.14–1.98) and 1.89 ± 0.31 (1.48–2.58) mg/kg BM for the CAF and GUA treatments, respectively, both of which are relatively low doses of caffeine.

2.3.3. Cognitive and Mood Assessments Administration

All participants arrived at the laboratory at approximately the same time in the morning following an overnight fast. The baseline cognitive tests were performed in approximately 10 min for all the participants, directly before and 60 min after capsule ingestion, under seated resting conditions in a thermally neutral controlled laboratory (23 °C, 40% RH). The computerized cognitive tasks were the Simon Task and the 2N-Back Task. For the exercise subgroup, mood scales and surveys were also completed directly after the cognitive tests and 20 min after the completion of a fatigue-inducing 75 min cycling bout.

2.4. *Experimental Cognitive and Mood Assessments*

2.4.1. Simon Task

The Simon Task was programmed using PsychoPy. The Simon Task is commonly used to assess response inhibition and attention [36]. Participants are instructed to press the left arrow key for a red square and right arrow key for a blue square, while ignoring the position of the square on the screen (left or right), while responding as quickly and accurately as possible. The primary outcome measures were accuracy (ACC) and response time (RT). ACC was the percentage of correct responses out of a total 80 responses possible. RT was the time from stimulus presentation until an arrow key was pressed.

2.4.2. 2N-Back Task

The 2N-Back Task was also developed on PsychoPy. The 2N-Back Task is a commonly used cognitive task to assess working memory [37]. Participants viewed a continuous string of letters (A–F) and indicated whether the current letter matched the letter shown two letters prior. The primary outcome measures were ACC and RT. ACC was expressed as a percentage of the total correct responses, in which the space key was pressed corresponding to a letter match. A total of 80 responses were collected. RT was measured as the time from the correctly matched letter stimuli presentation to space key press.

2.4.3. The Brunel Mood Scale

The Brunel Mood scale (BRUMS) is a self-reported survey with 24 item ratings using a five-point Likert scale [38]. The subscales (anger, confusion, depression, fatigue, tension, and vigor) are derived from the sum of corresponding item ratings in the range of 0–16, with a higher score denoting a higher feeling for that particular mood attribute.

2.4.4. The NASA Task Load Index

The NASA Task Load Index is a self-reported survey with six questions [39] corresponding to the perceived level of mental workload, with higher ratings reflecting a higher perception of that type of mental workload. The workload types include mental demand, physical demand, temporal demand, performance, effort, and frustration.

2.4.5. Motivation and Energy Visual Analog Scales

The Motivation and Energy Visual Analog Scales is a self-reported survey with seven questions and corresponding items [40]. The mental and physical activities items include energy, fatigue, vigor, exhaustion, pep, worn out, and an overall motivation.

2.5. Experimental Physiological Assessments

Heart Rate Variability

Heart rate variability (HRV) was recorded for five minutes at the starting points of pre-ingestion, post-ingestion, and post-exercise in the exercise subgroup using a chest monitor (H10, Polar) connected to the HRV Elite APP, previously validated in another study [41]. HRV was recorded using the root mean square of successive differences between normal heartbeats (RMSSD). Increased resting RMSSD is a potential indicator of psychological resiliency and flexibility, indicating an increased ability to effectively adapt to altering demands and stressors [42].

2.6. Statistical Analysis

Analyses were performed using IBM SPSS software (version 29). A two-factor analysis of variance with repeated measures (supplement × time) was utilized to determine differences among treatments at baseline (prior to ingestion), post-ingestion, and post-exercise (in the exercise sub-group). If a significant difference was observed, pairwise comparisons were analyzed with Bonferroni post hoc tests. Statistical significance was denoted by an alpha level of $p < 0.05$.

3. Results

3.1. Simon Task Performance

For all participants ($n = 20$; Figure 2A), there were no differences in the Simon Task ACC for treatment, time, or time-by-treatment interaction ($p > 0.05$), or net change in the Simon Task ACC from pre-ingestion to post-ingestion (Figure 2B). There were no differences for treatment effect ($p = 0.433$), time effect ($p = 0.066$) or time-by-treatment interaction effects ($p = 0.613$) in the Simon Task RT (Figure 2C). No differences were observed among the treatments for net change in the Simon Task RT from pre-ingestion to post-ingestion (Figure 2D).

In the exercise sub-group ($n = 11$), there were no significant treatment differences for net change scores in the Simon Task from baseline, following physical fatigue (cycling test) after ingesting the three supplements ~3 h earlier ($p = 0.893$, Table 1). Although RT became faster relative to baseline, there were no treatment differences due to GUA, CAF, and PLA ($p = 0.535$).

Table 1. Net change (±SD) in ACC and RT (Post Exercise vs. Pre-Ingestion) for the Simon and 2N-Back Tasks in the exercise subgroup ($n = 11$) for placebo, caffeine, and Guarana.

	Placebo	Guarana	Caffeine
ΔSimon ACC (%)	−0.57 ± 1.71	−0.23 ± 2.61	−0.57 ± 3.46
ΔSimon RT (s)	−0.02 ± 0.03	−0.03 ± 0.02	−0.04 ± 0.06
Δ2N-Back ACC (%)	1.93 ± 2.12	1.82 ± 3.18	−0.68 ± 3.89
Δ2N-Back RT (s)	−0.10 ± 0.10	−0.10 ± 0.10	−0.09 ± 0.15

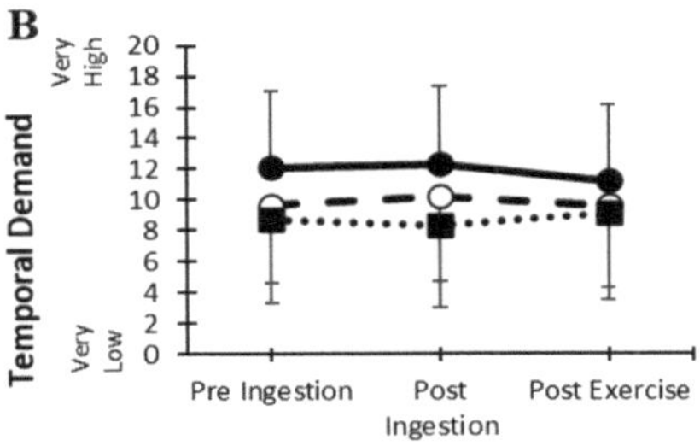

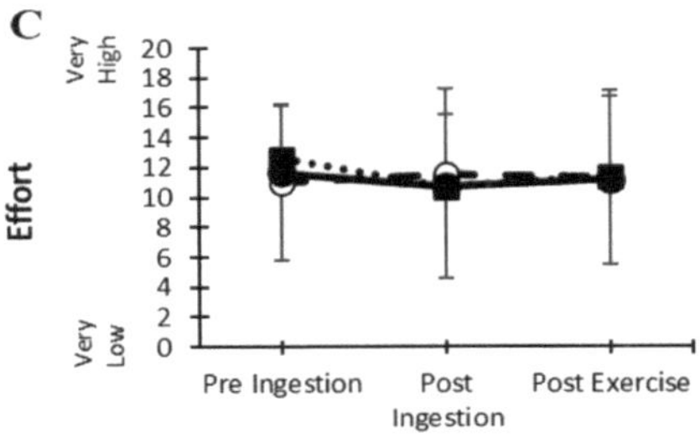

Figure 4. Mean (±SD) NASA Task Load Index for mental demand (**A**), temporal demand (**B**), and effort (**C**) over time among treatments (exercise subgroup $n = 11$).

3.4. Brunel Mood Scale Scores

In the exercise subgroup, there were no significant treatment or time-by-treatment interaction effects for all mood sub-score ratings ($p > 0.05$) for anger, confusion, depression, fatigue, tension, and vigor. There was a significant time effect ($p = 0.001$), but only for fatigue ratings. Post hoc analysis shows that post-ingestion effects were consistently lower than at pre-ingestion and post-exercise effects ($p = 0.006$ and $p = 0.010$, respectively).

3.5. Motivation and Energy Visual Analog Ratings

As presented in Figure 5, there were no treatment, time, or time-by-treatment interaction effects for the following: fatigue, energy, vigor, exhaustion, and motivation ($p > 0.05$). For the mentally worn out item, there was only a time effect ($p = 0.024$) with higher post-exercise ratings compared to pre-ingestion ones ($p = 0.047$). There was a treatment-by-time interaction effect ($p = 0.030$) for mental pep (Figure 5F). Pre-ingestion for GUA was lower than pre-ingestion than PLA ($p = 0.032$), which translated into comparatively higher post-ingestion and post-exercise scores ($p = 0.006$ and $p = 0.018$, respectively).

As expected, the time effect for physical fatigue ($p = 0.001$, Figure 5A), mentally worn out ($p = 0.002$, Figure 5C), and exhaustion ($p = 0.001$) had higher post-exercise ratings than the pre-ingestion ($p = 0.001$, $p = 0.031$, and $p = 0.004$, respectively) and post-ingestion levels ($p = 0.002$, $p = 0.027$, and $p = 0.006$, respectively). There were no treatment, time, or time-by-treatment interaction effects for physical pep, energy, and vigor ($p > 0.05$). However, (Figure 5A), there was a treatment-by-time interaction ($p = 0.001$) for physical fatigue. At pre-ingestion, GUA had higher physical fatigue than CAF ($p = 0.045$). Post-exercise ratings for PLA and CAF were higher in physical fatigue than pre-ingestion ($p = 0.001$ and $p = 0.001$, respectively) and post-ingestion ratings ($p = 0.001$ and $p = 0.006$, respectively). For physical exhaustion, there was a treatment-by-time interaction effect ($p = 0.029$) with post-exercise GUA and CAF being higher than pre-ingestion ($p = 0.044$ and $p = 0.004$, respectively) and post-ingestion levels, but for only CAF ($p = 0.003$).

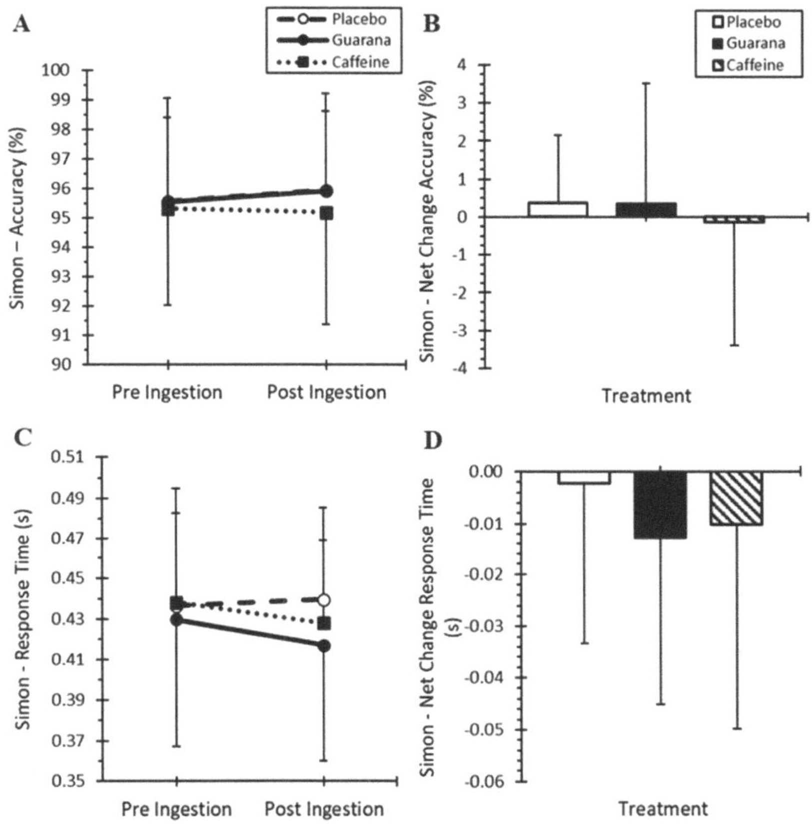

Figure 2. Mean (±SD) Simon Task performance for accuracy (**A**), net change in accuracy (**B**), response time (**C**), and net change in response time (**D**) in all participants (n = 20) among treatments (placebo, caffeine, and Guarana).

3.2. 2N-Back Task Performance

There were no differences in the 2N-Back ACC (Figure 3A) for treatment ($p = 0.962$) or time effects ($p = 0.169$); however, there was a significant time-by-treatment interaction ($p = 0.029$). For PLA, ACC was higher ($p = 0.033$) at post-ingestion (93.4 ± 6.1%) compared to pre-ingestion (90.6 ± 7.2%). Net change in ACC (Figure 3B) differed by treatments ($p = 0.029$) as PLA (+2.8 ± 5.4%) was improved ($p = 0.019$) versus CAF (−1.1 ± 3.1%). There were no differences in RT among treatments ($p = 0.086$, Figure 3C) or time-by-treatment interaction effects ($p = 0.438$). However, there was an overall time effect for RT ($p = 0.001$) with slower RT pre-ingestion (0.70 ± 0.15 s) compared to post-ingestion (0.65 ± 0.14 s). Net change in RT (Figure 3D) was not different among the treatments.

In the exercise sub-group (n = 11), there were no significant treatment differences for net change scores in the 2N-Back Task from baseline to following physical fatigue (cycling test) after ingesting the three supplements ~3 h earlier ($p = 0.080$, Table 1). Although RT became faster relative to baseline, there were no treatment differences due to GUA, CAF and PLA ($p = 0.963$).

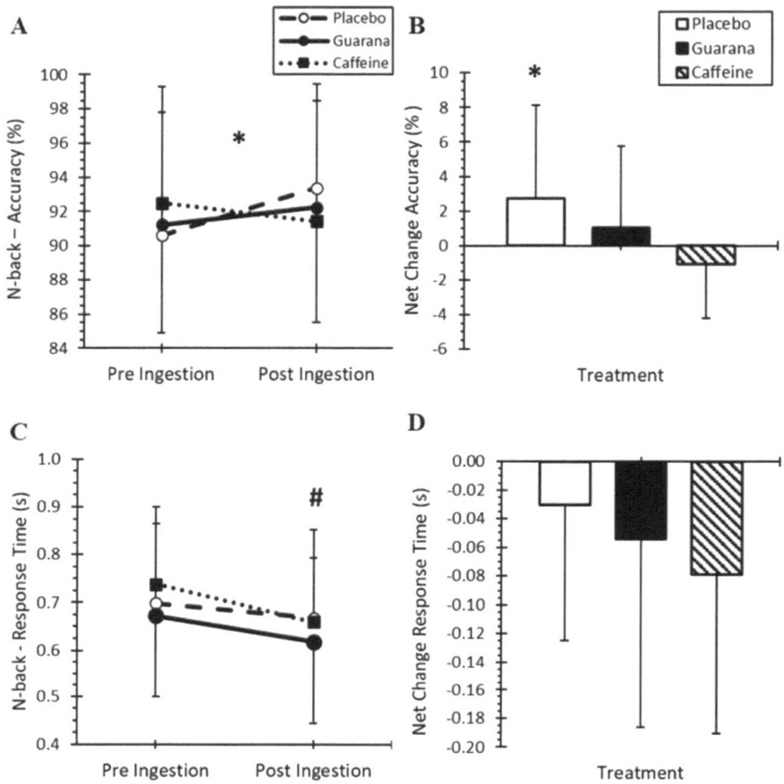

Figure 3. Mean (±SD) 2N-Back Task performance for accuracy (**A**), net change in accuracy (**B**), response time (**C**), and net change in response time (**D**) among treatments. (**A**) * Significantly higher accuracy over time for placebo ($p = 0.033$) and (**B**) * Significantly higher for placebo compared to caffeine ($p = 0.019$). (**C**) # Significantly faster overall time effect ($p = 0.001$).

3.3. NASA Task Load Index Fatigue Scores

In the exercise subgroup, there were no significant treatment, time, or time-by-treatment interaction effects on all sub-score ratings ($p > 0.05$), regarding mental demand, physical demand, temporal demand, performance, effort, and frustration. The most closely related sub-scores to the mental workload of cognitive assessments include temporal demand, mental demand, and effort (Figure 4).

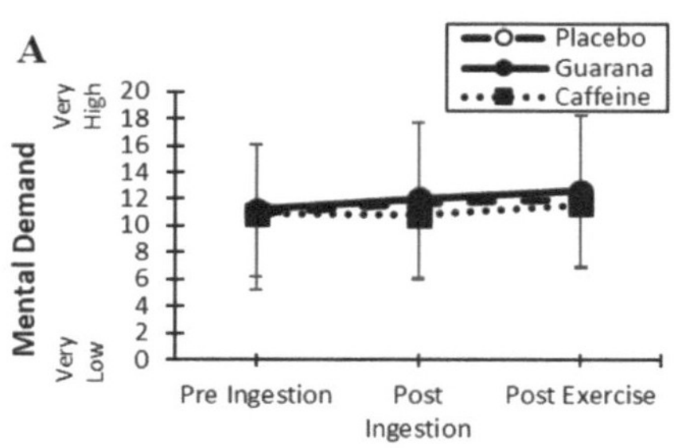

Figure 4. *Cont.*

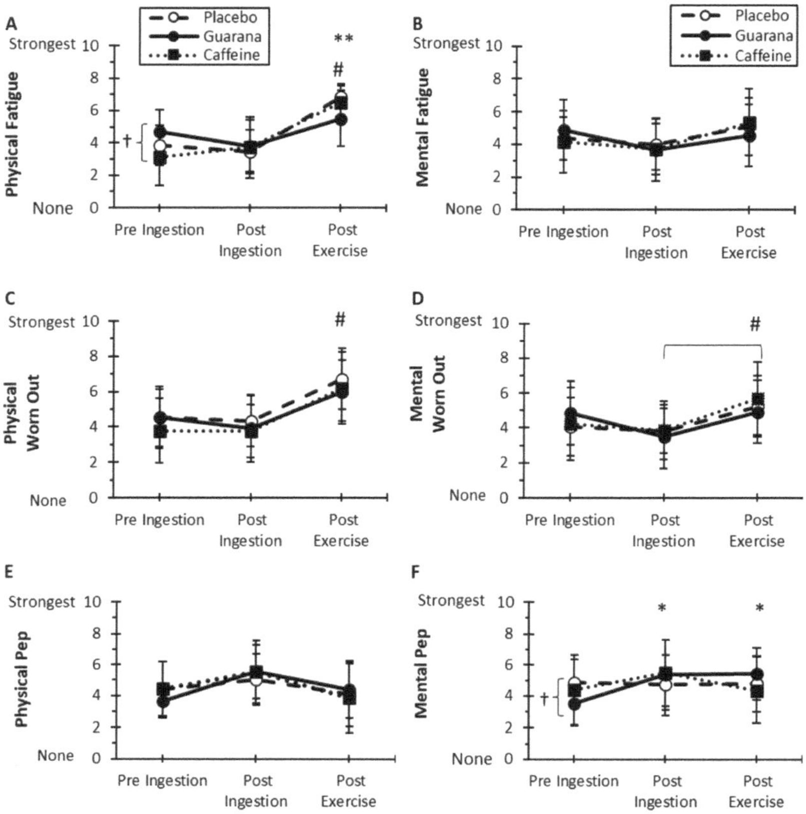

Figure 5. Mean (±SD) energy visual analog ratings for physical (**A**) and mental (**B**) fatigue, physical (**C**) and mentally (**D**) worn out, and physical (**E**) and mental (**F**) pep among treatments in exercise subgroup (n = 11). (**A**) # Post-exercise has a higher overall time effect than pre- and post-ingestion (p = 0.001 and p = 0.002, respectively). † Greater pre-ingestion effects for Guarana versus caffeine (p = 0.045). ** Placebo and caffeine have greater post-exercise versus pre-ingestion (p = 0.001 and p = 0.001, respectively) and post-ingestion effects (p = 0.001 and p = 0.006, respectively). (**C**) # Post-exercise has a higher overall time effect than pre-ingestion and post-ingestion (p = 0.031 and p = 0.027, respectively). (**D**) # Post-exercise has a higher overall time effect than post-ingestion (p = 0.047). (**F**) † Placebo was greater than Guarana at pre-ingestion (p = 0.032). * Post-ingestion (p = 0.006) and post-exercise (p = 0.018) for Guarana higher than pre-ingestion.

3.6. Heart Rate Variability Recordings

There were no significant treatment effects for HRV RMSSD post-ingestion (PLA = 61.2 ± 20.7, GUA = 61.6 ± 19.4, CAF = 62.3 ± 16.8 ms) or post-exercise (PLA = 25.5 ± 12.9, GUA = 23.0 ± 11.9, CAF = 24.5 ± 12.4 ms), nor time-by-treatment interaction ($p > 0.05$). As anticipated, due to the sympathetic activation with exercise, there was an overall time effect with lower RMSSD ($p < 0.001$) post-exercise (24.5 ± 12.4 ms) compared to pre-ingestion (56.9 ± 12.7 ms) and post-ingestion (61.7 ± 19.3 ms).

4. Discussion

The results indicate that natural Guarana seed extract did not consistently improve the cognitive or mood domains assessed either alone after ingestion or in combination with physical fatigue. To our knowledge, this is one of the first published investigations comparing the mental performance effects of Guarana to both a placebo control and a

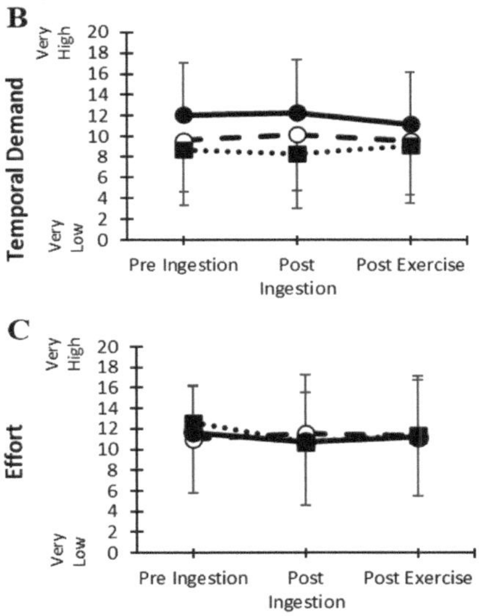

Figure 4. Mean (±SD) NASA Task Load Index for mental demand (**A**), temporal demand (**B**), and effort (**C**) over time among treatments (exercise subgroup n = 11).

3.4. Brunel Mood Scale Scores

In the exercise subgroup, there were no significant treatment or time-by-treatment interaction effects for all mood sub-score ratings ($p > 0.05$) for anger, confusion, depression, fatigue, tension, and vigor. There was a significant time effect ($p = 0.001$), but only for fatigue ratings. Post hoc analysis shows that post-ingestion effects were consistently lower than at pre-ingestion and post-exercise effects ($p = 0.006$ and $p = 0.010$, respectively).

3.5. Motivation and Energy Visual Analog Ratings

As presented in Figure 5, there were no treatment, time, or time-by-treatment interaction effects for the following: fatigue, energy, vigor, exhaustion, and motivation ($p > 0.05$). For the mentally worn out item, there was only a time effect ($p = 0.024$) with higher post-exercise ratings compared to pre-ingestion ones ($p = 0.047$). There was a treatment-by-time interaction effect ($p = 0.030$) for mental pep (Figure 5F). Pre-ingestion for GUA was lower than pre-ingestion than PLA ($p = 0.032$), which translated into comparatively higher post-ingestion and post-exercise scores ($p = 0.006$ and $p = 0.018$, respectively).

As expected, the time effect for physical fatigue ($p = 0.001$, Figure 5A), mentally worn out ($p = 0.002$, Figure 5C), and exhaustion ($p = 0.001$) had higher post-exercise ratings than the pre-ingestion ($p = 0.001$, $p = 0.031$, and $p = 0.004$, respectively) and post-ingestion levels ($p = 0.002$, $p = 0.027$, and $p = 0.006$, respectively). There were no treatment, time, or time-by-treatment interaction effects for physical pep, energy, and vigor ($p > 0.05$). However, (Figure 5A), there was a treatment-by-time interaction ($p = 0.001$) for physical fatigue. At pre-ingestion, GUA had higher physical fatigue than CAF ($p = 0.045$). Post-exercise ratings for PLA and CAF were higher in physical fatigue than pre-ingestion ($p = 0.001$ and $p = 0.001$, respectively) and post-ingestion ratings ($p = 0.001$ and $p = 0.006$, respectively). For physical exhaustion, there was a treatment-by-time interaction effect ($p = 0.029$) with post-exercise GUA and CAF being higher than pre-ingestion ($p = 0.044$ and $p = 0.004$, respectively) and post-ingestion levels, but for only CAF ($p = 0.003$).

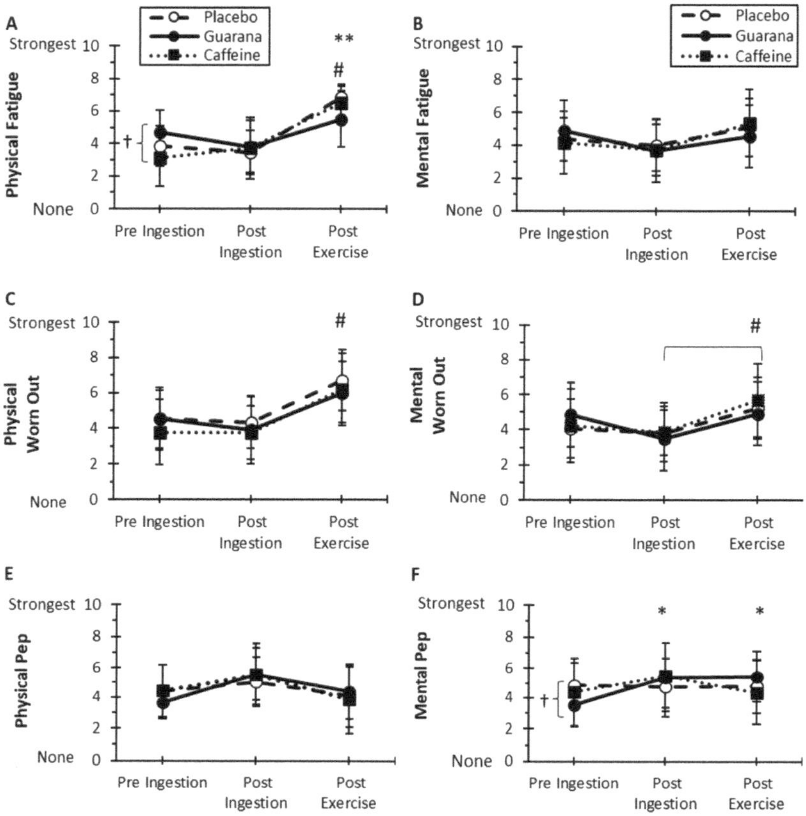

Figure 5. Mean (±SD) energy visual analog ratings for physical (**A**) and mental (**B**) fatigue, physical (**C**) and mentally (**D**) worn out, and physical (**E**) and mental (**F**) pep among treatments in exercise subgroup (n = 11). (**A**) # Post-exercise has a higher overall time effect than pre- and post-ingestion (p = 0.001 and p = 0.002, respectively). † Greater pre-ingestion effects for Guarana versus caffeine (p = 0.045). ** Placebo and caffeine have greater post-exercise versus pre-ingestion (p = 0.001 and p = 0.001, respectively) and post-ingestion effects (p = 0.001 and p = 0.006, respectively). (**C**) # Post-exercise has a higher overall time effect than pre-ingestion and post-ingestion (p = 0.031 and p = 0.027, respectively). (**D**) # Post-exercise has a higher overall time effect than post-ingestion (p = 0.047). (**F**) † Placebo was greater than Guarana at pre-ingestion (p = 0.032). * Post-ingestion (p = 0.006) and post-exercise (p = 0.018) for Guarana higher than pre-ingestion.

3.6. Heart Rate Variability Recordings

There were no significant treatment effects for HRV RMSSD post-ingestion (PLA = 61.2 ± 20.7, GUA = 61.6 ± 19.4, CAF = 62.3 ± 16.8 ms) or post-exercise (PLA = 25.5 ± 12.9, GUA = 23.0 ± 11.9, CAF = 24.5 ± 12.4 ms), nor time-by-treatment interaction ($p > 0.05$). As anticipated, due to the sympathetic activation with exercise, there was an overall time effect with lower RMSSD ($p < 0.001$) post-exercise (24.5 ± 12.4 ms) compared to pre-ingestion (56.9 ± 12.7 ms) and post-ingestion (61.7 ± 19.3 ms).

4. Discussion

The results indicate that natural Guarana seed extract did not consistently improve the cognitive or mood domains assessed either alone after ingestion or in combination with physical fatigue. To our knowledge, this is one of the first published investigations comparing the mental performance effects of Guarana to both a placebo control and a low caffeine dose after a fatiguing exercise along with HRV analysis. The only notable GUA supplement effect over time was an improved rating in one mental–visual analog scale (i.e., mental pep) both after ingestion and subsequent physical fatigue (52% and 54% improvement, respectively). However, this may have been due, in part, to differential ratings among the supplements at the baseline (prior to ingestion). Specifically, PLA had 39% higher mental pep ratings compared to GUA at pre-ingestion. As a result, a lower baseline for GUA in this one rating (which was not aligned with other mental fatigue ratings) makes this isolated result difficult to interpret on its own merits. One potential mechanism explaining greater mental alertness and energy from a low dose of caffeine (i.e., sympathetic activation) was not observed for either the CAF or GUA treatments based on HRV. Therefore, whether the lack of cognitive and mood performance differences with GUA is attributed to an insufficient dosage of caffeine remains unresolved.

Reported cognitive benefits due to caffeine are most frequently observed when taken in dosages > 200 mg [16]. Caffeine dosage at this minimum threshold or above has the potential to enhance memory consolidation [21], vigilance performance [22], ratings of alertness [22], and speed of encoding new information [22]. Despite the paucity of such research, claims have been made that lower doses of caffeine may also enhance performance, specifically on attention tasks compared to higher doses > 200 mg [17]. In summary, the dose–response effect on cognitive performance with caffeine remains uncertain [16]. Therefore, this study originally attempted to match the low caffeine dosage listed on the commercially available Guarana supplements at 100 mg to the same dose of caffeine alone. Unfortunately, the manufacturer's label incorrectly stated the caffeine content for GUA capsules (listed as 100 mg, later confirmed as 130 mg by NSF independent analysis). This discrepancy might be influenced by variable amounts of caffeine found in Guarana. Guarana seeds typically have 4–8% caffeine but that of Guarana extract may be higher (~20%) than coffee beans [18–20].

To induce a cognitive and mood effect with caffeine, several additional covariates must be considered, including participants' daily consumption habits, age, gender, body composition, disease, and genetic influences on the pharmacokinetics of caffeine [13,14]. These factors may influence how participants respond to caffeine, which could differentially modify the effect caffeine may have on various individuals [14]. Caffeine tends to significantly improve the cognitive performance of habitual caffeine consumers under acute ingestion for spatial memory tasks and rapid visual information processing tasks compared to non-habitual caffeine drinkers [15]. The habitual caffeine intake was not recorded for all participants; however, no participants in the exercise subgroup had daily consumption above an average caffeine intake (~250 mg per day).

This present study failed to align with some research findings that the benefits obtained after consuming Guarana are associated with greater cognitive performance improvements than the caffeine content alone might suggest [43]. An earlier meta-analysis [27] from our group indicated that acute Guarana ingestion may influence specific response time outcomes with a small magnitude of effect, but not the accuracy in various cognitive performance assessments. In contrast, the present study found no difference in RT among treatments in cognitive measures involving attention and working memory. Although there was a positive net change in ACC in one task (2N-Back) for PLA versus CAF, this appears to be driven primarily by three participants with apparently large improvements over time (10–11%). This suggests a potential task-learning effect among these participants that cannot be attributed to a treatment effect. No net change in ACC for the Simon Task was observed for any treatments, as approximately 95% of responses were correct, indicating that this task had a ceiling effect and likely lacked the sensitivity to produce observable differences among treatments.

In this present study, the lack of discernible differences between treatments in the Simon and 2N-Back Tasks indicates that GUA had no beneficial effects on the respective response inhibition and working memory parameters assessed under either the normal or physically fatigued states. This conflicts with other individual studies compiled earlier [27] which found that a single dose of 37.5 mg and 75 mg Guarana increased the secondary memory accuracy of activities in Cognitive Drug Research (CDR) Computerized Assessment Battery among healthy young adults [28]. In relation to memory improvements, another study [29] also found that participants who took 75 mg of Guarana displayed improved scores in secondary memory activities of the CDR Computerized Assessment Battery at 150 min after ingestion compared to the placebo. In the same study, improvements in accuracy for other working memory parameters assessed by Serial Sevens Subtraction Task were found with 75 mg Guarana at 360 min after ingestion compared to the placebo [29]. However, a few studies [34,44] have also supported that Guarana ingestion does not always have a positive impact on cognitive performance, which is more aligned with our present study results. In healthy young adults, it was observed that 222 mg of Guarana in a vitamin and mineral complex had no treatment differences in response time measured by the Choice Reaction Time Task at 30, 75, and 150 min after ingestion compared to a placebo [34]. In the same study, no treatment differences were found in the working memory accuracy and response time parameters measured by Delayed Word Recall Tasks at 30, 75, and 150 min after ingestion compared to a placebo [34]. In another study, it was observed that the same 222 mg of Guarana in a vitamin and mineral complex had no between-treatment differences in score and accuracy for working memory parameters measured by the Serial Threes and Sevens Subtraction Tasks up to 80 min after ingestion compared to a placebo [44].

According to other studies, several elements of mood and fatigue perception may be positively impacted following acute Guarana ingestion [28,45]. A single dose of 300 mg Guarana increased alertness among young adults in the Bond–Lader Mood Assessment [28]. Similarly, another study found that a single 100 mg dose of Guarana dissolved in decaffeinated coffee improved alertness ratings 150 min after ingestion in young women, as assessed by the Eighteen Bipolar Visual Analogue Scale [45]. In contrast, male adults ingesting a single dose of 222 mg Guarana had no treatment differences in alertness, calmness, and content ratings in the Bond–Lader Mood Assessment up to 150 min after ingestion [34], which is in alignment with the present study. No difference among treatments was found in Brunel Mood Scale 60 min following ingestion and exercise. Another study examining acute mental fatigue following the ingestion of 222 mg GUA reported reduced mental fatigue ratings in healthy young volunteers up to an hour post-ingestion compared to the placebo [44]. In contrast, the present study lacked any significant treatment differences for mental demand and effort measured by the NASA Task Load and Motivation and Energy Visual Analog Scales. Only in GUA were there improved feelings of mental pep after ingestion and physical fatigue in the exercise subgroup. However, there was no impact on the other corroborating survey items for mental fatigue with GUA. This lack of mental fatigue benefits aligns with another study that found that 222 mg GUA in a vitamin and mineral complex lacked any treatment differences in concentration and mental stamina ratings as measured by an energy visual analog scale [34].

This present study has reported no treatment differences for HRV at various time points after ingestion and exercise. This is in conflict with another study that reported that 300 mg GUA in healthy caffeine consumers had a lesser impact on HRV compared to a significantly lower HRV for CAF and PLA 60–90 min after ingestion [25]. However, we observed an expected time effect for all treatments post-exercise with lower HRV compared to pre-ingestion and post-ingestion. This time effect was similar to other studies [46,47], noting that the reduced HRV after exercise due to changes in vagal tone exerting an influence on heart rate. Activation of the sympathetic nervous system to meet the physiological demand of exercise usually correlates with a decrease from the baseline HRV levels after exercise [42]. Therefore, the lack of differences between GUA and CAF compared to PLA suggests that these treatments were insufficient to impact the autonomic nervous system response to physical exercise.

Lastly, other studies have suggested potential benefits due to other physiological mechanisms involving additional bioactive compounds found in Guarana [24,48–50]. Unlike other caffeinated products, Guarana also naturally contains flavonoids (e.g., catechins and epicatechins) and proanthocyanidins [24]. Flavonoids are proposed to be strong antioxidants, scavenging and neutralizing dangerous reactive oxygen species and free radicals in the brain [48]. This is significant because neuronal cell damage brought on by oxidative stress has been linked to cognitive decline and neurodegenerative disorders [48]. Flavonoids shield neurons and support general cognitive function by lowering oxidative stress [49]. Findings from a small selection of studies with randomized, controlled, human trials suggest a positive correlation between flavonoid consumption and cognitive function [49]. Proanthocyanidins can control the activity of inflammatory pathways and have anti-inflammatory effects, maintaining cognitive function by decreasing neuroinflammation [50]. However, additional comprehensive investigations are required to link these findings and their application to cognitive and mood benefits based on acute Guarana ingestion.

The inconsistency in findings may be attributable to differences in research design, supplement doses, GUA sources, participants, and the particular cognitive and mood tasks performed. These contradictory findings point to the need for additional research to determine the cognitive and mood effects associated with Guarana on working memory, attention, response inhibition, and mental fatigue. There are several limitations in the current study. As a result of using convenience sampling, there were only three females recruited, making it impractical to examine sex-related differences. Although our sample size was typical for CAF studies [51], it may have been underpowered to detect differences across cognitive and mood outcome measures. Due to the lack of access to equipment and survey/scales not being translated to Portuguese, only certain assessments were recorded in a separate international laboratory for the non-exercise subgroup.

5. Conclusions

Novel findings of this present study indicate that Guarana seed extract did not consistently improve cognitive and mood domains following acute ingestion in comparison to either a low dose (100 mg) of caffeine or placebo. This suggests Guarana seed extract (500 mg) with a naturally low dose of caffeine ($\leq$130 mg) cannot be categorized as a mood- or cognitive-enhancing supplement. Secondly, we also found limited mental performance benefits with a low caffeine dose for individuals who have a below-average habitual caffeine intake. Following physical fatigue, this non-significant result persisted although there was higher mental pep observed with Guarana, which appears unrelated to changes in vagal modulation. Whether Guarana seed extract confers additional mental related benefits beyond its caffeine content cannot be ascertained, indicating that additional investigations are warranted.

Author Contributions: Conceptualization, M.M.-S. and E.M.P.; methodology, M.M.-S.; formal analysis, A.H.; investigation, E.M.P., B.P.H. and A.H.; writing—original draft preparation, T.N.T., E.M.P. and M.M.-S.; writing—review and editing, T.N.T. and M.M.-S.; visualization, A.H.; project administration, A.H. and B.P.H. All authors have read and agreed to the published version of the manuscript.

Funding: The Fulbright Brasil (Junior Scholar Award—2021) and Pro-Rectory of Research from Federal University of Pará (04/2023) provided travel support to the author E.M.P. for research collaboration in the United States.

Institutional Review Board Statement: The study was conducted in accordance with the Declaration of Helsinki and approved by the Institutional Review Board of the Georgia Institute of Technology (protocol number: H22046 approved on 23 February 2022). Approved by Federal University of Pará ethics committee under the protocol number: 63186822.4.0000.0018 approved on 11 November 2022.

Informed Consent Statement: Informed consent was obtained from all subjects involved in the study.

Data Availability Statement: Data are unavailable due to privacy restrictions across the two institutions in two countries.

Acknowledgments: Technical support and donation of time to analyze the Guarana supplement for caffeine was performed by Donald Harber at the National Sanitation Foundation, Ann Arbor, MI, USA.

Conflicts of Interest: The authors declare no conflicts of interest.

References

1. Harvey, P.D. Domains of cognition and their assessment. *Dialogues Clin. Neurosci.* **2019**, *21*, 227–237. [CrossRef] [PubMed]
2. Tyng, C.M.; Amin, H.U.; Saad, M.N.M.; Malik, A.S. The influences of emotion on learning and memory. *Front. Psychol.* **2017**, *8*, 1454. [CrossRef] [PubMed]
3. Tran, Y.; Craig, A.; Craig, R.; Chai, R.; Nguyen, H.T. The influence of mental fatigue on brain activity: Evidence from a systematic review with meta-analyses. *Psychophysiology* **2020**, *57*, e13554. [CrossRef] [PubMed]
4. Hakim, H.; Khemiri, A.; Chortane, O.G.; Boukari, S.; Chortane, S.G.; Bianco, A.; Marsigliante, S.; Patti, A.; Muscella, A. Mental fatigue effects on the produced perception of effort and its impact on subsequent physical performances. *Int. J. Environ. Res. Public Health* **2022**, *19*, 10973. [CrossRef] [PubMed]
5. Madireddy, S. Most effective combination of nutraceuticals for improved memory and cognitive performance in the house cricket, Acheta domesticus. *Nutrients* **2021**, *13*, 362. [CrossRef] [PubMed]
6. Childs, E. Influence of energy drink ingredients on mood and cognitive performance. *Nutr. Rev.* **2014**, *72*, 48–59. [CrossRef]
7. Frary, C.D.; Johnson, R.K.; Wang, M.Q. Food sources and intakes of caffeine in the diets of persons in the United States. *J. Am. Diet. Assoc.* **2005**, *105*, 110–113. [CrossRef] [PubMed]
8. Spaeth, A.M.; Goel, N.; Dinges, D.F. Cumulative neurobehavioral and physiological effects of chronic caffeine intake: Individual differences and implications for the use of caffeinated energy products. *Nutr. Rev.* **2014**, *72*, 34–47. [CrossRef]
9. Hung, N.; Akhter, S.; Miao, Y. Pathways and mechanism of caffeine binding to human adenosine A2A receptor. *Front. Mol. Biosci.* **2021**, *8*, 673170.
10. Fiani, B.; Zhu, L.; Musch, B.; Briceno, S.; Andel, R.; Sadeq, N.; Ansari, A.Z. The neurophysiology of caffeine as a central nervous system stimulant and the resultant effects on cognitive function. *Cureus* **2021**, *13*, 15032.
11. Voskoboinik, A.; Koh, Y.; Kistler, P.M. Cardiovascular effects of caffeinated beverages. *Trends Cardiovasc. Med.* **2019**, *29*, 345–350. [CrossRef] [PubMed]
12. Grgić, J.; Del Coso, J. Ergogenic effects of acute caffeine intake on muscular endurance and muscular strength in women: A meta-analysis. *Int. J. Environ. Res. Public Health* **2021**, *18*, 5773. [CrossRef] [PubMed]
13. Nehlig, A. Interindividual differences in caffeine metabolism and factors driving caffeine consumption. *Pharmacol. Rev.* **2018**, *70*, 384–411. [CrossRef] [PubMed]
14. Yang, A.H.; Palmer, A.A.; de Wit, H. Genetics of caffeine consumption and responses to caffeine. *Psychopharmacology* **2010**, *211*, 245–257. [CrossRef] [PubMed]
15. Haskell, C.F.; Kennedy, D.O.; Wesnes, K.; Scholey, A.B. Cognitive and mood improvements of caffeine in habitual consumers and habitual non-consumers of caffeine. *Psychopharmacology* **2005**, *179*, 813–825. [CrossRef] [PubMed]
16. Zhang, R.; Madan, C.R. How does caffeine influence memory? Drug, experimental, and demographic factors. *Neurosci. Biobehav. Rev.* **2021**, *131*, 525–538. [CrossRef] [PubMed]
17. Bryant, C.; Farmer, A.; Tiplady, B.; Keating, J.; Sherwood, R.; Swift, C.G.; Jackson, S.H.D. Psychomotor performance: Investigating the dose-response relationship for caffeine and theophylline in elderly volunteers. *Eur. J. Clin. Pharmacol.* **1998**, *54*, 461–468. [CrossRef] [PubMed]
18. Torres, E.B.; Pinaffi-Langley, A.C.C.; De Souza Figueira, M.; Cordeiro, K.S.; Negrão, L.D.; Soares, M.J.; da Silva, C.P.; Alfino, M.C.Z.; Sampaio, G.R.; de Camargo, A.C. Effects of the consumption of guarana on human health: A narrative review. *Compr. Rev. Food Sci. Food Saf.* **2021**, *21*, 272–295. [CrossRef]
19. Schimpl, F.C.; Da Silva, J.A.G.; De Carvalho Gonçalves, J.F.; Mazzafera, P. Guarana: Revisiting a highly caffeinated plant from the Amazon. *J. Ethnopharmacol.* **2013**, *150*, 14–31. [CrossRef]
20. Olechno, E.; Puścion-Jakubik, A.; Zujko, M.E.; Socha, K. Influence of various factors on caffeine content in coffee brews. *Foods* **2021**, *10*, 1208. [CrossRef]
21. Borota, D.; Murray, E.; Keceli, G.; Chang, A.; Watabe, J.M.; Ly, M.; Toscano, J.P.; Yassa, M.A. Post-study caffeine administration enhances memory consolidation in humans. *Nat. Neurosci.* **2014**, *17*, 201–203. [CrossRef] [PubMed]
22. Smith, A.; Sutherland, D.E.; Christopher, G. Effects of repeated doses of caffeine on mood and performance of alert and fatigued volunteers. *J. Psychopharmacol.* **2005**, *19*, 620–626. [CrossRef] [PubMed]
23. Da Silva, G.S.; Canuto, K.M.; Ribeiro, P.R.V.; de Brito, E.S.; Nascimento, M.M.; Zocolo, G.J.; de Jesus, R.M. Chemical profiling of guarana seeds (*Paullinia cupana*) from different geographical origins using UPLC-QTOF-MS combined with chemometrics. *Food Res. Int.* **2017**, *102*, 700–709. [CrossRef] [PubMed]
24. Silva, C.A.; Sampaio, G.R.; Freitas, R.A.M.S.; Da Silva Torres, E.A.F. Polyphenols from guaraná after in vitro digestion: Evaluation of bioaccessibility and inhibition of activity of carbohydrate-hydrolyzing enzymes. *Food Chem.* **2018**, *267*, 405–409. [CrossRef] [PubMed]

25. Pomportes, L.; Davranche, K.; Brisswalter, I.; Hays, A.; Brisswalter, J. Heart rate variability and cognitive function following a multi-vitamin and mineral supplementation with added guarana (*Paullinia cupana*). *Nutrients* **2014**, *7*, 196–208. [CrossRef] [PubMed]
26. Pomportes, L.; Brisswalter, J.; Hays, A.; Davranche, K. Effects of carbohydrate, caffeine, and guarana on cognitive performance, perceived exertion, and shooting performance in high-level athletes. *Int. J. Sports Physiol. Perform.* **2019**, *14*, 576–582. [CrossRef] [PubMed]
27. Hack, B.; Penna, E.M.; Talik, T.; Chandrashekhar, R.; Millard-Stafford, M.L. Effect of guarana (*Paullinia cupana*) on cognitive performance: A systematic review and meta-analysis. *Nutrients* **2023**, *15*, 434. [CrossRef] [PubMed]
28. Haskell, C.F.; Kennedy, D.O.; Wesnes, K.; Milne, A.; Scholey, A.B. A double-blind, placebo-controlled, multi-dose evaluation of the acute behavioural effects of guaraná in humans. *J. Psychopharmacol.* **2006**, *21*, 65–70. [PubMed]
29. Kennedy, D.O.; Haskell, C.F.; Wesnes, K.; Scholey, A.B. Improved cognitive performance in human volunteers following administration of guarana (*Paullinia cupana*) extract: Comparison and interaction with Panax ginseng. *Pharmacol. Biochem. Behav.* **2004**, *79*, 401–411. [CrossRef]
30. Staiano, W.; Bonet, L.R.S.; Romagnoli, M.; Ring, C. Mental fatigue impairs repeated sprint and jump performance in team sport athletes. *J. Sci. Med. Sport* **2023**, *26*, 1016. [CrossRef]
31. Van Cutsem, J.; Marcora, S.M.; De Pauw, K.; Bailey, S.; Meeusen, R.; Roelands, B. The effects of mental fatigue on physical performance: A systematic review. *Sports Med.* **2017**, *47*, 1569–1588. [CrossRef]
32. Grgić, J.; Grgic, I.; Pickering, C.; Schoenfeld, B.J.; Bishop, D.J.; Pedisic, Z. Wake up and smell the coffee: Caffeine supplementation and exercise performance—An umbrella review of 21 published meta-analyses. *Br. J. Sports Med.* **2019**, *54*, 681–688. [CrossRef]
33. Gurney, T.; Bradley, N.; Izquierdo, D.; Ronca, F. Cognitive effects of guarana supplementation with maximal intensity cycling. *Br. J. Nutr.* **2022**, *130*, 253–260. [CrossRef]
34. Veasey, R.C.; Haskell-Ramsay, C.F.; Kennedy, D.N.; Wishart, K.; Maggini, S.; Fuchs, C.J.; Stevenson, E.J. The effects of supplementation with a vitamin and mineral complex with guaraná prior to fasted exercise on affect, exertion, cognitive performance, and substrate metabolism: A randomized controlled trial. *Nutrients* **2015**, *7*, 6109–6127. [CrossRef] [PubMed]
35. Penna, E.M.; Harp, A.; Hack, B.; Talik, T.N.; Millard-Stafford, M. Guarana (*Paullinia cupana*) but not low-dose caffeine improves cycling time-trial performance versus placebo. *Int. J. Sport Nutr. Exerc. Metab.* **2024**, *34*, 30–37. [CrossRef] [PubMed]
36. Simon, J.; Rudell, A.P. Auditory S-R compatibility: The effect of an irrelevant cue on information processing. *J. Appl. Psychol.* **1967**, *51*, 300–304. [CrossRef]
37. Kirchner, W.K. Age differences in short-term retention of rapidly changing information. *J. Exp. Psychol.* **1958**, *55*, 352–358. [CrossRef] [PubMed]
38. Terry, P.C.; Lane, A.M. *User Guide to Brunel Mood Scale*; University of Southern Queensland: Toowoomba, Australia, 2010.
39. Hart, S.G.; Staveland, L.E. Development of NASA-TLX (Task Load Index): Results of empirical and theoretical research. *Adv. Psychol.* **1988**, *52*, 139–183.
40. Maridakis, V.; O'Connor, P.J.; Tomporowski, P.D. Sensitivity to change in cognitive performance and mood measures of energy and fatigue in response to morning caffeine alone or in combination with carbohydrate. *Int. J. Neurosci.* **2009**, *119*, 1239–1258. [CrossRef]
41. Himariotis, A.T.; Coffey, K.F.; Noël, S.; Cornell, D.J. Validity of a smartphone application in calculating measures of heart rate variability. *Sensors* **2022**, *22*, 9883. [CrossRef]
42. Shaffer, F.; Ginsberg, J.P. An overview of heart rate variability metrics and norms. *Front. Public Health* **2017**, *5*, 258. [CrossRef] [PubMed]
43. Kennedy, D.N.; Wightman, E.L. Mental performance and sport: Caffeine and co-consumed bioactive ingredients. *Sports Med.* **2022**, *52*, 69–90. [CrossRef] [PubMed]
44. Kennedy, D.O.; Haskell, C.F.; Robertson, B.; Reay, J.; Brewster-Maund, C.; Luedemann, J.; Scholey, A.B. Improved cognitive performance and mental fatigue following a multi-vitamin and mineral supplement with added guaraná (*Paullinia cupana*). *Appetite* **2008**, *50*, 506–513. [CrossRef] [PubMed]
45. Meyer, K.; Ball, P. Psychological and cardiovascular effects of guarana and yerba mate: A comparison with coffee. *Interam. J. Psychol.* **2004**, *38*, 87–94.
46. Michael, S.; Graham, K.; Davis, G.M. Cardiac autonomic responses during exercise and post-exercise recovery using heart rate variability and systolic time intervals—A review. *Front. Physiol.* **2017**, *8*, 301. [CrossRef] [PubMed]
47. Mongin, D.; Chabert, C.; Extremera, M.G.; Hue, O.; Courvoisier, D.S.; Carpena, P.; Galvan, P.A.B. Decrease of heart rate variability during exercise: An index of cardiorespiratory fitness. *PLoS ONE* **2022**, *17*, e0273981. [CrossRef] [PubMed]
48. Spencer, J.P.E. Flavonoids and brain health: Multiple effects underpinned by common mechanisms. *Genes Nutr.* **2009**, *4*, 243–250. [CrossRef] [PubMed]
49. Macready, A.L.; Kennedy, O.B.; Ellis, J.A.; Williams, C.M.; Spencer, J.P.E.; Butler, L.T. Flavonoids and cognitive function: A review of human randomized controlled trial studies and recommendations for future studies. *Genes Nutr.* **2009**, *4*, 227–242. [CrossRef] [PubMed]

50. Yang, L.; Xian, D.; Xiong, X.; Lai, R.; Song, J.; Zhong, J. Proanthocyanidins against oxidative stress: From molecular mechanisms to clinical applications. *BioMed Res. Int.* **2018**, *2018*, 8584136. [CrossRef]
51. Conger, S.A.; Tuthill, L.M.; Millard-Stafford, M. Does caffeine increase fat metabolism? A systematic review and meta-analysis. *Int. J. Sport Nutr. Exerc. Metab.* **2023**, *33*, 112–120. [CrossRef]

nutrients

MDPI

Article

Biomarkers Associated with Depression Improvement in Veterans with Gulf War Illness Using the Low-Glutamate Diet

Amy A. Maury [1] and Kathleen F. Holton [2,3,*]

[1] Department of Neuroscience, American University, Washington, DC 20016, USA; am6140a@american.edu
[2] Department of Health Studies, American University, Washington, DC 20016, USA
[3] Center for Neuroscience and Behavior, American University, Washington, DC 20016, USA
* Correspondence: holton@american.edu

Abstract: Gulf War Illness (GWI) is a chronic multi-symptom neurological disorder affecting veterans of the Gulf War that is commonly comorbid with depression. A secondary data analysis was conducted to examine serum homocysteine and inflammatory cytokines (IFN-γ, IL-6, IL-1β, TNF-α) as potential biomarkers of depression improvement among veterans with GWI after a one-month dietary intervention aimed at reducing excitotoxicity and increasing micronutrients. Analyses, including multiple linear and logistic regression, were conducted in R studio. Dietary adherence was estimated using a specialized excitotoxin food frequency questionnaire (FFQ), and depression was measured using the Center for Epidemiologic Studies Depression (CES-D) scale. After one month on the diet, 52% of participants reported a significant decrease in depression ($p < 0.01$). Greater dietary adherence (FFQ) was associated with increased likelihood of depression improvement; OR (95% CI) = 1.06 (1.01, 1.11), ($p = 0.02$). Reduced homocysteine was associated with depression improvement after adjusting for FFQ change ($\beta = 2.58$, $p = 0.04$), and serum folate and vitamin B12 were not mediators of this association. Reduction in IFN-γ was marginally associated with likelihood of depression improvement (OR (95% CI) = 1.11 (0.00, 1.42), ($p = 0.06$)), after adjustment for potential confounders. Findings suggest that homocysteine, and possibly IFN-γ, may serve as biomarkers for depression improvement in GWI. Larger trials are needed to replicate this work.

Keywords: depression; dietary intervention; low-glutamate diet; Gulf War Illness; homocysteine; inflammatory cytokines; biomarkers

Citation: Maury, A.A.; Holton, K.F. Biomarkers Associated with Depression Improvement in Veterans with Gulf War Illness Using the Low-Glutamate Diet. *Nutrients* **2024**, *16*, 2255. https://doi.org/10.3390/nu16142255

Academic Editors: Roser Granero and Gemma Guillazo-Blanch

Received: 11 June 2024
Revised: 8 July 2024
Accepted: 10 July 2024
Published: 13 July 2024

1. Introduction

Gulf War Illness (GWI) is a multi-symptom disorder characterized by widespread chronic pain, fatigue, headaches/migraines, cognitive dysfunction, and mood symptoms such as depression, anxiety, and post-traumatic stress disorder (PTSD). Of these, depression occurs in approximately one third of Gulf War veterans and is thought to contribute greatly to their decreased quality of life [1]. Deployed veterans of the Gulf War (GW) (1990–1991) are more than twice as likely as their non-deployed counterparts to experience depression, often comorbid with Gulf War Illness (GWI) [2,3]. Moreover, female veterans of the Gulf War have a significantly higher risk of suicide as compared to female non-Gulf War veterans and as compared with the general female U.S. population [4].

We have previously reported significant improvements in depression as a comorbid condition of GWI after one month on the low-glutamate diet ($p < 0.001$) [5]. The low-glutamate diet eliminates or significantly reduces foods containing excitotoxins, including free (unbound) glutamate and aspartate, while increasing whole foods that are high in nutrients known to be protective against excitotoxicity, including vitamins B2, B6, C, D, and E, omega-3 fatty acids, and the minerals magnesium and zinc. The glutamatergic system is thought to be dysregulated in depression [6]. Moreover, veterans of the Gulf War may have a higher susceptibility to dietary excitotoxins resulting from a compromised blood–brain barrier (BBB) as a result of neurotoxic exposures, head injuries, chronic stressors, and other insults related to military action [7]. Thus, a significant reduction in dietary excitotoxins may be able to reduce the chronic overactivation of the NMDA glutamate receptors thought to contribute to depression symptoms [8].

Previous studies have suggested that homocysteine and inflammatory cytokines may be potential biomarkers of interest for depression. Elevated homocysteine has been associated with depression in prior research [9–12]. It acts as a direct agonist of the NMDA-receptor, leading to dysregulated glutamatergic neurotransmission [9,13], and may worsen BBB permeability [12,14]. Further, insufficient levels of folate (B9) and/or vitamin B12 may result in elevated serum homocysteine via the methylation cycle. Similarly, depression is also associated with circulating inflammatory cytokines [15–18]. Recent studies have shown a causative relationship between inflammatory cytokines and the etiology of depression [19] and that those with inflammation-associated depression are more likely to experience treatment resistance [20].

The comprehensive dietary approach using the low-glutamate diet may be uniquely suited to improve dysregulated metabolic and immune pathways known to contribute to depression. Thus, the objective of this research was to understand whether homocysteine and/or the inflammatory cytokines IFN-γ, TNF-α, IL-6, and IL-1β, may be associated with depression improvement in veterans with GWI after one month on the low-glutamate diet.

2. Materials and Methods

2.1. Participants

This research used data from a prior completed randomized controlled clinical trial (NCT#03342482). A detailed consort flow diagram and recruitment information have been published previously [21]. The methods will be described here briefly. All participants were veterans of the U.S. Armed Forces, deployed to the Persian Gulf during the Gulf War (1990–1991), and were diagnosed with Gulf War Illness (GWI) based on both the Kansas case definition [22] and the CDC criteria [23]. Forty veterans with GWI were recruited from across the United States. To qualify, they had to be under 75 years old, have maintained stable medication usage for the last 3 months or more, have been actively deployed in the Gulf War, and be willing to change their diet while also discontinuing the use of alcohol, marijuana, and/or dietary supplements. Excluded subjects were those currently on active duty, active nicotine users, those who have been diagnosed with a seizure disorder (past or current) or substance use disorder (past year), those who took medication affecting glutamatergic or GABAergic neurotransmission, and/or those with severe asthma requiring hospitalization. All medications were held constant throughout the study.

2.2. Ethical Approval and Consent

The study from which these data were evaluated was conducted according to the guidelines laid down in the Declaration of Helsinki, and all procedures involving human subjects/patients were approved by the American University Institutional Review Board (IRB-2017-301) on 12 May 2017 and the Human Research Protection Office of the Department of Defense (DOD) (HRPO Log NumberA-20203.a) prior to recruitment of subjects. Written informed consent was obtained from all subjects. The study was registered at ClinicalTrials.gov as study ID no: NCT03342482.

2.3. Procedures

For the primary study, at baseline and post-diet, fasting blood samples and anthropometric measurements were obtained. Questionnaires were collected including the CES-D depression measure and a specially designed excitotoxin food frequency questionnaire (FFQ) (Table S1). Excitotoxin FFQ scoring is completed by summing up the self-reported excitotoxic intake during the reported period, with a higher score representing more frequent consumption of excitotoxic foods. Results are reported at baseline and again post-diet to estimate exposure to dietary free glutamate and aspartate intake and to provide an estimate of dietary adherence.

Upon completion of baseline assessments, participants were randomized into two groups: a dietary intervention group (which started the diet immediately) or a waitlisted control group (which started the diet one month later). Once participants were scheduled to start the diet, they received a detailed 2-h dietary training via Skype with the Principal Investigator, Dr. Kathleen Holton, the creator of the low-glutamate diet. A binder of information was also provided that included a detailed list of food additives to avoid, shopping ideas, recipes, and a list of foods that are highest in each micronutrient. An emphasis was placed on consuming foods high in vitamins B2, B6, C, D, and E, omega-3 fatty acids, and minerals magnesium, and zinc, since these nutrients are protective against excitotoxicity and the related outcomes of oxidative stress and inflammation. All measures were again completed post-diet.

As a measure of depression symptoms, participants completed the Center for Epidemiological Studies Depression (CES-D) self-report measure at baseline and post-diet. The CES-D was designed for screening purposes for epidemiological studies of the general population but is not used for clinical diagnoses [24]. The measure includes 20 questions that use a Likert-type scale that considers current or recent mood state, asking "How often this past week did you...", and answers are rated 0 to 3. A score of (0) = rarely or none of the time (less than 1 day); (1) = some or a little of the time (1–2 days/week); (2) = occasionally/moderate amount of time (3–4 days/week); (3) = most or all of the time (5–7 days/week) [24]. Positive items are reverse-scored and answers are summed for a total score ranging from 0–60. A score greater than or equal to sixteen (16) is considered the threshold for depression.

Baseline and post-diet fasting blood samples were collected from participants using venous puncture. After being centrifuged, serum from the blood samples was extracted and aliquots were stored at −80 °C before shipping to the laboratories for analyses. Samples were tested for serum levels of homocysteine (μmoL/L), folate (ng/mL), vitamin B12 (pg/mL), and the cytokines IFN-γ, TNF-α, IL-6, and IL-1β (pg/mL). The cytokines were tested after thawing at INIM EM Papper Clinical Immunology Laboratory in Miami, FL using Quansys Biosciences custom 18-multiplex chemiluminescent assay (Quansys Biosciences, Logan, UT, USA) and plated in duplicate following the manufacturer protocols. Samples were tested for homocysteine at ZRT Laboratory in Beaverton, OR. The samples were plated in duplicate following protocols established by the manufacturer and, between plates, normalized using the internal controls run on each plate. Concentration calculations from standard curves that were created by a five-parameter weighted logistic regression were averaged for subsequent analyses.

2.4. Statistical Methods

While 40 participants participated in the primary study, this secondary analysis is based on the 33 participants ($n = 33$) who completed blood sample collection and the CES-D measures at their baseline and post-diet visits.

R Studio 2021.09.0 was used for all statistical analyses, and results were considered significant at $p < 0.05$. Corrections were not performed for multiple comparisons since the primary study was not powered specifically for these analyses. Linearity, independence, equality of error variance, and normality both visually and statistically were assessed for each biomarker variable.

Change scores were calculated for each biomarker variable by subtracting baseline concentrations from post-diet levels. The Shapiro–Wilk test of normality was used for each variable. For those that passed the test, baseline and post-diet paired t-tests were run, and Pearson correlations were evaluated for change in depression relative to change in each biomarker. For those variables that did not meet the test for normality, even after a power transformation, Spearman correlations were run. Multivariable linear regression was used to model the relation of change in each biomarker relative to change in depression score, after controlling for variables associated with depression, including age, sex, change in BMI, and dietary adherence measured by the excitotoxin FFQ.

Depression "improvement" was also assessed as a dichotomous variable, defined as either a reduction in the CES-D score by $\geq$30% or a post-diet CES-D score that changed from at or above the depression threshold of 16 [24,25] to below 16. Binary logistic regression was used to model the likelihood of depression improvement (odds ratios (OR) and 95% confidence interval (CI)) after adjustment for potential confounding factors, including age, sex, change in BMI, and dietary adherence measured by the excitotoxin FFQ. Biomarker variables were calculated using serum baseline levels minus post-diet levels for binary logistic regression.

Mediation analyses were conducted to explore whether folate and/or vitamin B12 would mediate the association between homocysteine and depression improvement since homocysteine production can be affected by dietary intake of folate and vitamin B12. These analyses were conducted using the R package "mediation" version 4.5.0 [26].

3. Results

3.1. Participant Demographics

Demographics of the 33 participants at the baseline visit are shown in Table 1. Study participants were predominantly Caucasian, with 67% of the sample being male, from four branches of the military, with an average age of 54 (6) years. At baseline, 76% of the study participants met the criteria for depression using the CES-D cut-off of 16 [24,25], with no differential observed based on sex (p = 0.67) or race (p = 0.68).

Table 1. Population description.

Demographic Variable (n = 33)	n (%)
Sex	
Female	11 (33%)
Male	22 (67%)
Race	
Caucasian	30 (91%)
Black/African American	3 (9%)
Military Branch	
Army	17 (52%)
Navy	6 (18%)
Air Force	5 (15%)
Marine Corp	5 (15%)
Depressed (CES-D)	
Yes	25 (76%)
No	8 (24%)
Antidepressant Medication *	
Yes	15 (45%)
No	18 (55%)
	Mean (SD)
Age (yrs.)	54.4 (5.7)
BMI (kg/mg^2)	31.8 (5.7)
FFQ score	70.0 (18.8)
CES-D Score	28.6 (14.0)

* The following medications were reported by participants (all were held constant throughout the study): duloxetine, venlafaxine, sertraline, escitalopram, trazadone, and bupropion.

At baseline, there was no significant difference in depression scores between those taking antidepressant medication and those who were not taking medication (p = 0.30) and the mean CES-D scores for both groups were in the range that indicated depression (M = 32 (14) and M = 26 (14), respectively).

Biomarkers were compared at baseline to assess any differences based on depression symptom severity according to the CES-D cut-off (see Table 2). At baseline, serum homocysteine was the only biomarker to show a significant difference based on depression symptom score. Those who were depressed, based on the CES-D, had a median homocysteine level of 11 (5.7) μmol/L as compared to 9 (2.3) μmol/L for those not meeting the cut-off for depression ($p = 0.03$).

Table 2. Characteristics of subjects with depression at baseline.

Variable	Depressed * Yes *n* (%)	Depressed * No *n* (%)	*p*-Value **
	25 (76%)	8 (24%)	
Sex			0.67
Female	9 (82%)	2 (18%)	
Male	16 (73%)	6 (27%)	
Race			0.68
Caucasian (91%)	23 (76%)	7 (23%)	
Black/African American (9%)	2 (67%)	1(33%)	
	Median (IQR)		*p*-value **
Age (years)	53 (6)	57.5 (6)	0.34
BMI at baseline (kg/mg^2)	31.0 (8.7)	31.2 (5.1)	0.58
FFQ at baseline	76 (19)	56 (27)	0.64
Homocysteine (μmoL/L)	11.3 (5.7)	9.0 (2.3)	**0.03**
Folate (ng/mL)	13.5 (9.9)	16.3 (7.6)	0.34
Vitamin B12 (pg/mL)	559 (301)	763 (461)	0.40
Cytokines:			
TNF-α (pg/mL)	2.6 (4.9)	1.8 (1.7)	0.30
IFN-γ (pg/mL)	13.9 (7.0)	10.5 (4.3)	*0.10*
IL-6 (pg/mL)	2.4 (1.8)	3.1 (1.9)	0.27
IL-1β (pg/mL)	11.2 (4.3)	11.0 (3.1)	0.92

* "Depressed" at baseline is defined as a score of ≥16 using CES-D. ** Mann–Whitney. Bold font indicates significant difference. Italics indicates marginally significant differences based on alpha 0.05.

Notably, a higher range of serum homocysteine levels was evident in the subjects who met the cut-off score for depression, reaching as high as 22 μmol/L, whereas those who scored <16 on the CES-D scale peaked at 11 μmol/L (see Figure 1).

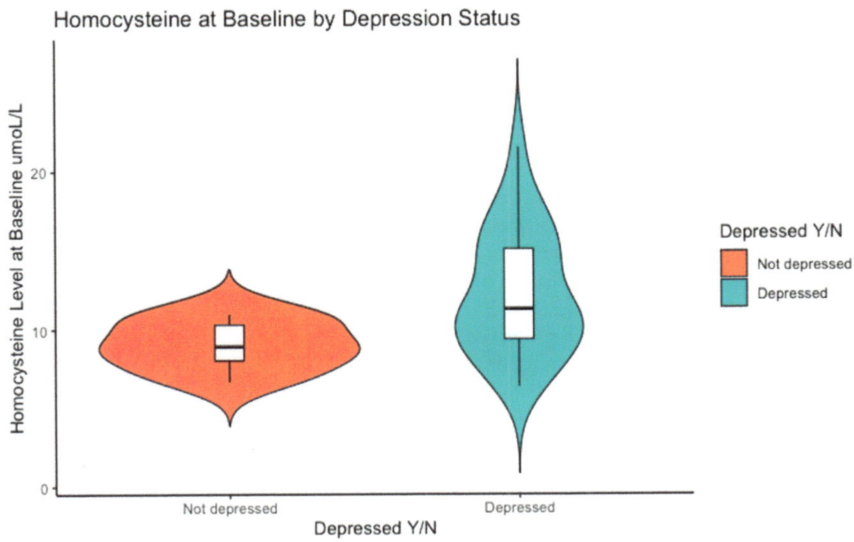

Figure 1. Baseline median concentration of serum homocysteine. The non-depressed group had a median value of Hcy of 9 μmol/L versus 11 μmol/L in the depressed sub-group, $p = 0.03$.

The baseline levels of the cytokines IFN-γ, TNF-α, IL-6, and IL1-β did not show significant differences when comparing groups with scores above versus below the threshold for depression. However, median serum IFN-γ was 13.9 (7) pg/mL in the depressed group versus 10.5 (4.3) pg/mL for those below the depression score threshold, a marginally significant difference ($p = 0.10$). An extreme outlier was observed for IFN-γ in one non-depressed subject who had a very high serum level that was 2.8 SDs above the mean. A sensitivity analysis was completed to evaluate the level of influence of this outlier on the overall results. After removal of the outlier, there was a significant difference in median baseline serum concentrations of IFN-γ in those who were depressed compared to those who were not depressed at baseline (13.9 pg/mL versus 9.9 pg/mL, respectively ($p = 0.02$)).

3.2. Change in Depression Score and Biomarkers after 1-month Dietary Intervention

Of the 25 participants who scored in the range for depression at baseline, 96% had a reduction in depression-symptom score by an average of 40% after one month on the low-glutamate diet. Participant dietary adherence was high based on the reported reduced intake of excitotoxic foods from baseline to post-diet, measured by the specialized excitotoxin FFQ score ($p < 0.001$). Table 3 shows the change in all measures from pre-diet to post-diet.

Table 3. Changes from baseline to post-diet ($n = 33$).

	Pre-Diet (Baseline)	Post-Diet	*p*-Value *
	Mean (SD)		
CES-D Score	28.6 (14.1)	18.5 (12)	**<0.001**
Dietary Adherence (Excitotoxin FFQ)	70.0 (18.8)	7.3 (9.0)	**<0.001**
Homocysteine (µmoL/L)	11.5 (3.7)	11.5 (3.4)	0.85
Folate (ng/mL)	14.7 (6.3)	13.0 (5.4)	**0.04**
TNF-α (pg/mL)	3.1 (2.7)	3.9 (3.3)	0.30
IFN-γ (pg/mL)	13.7 (5.6)	11.4 (4.3)	*0.08*
	Median (IQR)		*p*-value †
Vitamin B12 (pg/mL)	572 (333)	574 (445)	0.72
IL-6 (pg/mL)	2.9 (1.5)	2.6 (0.9)	1.00
IL1-β (pg/mL)	11.2 (4.3)	9.9 (3.2)	0.78

* Paired samples *t*-test. † Wilcoxon signed-rank test. Bold font indicates significant difference; italic text indicates marginally significant differences based on alpha of 0.05.

After one month on the low-glutamate diet, participants had a significant reduction in depression scores as measured by the CES-D, and this was true whether or not participants were taking antidepressant medication (see Figure 2).

No significant reductions were observed for homocysteine or the inflammatory cytokines after one month on the low-glutamate diet; however, IFN-γ was marginally reduced ($p = 0.08$). The cytokine TNF-α did not reach a level of significance in paired tests; however, the decrease in TNF-α concentrations was strongly correlated with excitotoxin FFQ dietary adherence (see Figure 3), indicating that as consumption of dietary excitotoxins is reduced, TNF-α levels are lowered.

The median serum folate concentration was significantly reduced from the dietary intervention ($p = 0.04$), but there was no evidence of dietary deficiency or insufficiency in folate either at baseline or post-diet. The reduction in folate was likely due to participants not adequately incorporating natural food sources of folate (e.g., green leafy vegetables, beans, etc.) as they reduced their intake of processed foods, which tend to be fortified with folic acid.

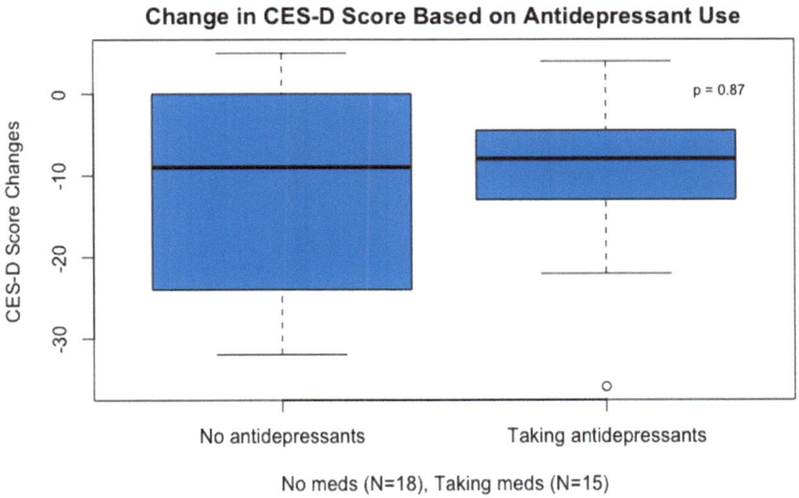

Figure 2. The change in mean depression scores for those subjects who did not take antidepressant medication (11-point mean drop on the CES-D scale) was similar to the change for those not taking medication (10-point drop). It should be noted that one participant's score was an outlier (in the medication group), with a greater than 30-point reduction in their CES-D score.

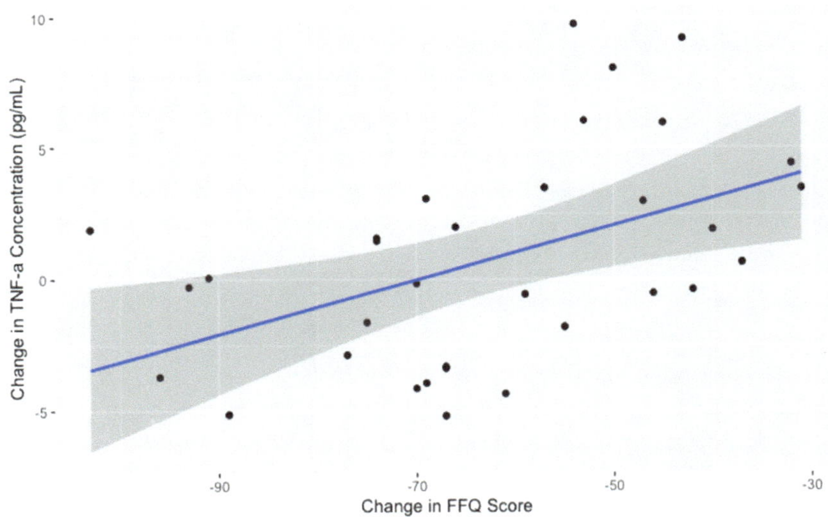

Figure 3. TNF-α and dietary adherence, measured as change in the excitotoxin FFQ ($r = 0.50$, $p < 0.01$). Greater reduction in free glutamate/aspartate in the diet was positively correlated with reduced serum TNF-α. The black dots represent individual participant excitotoxin FFQ score change (x-axis) and TNF-α blood concentration change (pg/mL) (y-axis). The blue line represents the smoothed trend line, with the 95% confidence interval shaded in gray.

3.3. Binary Measure of Depression Improvement

To better understand the biomarker changes that may have been associated with depression improvement, a binary measure was created based on either a reduction in CES-D score by 30% or a drop to below the cut-off of 16. By this measure, 52% of the study participants were considered "improved" ($p = 0.02$) after one month on the low-glutamate diet (see Figure 4).

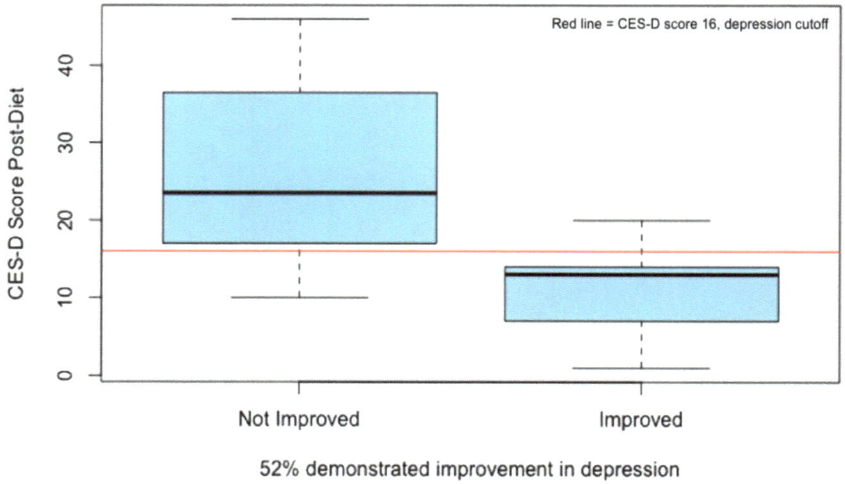

Figure 4. Post-diet CES-D scores based on a binary variable for depression improvement. A total of 52% of participants ($n = 17$) demonstrated ≥30% improvement in CES-D score and/or dropped below the threshold for depression (score of 16) indicated by the red line [27].

Using the binary measure for depression improvement, Table 4 compares serum homocysteine, vitamin, and cytokine measures between those who did and did not experience improvement in depression scores after one month on the low-glutamate diet.

Table 4. Characteristics of depression improvement.

Variable	Depression Improved [1]		
	Yes	No	
	17 (52%)	16 (48%)	
	Median (IQR)		*p*-Value [†]
Age (years)	54 (8.0)	53 (7.5)	0.34
BMI Change (kg/mg^2)	−0.47 (0.85)	−0.41 (1.0)	0.94
Excitotoxin FFQ Change	−70.0 (10)	−54.5 (18)	**<0.01**
Homocysteine Change (μmoL/L)	−0.60 (1.5)	0.55 (1.3)	*0.10*
Folate Change (ng/mL)	−0.70 (4.6)	−4.4 (6.4)	*0.07*
Vitamin B12 Change (ng/mL)	−1.0 (217)	−15.5 (140)	0.80
Cytokine Change:			
TNF-α (pg/mL)	−0.29 (4.9)	1.9 (4.6)	0.20
IFN-γ (pg/mL)	−5.0 (11.8)	0.31 (8.3)	*0.08*
IL-6 (pg/mL)	0.01 (1.5)	0.20 (2.1)	0.82
IL1-β (pg/mL)	0.67 (6.2)	−0.39 (3.4)	0.89

[1] Depression improvement is defined as a ≥30% reduction in CES-D scores and/or a drop from at or above the threshold for depression (score of 16) to below the threshold. [†] Wilcoxon rank-sum test. Bold font indicates significant difference; italic font indicates marginally significant difference based on alpha of 0.05.

The reduction in dietary intake of excitotoxic foods was notably greater among those who had depression improvement, indicating a larger reduction in self-reported consumption of foods containing free glutamate and aspartate during the one-month intervention period ($p < 0.01$). Notably, serum homocysteine levels appeared to be reduced in those who had depression improvement, but increased in those who did not, though this did not reach statistical significance ($p = 0.10$). The cytokine IFN-γ also appeared to be more reduced in those who experienced depression symptom improvement compared to those who did not, but again, this biomarker change was shy of statistical significance ($p = 0.08$).

3.4. Modeling Results

A multivariable linear regression analysis showed that there was a significant association between change in total homocysteine and change in CES-D depression score after one month on the low-glutamate diet, after adjustment for potential confounding factors, (ß = 2.58, $p = 0.04$), F-statistic = 2.54 (5,27), $p = 0.05$, $R^2 = 0.32$, with the proposed model:

$$\text{CES-D Change} = 17.8 + 2.58 * \text{Hcy Change} + 0.20 * \text{FFQ Change} + 4.97 * \text{Sex} - 0.32 * \text{Age} - 2.11 * \text{BMI Change} \quad (1)$$

Folate and vitamin B12 were assessed for potential mediating effects on this linear relationship. While the direct effect of folate as a predictor had a marginally significant impact on homocysteine change (F = 3.345 (1, 31), ($p = 0.08$)), formal mediation was not supported since homocysteine change remained significant regardless of folate being included in the model. Furthermore, formal mediation by vitamin B12 was not observed since depression symptom improvement could not be attributed to changes associated with vitamin B12.

Logistic regression modeling was also used to assess the likelihood of depression improvement. The change in serum level of homocysteine was not associated with a significantly increased likelihood of depression improvement in logistic regression modeling: OR (95% CI) = 1.37 (−0.16, 0.79), ($p = 0.20$). However, a greater reduction in serum IFN-γ levels after one month on the low-glutamate diet was marginally associated with a higher likelihood of depression improvement: OR (95% CI) = 1.11 (0.00, 1.42), ($p = 0.06$) after controlling for age, sex, race, BMI change, and FFQ change.

4. Discussion

Biomarkers are needed to better understand and monitor the metabolic and immunoinflammatory changes that relate to depression symptom changes. This study showed that homocysteine and the inflammatory cytokine IFN-γ may serve as potential biomarkers for depression improvement among veterans with GWI.

There appeared to be strong adherence to the low-glutamate diet shown by the self-reported significant reduction in excitotoxic food intake. A greater reduction in excitotoxic food intake, as indicated by the excitotoxin FFQ change score, predicted greater depression improvement [28]. This is in alignment with animal research investigating the effect of glutamate on depression-like behavior. A rodent study demonstrated that exogenous glutamate delivered via food consumption, gavage, or intravenous administration resulted in behavioral changes and elevated symptoms of stress-induced depression behavior [6].

Homocysteine is directly related to glutamatergic dysregulation, where it has the ability to directly agonize the NMDA glutamate receptor [29], which can lead to depression symptoms [11,30]. Baseline serum homocysteine levels in our study reflected this relationship, with significantly higher levels of serum homocysteine in depressed subjects as compared to those without depression. Further, after one month on the low-glutamate diet, reduction in serum homocysteine was significantly associated with a reduction in the CES-D score.

Serum levels of homocysteine above 10 µmol/L have been associated with depression in several studies [13], including the Rotterdam Study involving 3,884 elderly subjects who were screened for depression using the CES-D [31]. In another study, median homocysteine levels of 14.7 µmol/L were found in 89 depressed adolescents and children, compared to 43 controls with levels of 10.2 µmol/L ($p < 0.001$) [32]. Moreover, higher serum homocysteine levels increase the odds of having depression, with the highest odds at levels above 15 mmol/L, according to the Hordaland Homocysteine Study involving 5948 adult subjects [33]. Elevated concentrations of homocysteine were also found to be a risk factor for depression in a two-year longitudinal study involving 732 Korean adults, wherein no interaction was evident between folate and vitamin B12 with homocysteine, and there was little evidence of confounding factors such as disability, cardiovascular disease, or lifestyle factors [34].

However, not all studies are consistent with these findings. In order to control for confounding factors related to homocysteine, a twin study involving U.S. veterans of the Vietnam War who were discordant for depression (n = 55 pairs) found no differences in homocysteine concentrations in the twin pairs based on depression status [30]. The researchers concluded that homocysteine levels were incidental to confounders, including high stress, reduced exercise, or other causes not directly associated with depression; however, a significant between-pair effect was observed, with higher depression scores (based on the Beck Depression Inventory (BDI)) being associated with higher homocysteine levels at the pair-level ($p < 0.001$) [30]. The Rotterdam Study also identified cardiovascular risk and functional disabilities as confounders for elevated homocysteine in depressed subjects [31].

Elevated levels of homocysteine are also associated with age, sex, race, high stress, and genetic abnormalities that cause homocystinuria; however, supplements of folate and SAM alone have been successfully used as therapeutic treatments for depression, suggesting that disrupted cellular methylation can be improved with dietary change and result in symptom improvement for certain depression sub-types [13].

Our study did not support the role of either folate or vitamin B12 as mediators for homocysteine change with depression improvement. No deficiency or insufficiency of either vitamin was evident at baseline or post-diet; therefore, the observed reduction in homocysteine post-diet should not be attributed to changes in serum folate or vitamin B12.

Serum levels of the cytokine IFN-γ were significantly reduced post-diet, and the levels of TNF-α also trended downward and strongly correlated with a greater reduction in consumption of excitotoxic foods, as measured by excitotoxin FFQ score change. Reduced cytokine levels may have influenced the activation of the kynurenine pathway. Dysregulation of the kynurenine pathway is a known factor contributing to the pathophysiology of depression. The inflammatory cytokines IFN-γ and TNF-α are suggested inducers for the kynurenine pathway that stimulate the expression of the enzyme indoleamine 2,3 di-oxygenase (IDO), which catabolizes tryptophan [35,36]. Activation of the kynurenine pathway shunts tryptophan away from the synthesis of serotonin and melatonin, and towards the production of kynurenine, which produces downstream metabolites, including neurotoxic quinolinic acid (QA), which can over-activate the NMDA glutamate receptor [37,38]. Evidence for the association between increased levels of the cytokine TNF-α and IDO has been found in rodent studies of stress-induced depression, where stress caused the upregulation of IDO in the cortex [36]. Upon the administration of an antidepressant, reduced symptoms of depression were accompanied by a reduction in both IDO and TNF-α levels in the frontal cortex [36]. Even stronger data suggest an association between IFN-γ and activation of IDO, with IFN-γ actually being used as an inducer of IDO in animal studies [35,39–41]. Moreover, there are strong data to suggest that IFN-γ treatment is an inducer of depression in cancer patients [42].

This is the first known study to evaluate changes in homocysteine and inflammatory cytokines relative to improvement in depression in veterans with Gulf War Illness. One of the strengths of this study was that females represented one third of participants in the study (33%). This is important since the Gulf War had a higher ratio of females than any prior military action and since female deployed veterans of the Gulf War have shown a higher risk of suicide than non-deployed Gulf War female veterans [4]. Participants also represented a wide range of geographical areas of the United States. There was evidence of adequate adherence to dietary protocols achieved by the participants as indicated by the change in the excitotoxin FFQ scores from baseline to post-diet ($p < 0.001$).

5. Limitations and Future Directions

This study was limited by its small sample size, which reduced statistical power for these analyses, and limited diversity of the sample. Future research should include a more ethnically and gender diverse sample. The balance of depressed versus non-depressed subjects was not equal due to this not being a criterion for entry into the study. Moreover, psychotherapeutic treatments were not assessed during the dietary intervention period, though participants were asked to keep their psychotherapy stable across the study period, similar to keeping their medication use stable. Also, many participants in this study had a BMI in the range of obesity (BMI > 30 kg/m^2), which limits our ability to extrapolate these findings to normal-weight individuals. To analyze the potential confounding effect of obesity on the chronic release of inflammatory cytokines, future research should include participants not exhibiting obesity as a comorbid condition [43]. Future research could also include collection of the blood level of vitamins B6 and riboflavin (B2) to verify whether dietary nutrient composition may have improved the efficiency of the metabolic pathways of one-carbon metabolism. A measure of quinolinic acid produced by activation of the kynurenine pathway would also be pertinent to future research, as it may indicate whether inflammatory mechanisms are leading tryptophan metabolism away from the production of serotonin and melatonin, and toward the kynurenine pathway. A measure of plasma glutamate should also be included to verify whether dietary intake changes are correlated with a change in plasma levels of free glutamate, so that self-reported excitotoxin FFQ scores are not relied upon as the sole measure of dietary adherence.

6. Conclusions

This study demonstrated that serum homocysteine and the cytokine IFN-γ may serve as possible biomarkers for depression improvement in GWI using a low-glutamate diet. Both biomarkers were elevated at baseline in subjects with depression. Changes in serum homocysteine levels were significantly associated with CES-D score reduction, and the cytokine IFN-γ was marginally able to predict depression improvement after one month on the low-glutamate diet. Future larger-scale research is needed to better understand the metabolic and inflammatory mechanisms associated with depression in Gulf War veterans and to assess the viability and reliability of biomarkers as a tool to evaluate depression improvement. If results from future larger clinical trials confirm the use of the low-glutamate diet for depression improvement among veterans with Gulf War Illness, this diet could be used in the future as an adjunct clinical treatment for depression in this group. These results also suggest that future clinical trials to test this dietary approach as a treatment for depression alone may also be warranted.

Supplementary Materials: The following supporting information can be downloaded at https://www.mdpi.com/article/10.3390/nu16142255/s1, Table S1: Excitotoxin Food Frequency Questionnaire.

Author Contributions: Conceptualization, A.A.M. and K.F.H.; methodology, A.A.M. and K.F.H.; software, A.A.M.; validation, A.A.M. and K.F.H.; formal analysis, A.A.M.; investigation, K.F.H.; resources, A.A.M. and K.F.H.; data curation, A.A.M. and K.F.H.; writing—original draft preparation, A.A.M.; writing—review and editing, A.A.M. and K.F.H.; visualization, A.A.M.; supervision, K.F.H.; project administration, K.F.H.; funding acquisition, K.F.H. All authors have read and agreed to the published version of the manuscript.

Funding: The original research from which this secondary analysis was completed was funded by the U.S. Army Medical Research Acquisition Activity, 820 Chandler Street, Fort Detrick, MD 21702-5014, which is the awarding and administering acquisition office. This work was supported by the Office of the Assistant Secretary of Defense for Health Affairs, through the Gulf War Illness Research Program under Award No. W81XWH-17-1-0457. Opinions, interpretations, conclusions, and recommendations are those of the author(s) and are not necessarily endorsed by the Department of Defense.

Institutional Review Board Statement: This study was conducted in accordance with the Declaration of Helsinki and approved by the Institutional Review Board of American University (IRB-2017-301) and the Human Research Protection Office of the Department of Defense (DOD) (HRPO Log NumberA-20203.a) for studies involving humans, approval date 12 May 2017.

Informed Consent Statement: Informed consent was obtained from all subjects involved in the study.

Data Availability Statement: This study was registered at https://clinicaltrials.gov/study/NCT03342482 (accessed on 12 January 2021).

Conflicts of Interest: The authors declare no conflicts of interest. The funders had no role in the design of the study; in the collection, analyses, or interpretation of data; in the writing of the manuscript; or in the decision to publish the results.

References

1. Dursa, E.K.; Barth, S.K.; Schneiderman, A.I.; Bossarte, R.M. Physical and Mental Health Status of Gulf War and Gulf Era Veterans: Results from a Large Population-Based Epidemiological Study. *J. Occup. Environ. Med.* **2016**, *58*, 41–46. [CrossRef] [PubMed]
2. Blore, J.D.; Sim, M.R.; Forbes, A.B.; Creamer, M.C.; Kelsall, H.L. Depression in Gulf War Veterans: A Systematic Review and Meta-Analysis. *Psychol. Med.* **2015**, *45*, 1565–1580. [CrossRef] [PubMed]
3. Fiedler, N.; Ozakinci, G.; Hallman, W.; Wartenberg, D.; Brewer, N.T.; Barrett, D.H.; Kipen, H.M. Military Deployment to the Gulf War as a Risk Factor for Psychiatric Illness among US Troops. *Br. J. Psychiatry J. Ment. Sci.* **2006**, *188*, 453–459. [CrossRef] [PubMed]
4. Barth, S.K.; Kang, H.K.; Bullman, T. All-Cause Mortality Among US Veterans of the Persian Gulf War. *Public Health Rep.* **2016**, *131*, 822–830. [CrossRef] [PubMed]
5. Brandley, E.T.; Kirkland, A.E.; Baron, M.; Baraniuk, J.N.; Holton, K.F. The Effect of the Low Glutamate Diet on the Reduction of Psychiatric Symptoms in Veterans with Gulf War Illness: A Pilot Randomized-Controlled Trial. *Front. Psychiatry* **2022**, *13*, 926688. [CrossRef] [PubMed]
6. Onaolapo, A.Y.; Onaolapo, O.J. Dietary Glutamate and the Brain: In the Footprints of a Jekyll and Hyde Molecule. *NeuroToxicology* **2020**, *80*, 93–104. [CrossRef] [PubMed]
7. Joyce, M.R.; Holton, K.F. Neurotoxicity in Gulf War Illness and the Potential Role of Glutamate. *Neurotoxicology* **2020**, *80*, 60–70. [CrossRef] [PubMed]
8. Onaolapo, A.Y.; Onaolapo, O.J. Glutamate and Depression: Reflecting a Deepening Knowledge of the Gut and Brain Effects of a Ubiquitous Molecule. *World J. Psychiatry* **2021**, *11*, 297–315. [CrossRef]
9. Bottiglieri, T.; Laundy, M.; Crellin, R.; Toone, B.K.; Carney, M.W.; Reynolds, E.H. Homocysteine, Folate, Methylation, and Monoamine Metabolism in Depression. *J. Neurol. Neurosurg. Psychiatry* **2000**, *69*, 228–232. [CrossRef]
10. Gariballa, S. Testing Homocysteine-Induced Neurotransmitter Deficiency, and Depression of Mood Hypothesis in Clinical Practice. *Age Ageing* **2011**, *40*, 702–705. [CrossRef]
11. Moradi, F.; Lotfi, K.; Armin, M.; Clark, C.C.T.; Askari, G.; Rouhani, M.H. The Association between Serum Homocysteine and Depression: A Systematic Review and Meta-Analysis of Observational Studies. *Eur. J. Clin. Investig.* **2021**, *51*, e13486. [CrossRef] [PubMed]
12. Silva, V.; Oliveira, A.; D'Almeida, V. Homocysteine and Psychiatric Disorders. *J. Inborn Errors Metab. Screen.* **2017**, *5*, 232640981770147. [CrossRef]
13. Folstein, M.; Liu, T.; Peter, I.; Buell, J.; Arsenault, L.; Scott, T.; Qiu, W.W. The Homocysteine Hypothesis of Depression. *Am. J. Psychiatry* **2007**, *164*, 861–867. [CrossRef] [PubMed]
14. Erickson, M.A.; Dohi, K.; Banks, W.A. Neuroinflammation: A Common Pathway in CNS Diseases as Mediated at the Blood-Brain Barrier. *Neuroimmunomodulation* **2012**, *19*, 121–130. [CrossRef] [PubMed]
15. Dantzer, R.; O'Connor, J.C.; Lawson, M.A.; Kelley, K.W. Inflammation-Associated Depression: From Serotonin to Kynurenine. *Psychoneuroendocrinology* **2011**, *36*, 426–436. [CrossRef] [PubMed]
16. Miller, A.H.; Raison, C.L. The Role of Inflammation in Depression: From Evolutionary Imperative to Modern Treatment Target. *Nat. Rev. Immunol.* **2016**, *16*, 22–34. [CrossRef]
17. Pinto, E.F.; Andrade, C. Interferon-Related Depression: A Primer on Mechanisms, Treatment, and Prevention of a Common Clinical Problem. *Curr. Neuropharmacol.* **2016**, *14*, 743–748. [CrossRef] [PubMed]
18. Widner, B.; Ledochowski, M.; Fuchs, D. Interferon-Gamma-Induced Tryptophan Degradation: Neuropsychiatric and Immunological Consequences. *Curr. Drug Metab.* **2000**, *1*, 193–204. [CrossRef] [PubMed]
19. Harsanyi, S.; Kupcova, I.; Danisovic, L.; Klein, M. Selected Biomarkers of Depression: What Are the Effects of Cytokines and Inflammation? *Int. J. Mol. Sci.* **2022**, *24*, 578. [CrossRef]
20. Miller, A.H.; Maletic, V.; Raison, C.L. Inflammation and Its Discontents: The Role of Cytokines in the Pathophysiology of Major Depression. *Biol. Psychiatry* **2009**, *65*, 732–741. [CrossRef]
21. Holton, K.F.; Kirkland, A.E.; Baron, M.; Ramachandra, S.S.; Langan, M.T.; Brandley, E.T.; Baraniuk, J.N. The Low Glutamate Diet Effectively Improves Pain and Other Symptoms of Gulf War Illness. *Nutrients* **2020**, *12*, 2593. [CrossRef] [PubMed]
22. Fukuda, K.; Nisenbaum, R.; Stewart, G.; Thompson, W.W.; Robin, L.; Washko, R.M.; Noah, D.L.; Barrett, D.H.; Randall, B.; Herwaldt, B.L.; et al. Chronic Multisymptom Illness Affecting Air Force Veterans of the Gulf War. *JAMA* **1998**, *280*, 981–988. [CrossRef] [PubMed]
23. Mawson, A.R.; Croft, A.M. Gulf War Illness: Unifying Hypothesis for a Continuing Health Problem. *Int. J. Environ. Res. Public Health* **2019**, *16*, 111. [CrossRef] [PubMed]

24. Vilagut, G.; Forero, C.G.; Barbaglia, G.; Alonso, J. Screening for Depression in the General Population with the Center for Epidemiologic Studies Depression (CES-D): A Systematic Review with Meta-Analysis. *PLoS ONE* **2016**, *11*, e0155431. [CrossRef] [PubMed]
25. Weissman, M.M.; Sholomskas, D.; Pottenger, M.; Prusoff, B.A.; Locke, B.Z. Assessing Depressive Symptoms in Five Psychiatric Populations: A Validation Study. *Am. J. Epidemiol.* **1977**, *106*, 203–214. [CrossRef] [PubMed]
26. Tingley, D.; Teppei, H.; Mit, Y.; Keele, L.; State, P.; Imai, K. Mediation: R Package for Causal Mediation Analysis. *J. Stat. Softw.* **2014**, *59*, 1–38. [CrossRef]
27. Andresen, E.M.; Malmgren, J.A.; Carter, W.B.; Patrick, D.L. Screening for Depression in Well Older Adults: Evaluation of a Short Form of the CES-D (Center for Epidemiologic Studies Depression Scale). *Am. J. Prev. Med.* **1994**, *10*, 77–84. [CrossRef] [PubMed]
28. Quines, C.B.; Rosa, S.G.; Da Rocha, J.T.; Gai, B.M.; Bortolatto, C.F.; Duarte, M.M.M.F.; Nogueira, C.W. Monosodium Glutamate, a Food Additive, Induces Depressive-like and Anxiogenic-like Behaviors in Young Rats. *Life Sci.* **2014**, *107*, 27–31. [CrossRef]
29. Lipton, S.A.; Kim, W.-K.; Choi, Y.-B.; Kumar, S.; D'Emilia, D.M.; Rayudu, P.V.; Arnelle, D.R.; Stamler, J.S. Neurotoxicity Associated with Dual Actions of Homocysteine at the N-Methyl-d-Aspartate Receptor. *Proc. Natl. Acad. Sci. USA* **1997**, *94*, 5923–5928. [CrossRef]
30. Bremner, J.D.; Goldberg, J.; Vaccarino, V. Plasma Homocysteine Concentrations and Depression: A Twin Study. *J. Affect. Disord. Rep.* **2021**, *4*, 100087. [CrossRef]
31. Tiemeier, H.; van Tuijl, H.R.; Hofman, A.; Meijer, J.; Kiliaan, A.J.; Breteler, M.M.B. Vitamin B12, Folate, and Homocysteine in Depression: The Rotterdam Study. *Am. J. Psychiatry* **2002**, *159*, 2099–2101. [CrossRef]
32. Esnafoglu, E.; Ozturan, D.D. The Relationship of Severity of Depression with Homocysteine, Folate, Vitamin B12, and Vitamin D Levels in Children and Adolescents. *Child Adolesc. Ment. Health* **2020**, *25*, 249–255. [CrossRef]
33. Bjelland, I.; Tell, G.S.; Vollset, S.E.; Refsum, H.; Ueland, P.M. Folate, Vitamin B12, Homocysteine, and the MTHFR 677C→T Polymorphism in Anxiety and Depression: The Hordaland Homocysteine Study. *Arch. Gen. Psychiatry* **2003**, *60*, 618–626. [CrossRef] [PubMed]
34. Kim, J.-M.; Stewart, R.; Kim, S.-W.; Yang, S.-J.; Shin, I.-S.; Yoon, J.-S. Predictive Value of Folate, Vitamin B12 and Homocysteine Levels in Late-Life Depression. *Br. J. Psychiatry J. Ment. Sci.* **2008**, *192*, 268–274. [CrossRef] [PubMed]
35. Duda, W.; Curzytek, K.; Kubera, M.; Connor, T.J.; Fagan, E.M.; Basta-Kaim, A.; Trojan, E.; Papp, M.; Gruca, P.; Budziszewska, B.; et al. Interaction of the Immune-Inflammatory and the Kynurenine Pathways in Rats Resistant to Antidepressant Treatment in Model of Depression. *Int. Immunopharmacol.* **2019**, *73*, 527–538. [CrossRef]
36. Liu, Y.-N.; Peng, Y.-L.; Liu, L.; Wu, T.-Y.; Zhang, Y.; Lian, Y.-J.; Yang, Y.-Y.; Kelley, K.W.; Jiang, C.-L.; Wang, Y.-X. TNFα Mediates Stress-Induced Depression by Upregulating Indoleamine 2,3-Dioxygenase in a Mouse Model of Unpredictable Chronic Mild Stress. *Eur. Cytokine Netw.* **2015**, *26*, 15–25. [CrossRef]
37. Miura, H.; Ozaki, N.; Sawada, M.; Isobe, K.; Ohta, T.; Nagatsu, T. A Link between Stress and Depression: Shifts in the Balance between the Kynurenine and Serotonin Pathways of Tryptophan Metabolism and the Etiology and Pathophysiology of Depression. *Stress Amst. Neth.* **2008**, *11*, 198–209. [CrossRef] [PubMed]
38. Myint, A.M.; Kim, Y.K. Cytokine-Serotonin Interaction through IDO: A Neurodegeneration Hypothesis of Depression. *Med. Hypotheses* **2003**, *61*, 519–525. [CrossRef] [PubMed]
39. Dantzer, R. Role of the Kynurenine Metabolism Pathway in Inflammation-Induced Depression: Preclinical Approaches. *Curr. Top. Behav. Neurosci.* **2017**, *31*, 117–138. [CrossRef]
40. Sarkar, S.A.; Wong, R.; Hackl, S.I.; Moua, O.; Gill, R.G.; Wiseman, A.; Davidson, H.W.; Hutton, J.C. Induction of Indoleamine 2,3-Dioxygenase by Interferon-Gamma in Human Islets. *Diabetes* **2007**, *56*, 72–79. [CrossRef]
41. Taylor, M.W.; Feng, G.S. Relationship between Interferon-Gamma, Indoleamine 2,3-Dioxygenase, and Tryptophan Catabolism. *FASEB J. Off. Publ. Fed. Am. Soc. Exp. Biol.* **1991**, *5*, 2516–2522.
42. Castro, F.; Cardoso, A.P.; Gonçalves, R.M.; Serre, K.; Oliveira, M.J. Interferon-Gamma at the Crossroads of Tumor Immune Surveillance or Evasion. *Front. Immunol.* **2018**, *9*, 847. [CrossRef]
43. Miller, G.E.; Freedland, K.E.; Carney, R.M.; Stetler, C.A.; Banks, W.A. Pathways Linking Depression, Adiposity, and Inflammatory Markers in Healthy Young Adults. *Brain Behav. Immun.* **2003**, *17*, 276–285. [CrossRef]

nutrients

Article

The Effects of Testosterone on Hypothalamic and Serum Oxytocin Levels Are Affected by the Estrogen Milieu in Female Rats

Moeka Arata [1], Kou Tamura [1], Hidenori Aoki [1], Hiroki Noguchi [1], Asuka Takeda [1], Saki Minato [1], Shota Yamamoto [1,2], Riyo Kinouchi [1], Kanako Yoshida [1], Yuri Yamamoto [1], Takashi Kaji [1] and Takeshi Iwasa [1,*]

1 Department of Obstetrics and Gynecology, Institute of Biomedical Sciences, Tokushima University Graduate School, 3-18-15 Kuramoto-cho, Tokushima 770-8503, Japan; arata.moeka@tokushima-u.ac.jp (M.A.)
2 Department of Renal and Genitourinary Surgery, Graduate School of Medicine, Hokkaido University, Sapporo 060-0808, Japan
* Correspondence: iwasa.takeshi@tokushima-u.ac.jp; Tel.: +81-88-633-7177

Abstract: Previous studies have suggested that the effects of androgens on body weight (BW) and appetite are affected by the estrogen milieu in females; however, the mechanism underlying these effects remains unclear. We hypothesized that androgens may affect endogenous oxytocin (OT), which is a hypothalamic anorectic factor, and that these effects of androgens may be altered by the estrogen milieu in females. To investigate this hypothesis, in the present study, we examined the effects of testosterone on peripheral and central OT levels in ovariectomized female rats that did or did not receive estradiol supplementation. Ovariectomized female rats were randomly divided into non-estradiol-supplemented or estradiol-supplemented groups, and half of the rats in each group were concurrently supplemented with testosterone (i.e., rats were divided into four groups, $n = 7$ per each group). We also measured peripheral and central OT receptor (OTR) gene expression levels. As a result, we found that testosterone increased serum and hypothalamic OT levels and OT receptor mRNA levels in non-estradiol-supplemented rats, whereas it had no effects on these factors in estradiol-supplemented rats. In addition, testosterone reduced food intake, BW gain, and fat weight in non-estradiol-supplemented rats, whereas it did not have any effects on BW, appetite, or fat weight in estradiol-supplemented rats. These findings indicate that the effects of androgens on OT may be affected by the estrogen milieu, and elevated OT levels may be related to the blunting of appetite and prevention of obesity under estrogen-deficient conditions.

Keywords: oxytocin; estrogen; androgen

Citation: Arata, M.; Tamura, K.; Aoki, H.; Noguchi, H.; Takeda, A.; Minato, S.; Yamamoto, S.; Kinouchi, R.; Yoshida, K.; Yamamoto, Y.; et al. The Effects of Testosterone on Hypothalamic and Serum Oxytocin Levels Are Affected by the Estrogen Milieu in Female Rats. *Nutrients* **2024**, *16*, 2533. https://doi.org/10.3390/nu16152533

Academic Editor: Pilar Codoñer-Franch

Received: 28 May 2024
Revised: 30 July 2024
Accepted: 30 July 2024
Published: 2 August 2024

1. Introduction

Estrogen, a sex steroid hormone, has a variety of beneficial effects in women and is also involved in the maintenance of nutrient metabolism, i.e., it plays an important role in the regulation of food intake (FI) and preventing excessive body weight (BW) gain in women [1–3]. On the other hand, the roles of androgens in FI, energy metabolism, and BW regulation in women have not been fully investigated. Although several studies have indicated that androgens increase FI and fat weight in women of reproductive age [4–7], their effects in other women, e.g., post-menopausal women, remain unclear. Interestingly, it has been shown that androgens have favorable effects on metabolic maintenance in men. For example, testosterone, a representative androgen, has been suggested to play an important role in the prevention of excess weight gain and obesity. Thus, we hypothesized that the effects of androgens on female nutrient metabolism may depend on the estrogen milieu, i.e., they may have unfavorable effects in the presence of estrogen and favorable effects or less effectiveness in estrogen-deficient conditions. To further investigate this hypothesis, we compared the effects of testosterone on BW regulation in ovariectomized

(OVX) rats that did or did not receive estradiol supplementation. As a result, we found that testosterone promoted weight gain and obesity under estradiol-supplemented conditions but had inhibitory effects on weight gain and obesity under non-estrogen-supplemented conditions. These results support our hypothesis [1]. However, the neuroendocrine mechanisms underlying these estrogen-dependent differences in the effects of testosterone could not be determined in our experiments.

To examine these mechanisms, we focused on oxytocin (OT), which is a hormone involved in metabolism that is affected by sex steroid hormones. OT is an amino acid neuropeptide that is produced in the paraventricular nucleus of the hypothalamus and the supraoptic nucleus. It acts on G-protein-coupled OT receptors (OTRs) and influences several behaviors, including social behavior, reproduction, and lactation [8]. Recently, it has been revealed that OT plays an important role in BW and appetite regulation. OTR-deficient mice exhibited late-onset obesity accompanied by increased amounts of abdominal fat and impaired cold-induced thermogenesis [9]. In addition, the administration of OT has been shown to ameliorate metabolic and nutritional disorders, causing reductions in BW, appetite, and fat mass in many species, including humans [10–17]. These results indicate that both endogenous and exogenous OT have favorable effects on BW regulation and prevent obesity and adiposity in many species. Furthermore, our previous studies indicated that the effects of OT are affected by the gonadal steroid milieu, and that the effects of the gonadal steroid milieu on appetite and BW regulation may be mediated by OT [18–21]. Namely, hypothalamic and peripheral levels of OT in OVX rats were lower than those seen in OVX rats that received estradiol supplementation [20]. Similarly, serum OT levels in women of reproductive age were increased under hyperestrogenic conditions [21]. On the other hand, peripheral OT levels in female rats that received androgen supplementation were lower than those seen in intact female rats [10,18]. The administration of exogenous OT decreased FI, BW, and fat weight in the former (androgen-supplemented) rats [10,18]. In diseases such as PCOS, hyperandrogenism is known to increase the risk of obesity and nutritional metabolic diseases before menopause. In contrast, it has been suggested that these risks are reduced after menopause. In the present study, we hypothesized that androgens prevent overeating and obesity by increasing OT levels in postmenopausal women. On the other hand, it is hypothesized that these mechanisms are not invoked in the premenopausal period, making the risk of obesity and nutritional metabolic diseases more likely.

Based on our results, we hypothesized that the effects of testosterone on endogenous OT levels in females may be altered by the estrogen milieu, and that such diverse effects may be related to the abovementioned differences in the effects of testosterone on BW and appetite observed in our previous study. To investigate this hypothesis, in this study, we examined OT levels, FI, BW gain, and body fat in OVX female rats that received chronic testosterone administration with or without estradiol supplementation. In addition, peripheral and central OTR levels were also measured. This is because the mRNA expression levels of the OTR are greatly affected by female gonadal steroid hormones [21].

2. Materials and Methods

2.1. Animals

Eight-week-old Wistar female adult rats (200–230 g) were purchased from Charles River Laboratories Japan, Inc. (Kanagawa, Japan), and kept in a room under controlled light (12 h light, 12 h darkness; lights turned on at 08:00 and turned off at 20:00) and temperature (24 °C) conditions, with food and water provided ad libitum. In total, 28 rats were used in this study. All animal experiments were carried out according to the ethical standards of the institutional animal care and use committee of the University of Tokushima. Ovariectomy, tube implantation, and decapitation were carried out as in our previous study [1]. At 9 weeks of age, rats were ovariectomized bilaterally and housed individually after the surgery. The data and samples from these animals were already used for our previous study, and part of the data about body composition and samples were randomly selected for our present study. Thus, part of the results presented in this study, i.e., data about body composition, were included in our previous study. On the other hand, the main outcomes, i.e., OT, OTR, and hormone levels, were newly measured for our present study and not published previously.

2.2. *Effects of Chronic Testosterone Administration on Ovariectomized Rats That Did Not Receive Estradiol Supplementation (OVX)*

Four weeks after undergoing an ovariectomy (at 13 weeks of age), the rats were randomly assigned to a testosterone-treated (testosterone) or untreated (control) group ($n = 7$ per group). In the testosterone group, a silastic tube filled with crystalline testosterone (inner diameter: 3 mm, outer diameter: 5 mm, length of the filled part: 30 mm) (As One Co., Ltd., Tokyo, Japan) was implanted into each rat (De Vries et al., 1994 [22]). In the control group, an empty tube was implanted into each rat. At 16 days after the implantation procedure, the rats were sacrificed by decapitation after their BW and cumulative FI had been measured. The brain, blood, visceral fat (parametrial, perirenal, and mesenteric deposits), and subcutaneous fat (the inguinal deposit) were collected. The weights of the visceral fat and subcutaneous fat were measured, and tissue samples (around 300–400 mm^3) of the visceral (parametrial) and subcutaneous fat were dissected out. Serum and tissue samples were stored, and other tissue samples of visceral and subcutaneous fat were fixed as in our previous study [1].

2.3. *Effects of Chronic Testosterone Administration on Ovariectomized Rats That Received Estradiol Supplementation (OVX + E2)*

Four weeks after undergoing an ovariectomy (at 13 weeks of age), all of the rats were implanted with a silastic tube filled with crystalline estradiol (length of the filled part: 3 mm) (Le et al., 2014 [23]). At the same time, the rats were assigned to either the testosterone or control group, as described above ($n = 7$ per group). At 16 days after the implantation procedure, the rats were sacrificed by decapitation and the weight of each collected tissue was measured, and then samples were collected and stored or fixed, as described above.

2.4. *Hormone Assay*

Whole blood was centrifuged at 3000 rpm for 20 min at 4 °C, and the serum was sent to a commercial laboratory (SRL, Tokyo, Japan), where its OT levels were measured using a chemiluminescent enzyme immunoassay (ASKA Pharma Medical Co., Ltd., Kanagawa, Japan). The limit of detection for serum OT was 15 pg/mL.

2.5. *Quantitative Real-Time Polymerase Chain Reaction*

Whole hypothalamic explants were dissected from frozen brains, as described previously [18]. Total RNA was isolated and then cDNA was synthesized. PCR analysis was performed, and the mRNA expression levels of OT and the OTR were quantified. The mRNA expression levels were normalized to that of a housekeeping gene.

2.6. *Statistical Analyses*

All results are expressed as the means ± standard error of the mean (SEM). A Student's *t*-test for data with equal variances or a Mann–Whitney U test for data with high variance were used for statistical analyses. *p*-values < 0.05 were considered to be significant. Cohen's d (small effect = 0.2, medium effect = 0.5, large effect = 0.8) and r (small effect = 0.1, medium effect = 0.3, large effect = 0.5) are reported when analyses were undertaken by a Student's *t*-test and Mann–Whitney U test, respectively. Spearman's rank correlation coefficient was used for correlation analysis.

3. Results

3.1. Effects of Chronic Testosterone Administration on BW and FI in Ovariectomized Rats That Did (OVX + E2) or Did Not (OVX) Receive Estradiol Supplementation

In the OVX group, there were no significant differences in BW after implantation between the testosterone and control groups. Cumulative FI after implantation was significantly lower in the testosterone group than in the control group (Mann–Whitney U test: $p = 0.048$, U = 9, r = 0.53) (Figure 1A). In the OVX + E2 group, there were no significant differences in BW after implantation between the testosterone and control groups. Similarly, there were no significant differences in cumulative FI after implantation between the testosterone and control groups (Figure 1B).

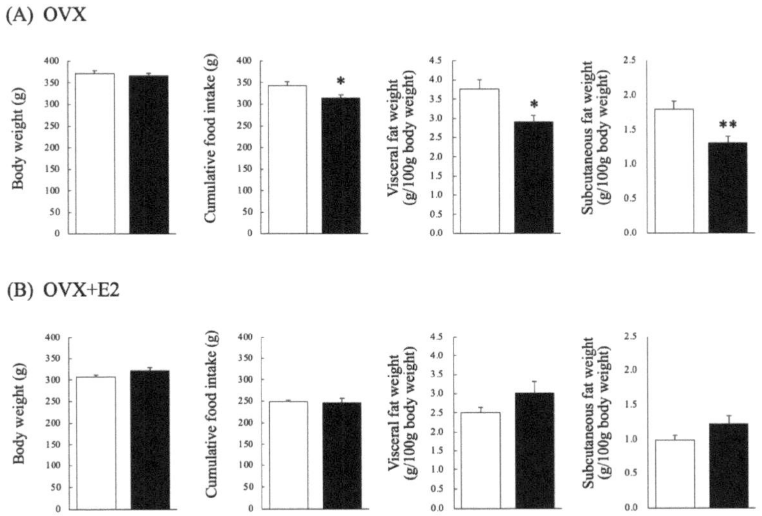

Figure 1. Body weight (BW), cumulative food intake (FI), visceral fat weight (g/100 g BW), and subcutaneous fat weight (g/100 g BW) in control (□) and testosterone-administered (■) female rats. The upper and lower rows show the results for ovariectomized rats that (**A**) did not (OVX) and (**B**) did (OVX + E2) receive estrogen supplementation, respectively. $n = 7$ per group. Data are expressed as means ± SEM. * $p < 0.05$, ** $p < 0.01$.

3.2. Effects of Chronic Testosterone Administration on Visceral Fat Weight and Subcutaneous Fat Weight in Ovariectomized Rats That Did (OVX + E2) or Did Not (OVX) Receive Estradiol Supplementation

In the OVX group, visceral fat weight (g/100 g BW) was significantly lower in the testosterone group than in the control group (Mann–Whitney U test: $p = 0.011$; U = 5, r = 0.67). Similarly, subcutaneous fat weight (g/100 g BW) was significantly lower in the testosterone group than in the control group (Student's t-test: $p < 0.01$; df = 12, t = 3.301, d = 1.60) (Figure 1A). In the OVX + E2 group, there were no significant differences in visceral fat weight (g/100 g BW) between the testosterone and control groups (Figure 1B).

3.3. Effects of Chronic Testosterone Administration on Serum OT Levels in Ovariectomized Rats That Did (OVX + E2) or Did Not (OVX) Receive Estradiol Supplementation

In the OVX group, the testosterone group exhibited significantly higher serum OT levels than the control group (Student's t-test: $p = 0.004$; df = 12, t = −3.607, d = 1.93) (Figure 2A). In the OVX + E2 group, there were no significant differences in serum OT levels between the testosterone and control groups (Figure 2B).

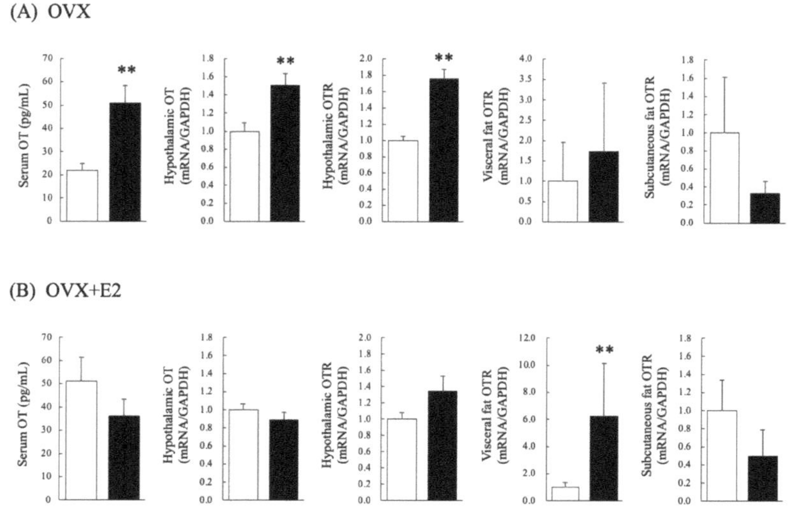

Figure 2. Serum OT concentrations, hypothalamic mRNA levels of OT and the OTR, and visceral and subcutaneous fat OTR mRNA levels in control (□) and testosterone-administered (■) female rats. The upper and lower rows show the results for ovariectomized rats that (**A**) did not (OVX) and (**B**) did (OVX + E2) receive estrogen supplementation, respectively. $n = 7$ per group. Data are expressed as means ± SEM. ** $p < 0.01$.

3.4. Effects of Chronic Testosterone Administration on Hypothalamic OT mRNA Levels, and Hypothalamic, Visceral Fat, and Subcutaneous Fat OTR mRNA Levels in Ovariectomized Rats That Did (OVX + E2) or Did Not (OVX) Receive Estradiol Supplementation

In the OVX group, hypothalamic mRNA levels of OT and the OTR were significantly higher in the testosterone group than in the control group (Student's *t*-test: hypothalamic OT: $p < 0.01$, df = 12, t = −3.137, d = 5.30; Mann–Whitney U test: hypothalamic OTR: $p < 0.01$, U = 0, r = 0.84) (Figure 2A). There were no significant differences in OTR mRNA levels in visceral or subcutaneous fat between the testosterone and control groups. In the OVX + E2 group, there were no significant differences in hypothalamic mRNA levels of OT and the OTR between the testosterone and control groups (Figure 2B). The testosterone group had significantly higher visceral fat OTR mRNA levels than the control group (Mann–Whitney U test: $p = 0.000$, U = 17, r = 0.15). Subcutaneous fat OTR mRNA levels of the testosterone and control groups did not differ significantly.

3.5. Correlations between Serum Testosterone Levels and Serum or Hypothalamic OT Levels in Ovariectomized Rats That Did (OVX + E2) or Did Not (OVX) Receive Estradiol Supplementation

In the OVX group, there was no correlation between serum testosterone and OT levels, or between serum testosterone levels and hypothalamic OT mRNA levels (Figure 3A). In the OVX + E2 group, there was no correlation between serum testosterone and OT levels, or between serum testosterone levels and hypothalamic OT mRNA levels (Figure 3B).

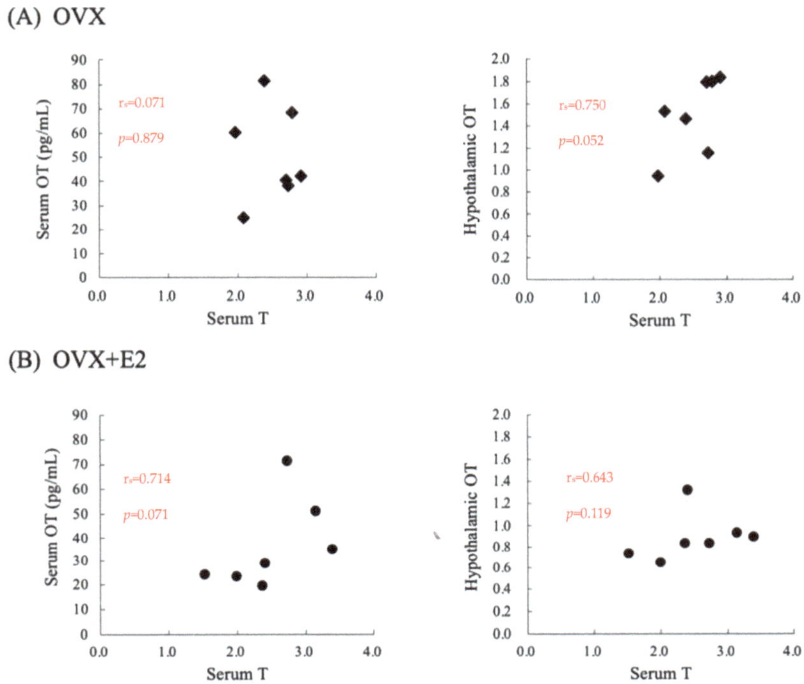

Figure 3. Correlations between serum testosterone levels and serum OT or hypothalamic OT mRNA levels. The upper and lower rows show the results for ovariectomized rats that (**A**) did not (OVX) and (**B**) did (OVX + E2) receive estrogen supplementation, respectively.

4. Discussion

Energy balance is closely related to reproductive function in most species. Estrogen and androgens (sex steroid hormones) are heavily involved in the regulation of FI, energy metabolism, and BW in mammals and humans [7]. Regarding estrogen, estrogen deficiency due to ovariectomy increases FI and BW in female animals, but these effects can be prevented by estradiol replacement, indicating that estrogen plays an important role in preventing hyperphagia and excess BW gain in females [7,24,25]. On the other hand, the roles of androgens in the regulation of FI, energy metabolism, and BW in females have not been fully evaluated; however, some studies have indicated that androgens may increase FI and promote adiposity in female animals and women of reproductive age [4–7], indicating that androgens may have effects that promote weight gain and obesity [7,24,25]. Interestingly, these effects of androgens on energy balance may be altered by the estrogen milieu, i.e., androgens increase FI, BW, and fat weight in the presence of estrogen, whereas they reduce these parameters in estrogen-deficient conditions [1]. However, the neuroendocrine mechanisms underlying the contradictory estrogen-dependent effects of androgens could not be determined in our previous studies.

In a previous study, we suggested that central and peripheral levels of OT, which are related to energy balance, are influenced by estrogen; namely, hypothalamic OT mRNA and serum OT levels are increased by estrogen in OVX female rats [20]. Similar results have been observed in human studies, i.e., serum OT levels were found to be increased under high estrogen conditions in women receiving ovarian stimulation [21]. Furthermore, it has been shown that estrogen increases OT levels via estrogen receptors (ERα) on OT-producing neurons [26–28]. Thus, we hypothesized that androgens may also affect central and peripheral OT levels, and these effects of androgens on OT may be altered by the estrogen milieu. In this study, we found that testosterone did not have any effects on serum

OT or hypothalamic OT or OTR mRNA levels under estrogen-supplemented conditions, whereas it increased both serum and hypothalamic levels of these factors under non-supplemented conditions. In addition, testosterone did not affect BW, FI, or visceral fat weight under estrogen-supplemented conditions. These findings indicate that the effects of androgens on OT may be affected by the estrogen milieu, and elevated OT levels may be related to the prevention of hyperphagia and obesity under estrogen-deficient conditions. Similar results were obtained in our previous study, in which the effects of testosterone on OT levels were evaluated in male rats, i.e., we found that testosterone increased serum OT and hypothalamic OTR mRNA levels and decreased body fat weight in male rats after orchidectomy [18]. The latter study supported our previous findings that androgens increase OT levels under estrogen-deficient conditions.

In the present study, testosterone increased visceral fat OTR mRNA levels under estrogen-supplemented conditions, whereas it did not affect visceral fat OTR mRNA levels under non-estrogen-supplemented conditions. These results regarding visceral fat levels of the OTR contradicted those concerning serum OT, hypothalamic OT, and OTR levels. Although we cannot confirm the reasons for this discrepancy, the following mechanisms might be related: Namely, testosterone may primarily act to increase OTR mRNA levels in visceral fat as seen in estrogen-supplemented conditions. However, testosterone may predominantly act to increase hypothalamic OT/OTR mRNA and serum OT levels in non-estrogen supplemented conditions, consequently, reducing visceral fat weight. In this condition, OTR mRNA levels in visceral fat may not be changed as one of the counter-regulations to prevent too much reduction in weight.

The limitations of this study are as follows: We did not find any correlation between serum testosterone levels and serum OT or hypothalamic OT mRNA levels in estrogen-supplemented or non-estrogen-supplemented conditions. We supposed that OT levels may increase when serum testosterone levels increase above a threshold level, but they may plateau if testosterone levels increase further. Future studies about the relationship between serum testosterone levels and central and peripheral OT/OTR levels should be investigated. Nonetheless, this is the first study to examine changes in the effects of testosterone on endogenous OT levels in female rats in the presence or absence of estrogen.

Also, comparisons are made between the OVX and OVX + E2 groups for this experiment. The OVX group is comparable to the OVX/E2 group as it has had ovariectomies and is, therefore, not affected by endogenous E2. In the present experiment, OT and OT receptor levels were examined to investigate the relationship between hormones and feeding factors, without focusing on the hypothalamus. Vasopressin V2 receptor (V2R) and arginine vasopressin (AVP) mRNA levels were not examined. Future research will examine the relationship with the hypothalamus.

5. Conclusions

In summary, testosterone increased OT levels and decreased FI, BW gain, and fat weight under estrogen-deficient conditions, whereas it did not affect OT levels or the aforementioned parameters under estrogen-supplemented conditions. Until now, the effects of androgens on metabolic functions in females and the mechanisms underlying these effects have remained unclear. The present study suggests that OT is a key factor in the pathophysiological roles of androgens in female metabolism.

Author Contributions: Conceptualization, T.I.; methodology, A.T., S.M., S.Y., T.K. and T.I.; validation, M.A. and T.I.; formal analysis, T.K. and T.I.; investigation, K.Y. and Y.Y.; writing—original draft preparation, M.A.; writing—review and editing, R.K. and T.I.; supervision, K.T., H.A. and H.N.; project administration, M.A.; funding acquisition, T.I. All authors have read and agreed to the published version of the manuscript.

Funding: This research received no external funding.

Institutional Review Board Statement: The animal study protocol was approved by the Ethics Committee of the University of Tokushima (protocol code T2022-102 and 24 January 2023 date of approval).

Informed Consent Statement: Not applicable.

Data Availability Statement: Data are contained within the article.

Acknowledgments: I would like to thank Tomotaka Nakagawa and Hiroaki Inui for useful discussions. I am grateful to Tomohiro Kagawa for collaboration on the early stages of this work. I wish to thank Atsuko Yoshida for advice on experimental design.

Conflicts of Interest: The authors declare no conflicts of interest.

References

1. Takeshi, I.; Matsuzaki, T.; Yano, K.; Yanagihara, R.; Tungalagsuvd, A.; Munkhzaya, M.; Mayila, Y.; Kuwahara, A.; Irahara, M. The Effects of Chronic Testosterone Administration on Body Weight, Food Intake, and Adipose Tissue Are Changed by Estrogen Treatment in Female Rats. *Horm. Behav.* **2017**, *93*, 53–61.
2. Butera Peter, C.; Beikirch, R.J. Central Implants of Diluted Estradiol: Independent Effects on Ingestive and Reproductive Behaviors of Ovariectomized Rats. *Brain Res.* **1989**, *491*, 266–273. [CrossRef] [PubMed]
3. Palmer, K.; Gray, J.M. Central vs. Peripheral Effects of Estrogen on Food Intake and Lipoprotein Lipase Activity in Ovariectomized Rats. *Physiol. Behav.* **1986**, *37*, 187–189. [CrossRef] [PubMed]
4. Lindén Hirschberg, A.; Naessén, S.; Stridsberg, M.; Byström, B.; Holte, J. Impaired Cholecystokinin Secretion and Disturbed Appetite Regulation in Women with Polycystic Ovary Syndrome. *Gynecol. Endocrinol.* **2004**, *19*, 79–87. [CrossRef] [PubMed]
5. Naessén, S.; Carlström, K.; Byström, B.; Pierre, Y.; Hirschberg, A.L. Effects of an Antiandrogenic Oral Contraceptive on Appetite and Eating Behavior in Bulimic Women. *Psychoneuroendocrinology* **2007**, *32*, 548–554. [CrossRef] [PubMed]
6. Lim, S.S.; Norman, R.J.; Clifton, P.M.; Noakes, M. Hyperandrogenemia, Psychological Distress, and Food Cravings in Young Women. *Physiol. Behav.* **2009**, *98*, 276–280. [CrossRef] [PubMed]
7. Hirschberg, A.L. Sex Hormones, Appetite and Eating Behaviour in Women. *Maturitas* **2012**, *71*, 248–256. [CrossRef]
8. Hannan, F.M.; Elajnaf, T.; Vandenberg, L.N.; Kennedy, S.H.; Thakker, R.V. Hormonal Regulation of Mammary Gland Development and Lactation. *Nat. Rev. Endocrinol.* **2023**, *19*, 46–61. [CrossRef] [PubMed]
9. Takayanagi, Y.; Kasahara, Y.; Onaka, T.; Takahashi, N.; Kawada, T.; Nishimori, K. Oxytocin Receptor-Deficient Mice Developed Late-Onset Obesity. *NeuroReport* **2008**, *19*, 951. [CrossRef]
10. Yamamoto, S.; Noguchi, H.; Takeda, A.; Arakaki, R.; Uchishiba, M.; Imaizumi, J.; Minato, S.; Kamada, S.; Kagawa, T.; Yoshida, A.; et al. Changes in Endogenous Oxytocin Levels and the Effects of Exogenous Oxytocin Administration on Body Weight Changes and Food Intake in Polycystic Ovary Syndrome Model Rats. *Int. J. Mol. Sci.* **2022**, *23*, 8207. [CrossRef]
11. Roberts, Z.S.; Wolden-Hanson, T.; Matsen, M.E.; Ryu, V.; Vaughan, C.H.; Graham, J.L.; Havel, P.J.; Chukri, D.W.; Schwartz, M.W.; Morton, G.J.; et al. Chronic Hindbrain Administration of Oxytocin Is Sufficient to Elicit Weight Loss in Diet-Induced Obese Rats. *Am. J. Physiol.-Regul. Integr. Comp. Physiol.* **2017**, *313*, R357–R371. [CrossRef] [PubMed]
12. Zhang, G.; Cai, D. Circadian Intervention of Obesity Development via Resting-Stage Feeding Manipulation or Oxytocin Treatment. *Am. J. Physiol.-Endocrinol. Metab.* **2011**, *301*, E1004–E1012. [CrossRef] [PubMed]
13. Maejima, Y.; Aoyama, M.; Sakamoto, K.; Jojima, T.; Aso, Y.; Takasu, K.; Takenosihita, S.; Shimomura, K. Impact of Sex, Fat Distribution and Initial Body Weight on Oxytocin's Body Weight Regulation. *Sci. Rep.* **2017**, *7*, 8599. [CrossRef] [PubMed]
14. Deblon, N.; Veyrat-Durebex, C.; Bourgoin, L.; Caillon, A.; Bussier, A.L.; Petrosino, S.; Piscitelli, F.; Legros, J.-J.; Geenen, V.; Foti, M.; et al. Mechanisms of the Anti-Obesity Effects of Oxytocin in Diet-Induced Obese Rats. *PLoS ONE* **2011**, *6*, e25565. [CrossRef] [PubMed]
15. Zhao, Z.; Gobrogge, K. Neurodevelopmental Model Explaining Associations between Sex Hormones, Personality, and Eating Pathology. *Brain Sci.* **2023**, *13*, 859. [CrossRef] [PubMed]
16. Nikolaenko, L.; Jia, Y.; Wang, C.; Diaz-Arjonilla, M.; Yee, J.K.; French, S.W.; Liu, P.Y.; Laurel, S.; Chong, C.; Lee, K.; et al. Testosterone Replacement Ameliorates Nonalcoholic Fatty Liver Disease in Castrated Male Rats. *Endocrinology* **2014**, *155*, 417–428. [CrossRef] [PubMed]
17. Erdenebayar, O.; Kato, T.; Kawakita, T.; Kasai, K.; Kadota, Y.; Yoshida, K.; Iwasa, T.; Irahara, M. Effects of Peripheral Oxytocin Administration on Body Weight, Food Intake, Adipocytes, and Biochemical Parameters in Peri- and Postmenopausal Female Rats. *Endocr. J.* **2021**, *68*, 7–16. [CrossRef] [PubMed]
18. Yamamoto, S.; Arakaki, R.; Noguchi, H.; Takeda, A.; Uchishiba, M.; Kamada, S.; Mineda, A.; Kon, M.; Kawakita, T.; Kinouchi, R.; et al. New Discoveries on the Interaction between Testosterone and Oxytocin in Male Rats—Testosterone-Mediated Effects of Oxytocin in the Prevention of Obesity. *Physiol. Behav.* **2023**, *266*, 114199. [CrossRef]
19. Iwasa, T.; Noguchi, H.; Tanano, R.; Yamanaka, E.; Takeda, A.; Tamura, K.; Aoki, H.; Sugimoto, T.; Sasada, H.; Maeda, T.; et al. Age-Dependent Changes in the Effects of Androgens on Female Metabolic and Body Weight Regulation Systems in Humans and Laboratory Animals. *Int. J. Mol. Sci.* **2023**, *24*, 16567. [CrossRef]

20. Tokui, T.; Kawakita, T.; Yanagihara, R.; Kamada, S.; Minato, S.; Takeda, A.; Imaizumi, J.; Yamamoto, Y.; Yoshida, K.; Kato, T.; et al. Effects of Gonadal Status and the Estrogen Milieu on Hypothalamic Oxytocin Gene Expression and Serum Oxytocin Levels in Female Rats. *Horm. Behav.* **2021**, *133*, 105005. [CrossRef]
21. Tachibana, A.; Yamamoto, Y.; Noguchi, H.; Takeda, A.; Tamura, K.; Aoki, H.; Minato, S.; Uchishiba, M.; Yamamoto, S.; Kamada, S.; et al. Changes in Serum Oxytocin Levels under Physiological and Supraphysiological Gonadal Steroid Hormone Conditions in Women of Reproductive Age: A Preliminary Study. *Nutrients* **2022**, *14*, 5350. [CrossRef] [PubMed]
22. De Vries, G.J.; Wang, Z.; Bullock, N.A.; Numan, S. Sex Differences in the Effects of Testosterone and Its Metabolites on Vasopressin Messenger RNA Levels in the Bed Nucleus of the Stria Terminalis of Rats. *J. Neurosci.* **1994**, *14*, 1789–1794. [CrossRef] [PubMed]
23. Le, T.Y.L.; Ashton, A.W.; Mardini, M.; Stanton, P.G.; Funder, J.W.; Handelsman, D.J.; Mihailidou, A.S. Role of Androgens in Sex Differences in Cardiac Damage During Myocardial Infarction. *Endocrinology* **2014**, *155*, 568–575. [CrossRef]
24. Asarian, L.; Geary, N. Sex Differences in the Physiology of Eating. *Am. J. Physiol. -Regul. Integr. Comp. Physiol.* **2013**, *305*, R1215–R1267. [CrossRef] [PubMed]
25. Blaustein, J.D.; Wade, G.N. Ovarian Influences on the Meal Patterns of Female Rats. *Physiol. Behav.* **1976**, *17*, 201–208. [CrossRef]
26. Heine, P.A.; Taylor, J.A.; Iwamoto, G.A.; Lubahn, D.B.; Cooke, P.S. Increased Adipose Tissue in Male and Female Estrogen Receptor-α Knockout Mice. *Proc. Natl. Acad. Sci. USA* **2000**, *97*, 12729–12734. [CrossRef] [PubMed]
27. Okura, T.; Koda, M.; Ando, F.; Niino, N.; Ohta, S.; Shimokata, H. Association of Polymorphisms in the Estrogen Receptor α Gene with Body Fat Distribution. *Int. J. Obes.* **2003**, *27*, 1020–1027. [CrossRef]
28. Gao, Q.; Mezei, G.; Nie, Y.; Rao, Y.; Choi, C.S.; Bechmann, I.; Leranth, C.; Toran-Allerand, D.; A Priest, C.; Roberts, J.L.; et al. Anorectic Estrogen Mimics Leptin's Effect on the Rewiring of Melanocortin Cells and Stat3 Signaling in Obese Animals. *Nat. Med.* **2007**, *13*, 89–94. [CrossRef]

nutrients

MDPI

Article

Food Addiction: Prevalence, Severity, and Impact on Vascular Stroke Risk Factors in a French Hospital-Based Sample

Bibi Aliya Seelarbokus [1,†], Yolaine Rabat [1,†], Christophe Lalanne [2], Igor Sibon [1,3,*] and Sylvie Berthoz [1,4]

1 Univ. Bordeaux, Institute for Cognitive and Integrative Neuroscience Aquitaine (INCIA), French National Centre for Scientific Research (CNRS), UMR5287, 33000 Bordeaux, France; bibi-aliya.aliya@u-bordeaux.fr (B.A.S.); yolaine.rabat@hotmail.fr (Y.R.); sylvie.berthoz-landron@inserm.fr (S.B.)
2 University Paris Cité, 75006 Paris, France; christophe.lalanne@aliquote.org
3 Neurovascular Unit, Bordeaux University Hospital, 33000 Bordeaux, France
4 Department of Psychiatry for Adolescents and Young Adults, Institut Mutualiste Montsouris, 75014 Paris, France
* Correspondence: igor.sibon@chu-bordeaux.fr; Tel.: +33-(0)5-56-79-55-20
† These authors contributed equally to this work.

Abstract: Background: Stroke ranks as the second leading cause of death and the third leading cause of disability in adults worldwide. While an unhealthy diet is an independent risk factor for stroke, its association with disordered eating behaviours on stroke remains overlooked. This exploratory study aimed to evaluate the prevalence and severity of addictive-like eating behaviours in stroke patients and their association with the main vascular stroke risk factors. Methods: First-ever minor or moderate stroke patients with the ability to complete self-report questionnaires were included. Addictive-like eating was assessed using the Yale Food Addiction Scale 2.0 (YFAS 2.0). The variables of interest were: (i) the proportion of patients meeting the diagnosis of food addiction (FA); (ii) FA symptoms count and severity; (iii) addictive-like eating profile severity. Their association with four main vascular risk factors (obesity, hypertension, dyslipidemia and diabetes) were tested using univariate and multivariate analyses. Results: Over a 4-month period, 101 patients (mean (standard deviation (SD)), 62.8 (13.7) years; males: 60.4%) were consecutively screened with the YFAS 2.0. Overall, 5% of the sample endorsed an FA diagnosis, and 38.6% screened positive for at least one of the symptom criteria, with the most frequently endorsed symptom being "Inability to cut down". Dyslipidemia was the only vascular risk factor associated with the FA diagnosis ($p = 0.043$, 95% CI [−0.21; 0.01]). However, the severity of the addictive profile was associated with dyslipidemia ($p = 0.016$, 95% CI [−2.16; −0.21]) and diabetes ($p = 0.038$, 95% CI [−1.77; 0.25]), but only independently with dyslipidemia ($p = 0.05$; OR = 1.25; 95% CI [1.00; 1.56]). There were significant associations between the number of vascular risk factors and the severity of Time spent, Tolerance, and Use despite adverse consequences of FA symptoms, both in univariate and multivariate analyses (all $p < 0.05$). The number of vascular risk factors and total number of FA symptoms were significantly associated in univariate analyses ($p = 0.007$) but not after adjusting for age ($p = 0.055$) or sex ($p = 0.083$). Conclusions: This study highlighted the potential importance of addictive-like behaviours in the secondary prevention of stroke. However, larger and longer-term studies investigating addictive-like eating in diverse samples of stroke patients are warranted to achieve precision medicine.

Keywords: food addiction; stroke; hypertension; obesity; diabetes; dyslipidaemia; disordered eating behaviour

Citation: Seelarbokus, B.A.; Rabat, Y.; Lalanne, C.; Sibon, I.; Berthoz, S. Food Addiction: Prevalence, Severity, and Impact on Vascular Stroke Risk Factors in a French Hospital-Based Sample. *Nutrients* **2024**, *16*, 4327. https://doi.org/10.3390/nu16244327

Academic Editor: Andrea Vania

Received: 25 November 2024
Revised: 6 December 2024
Accepted: 12 December 2024
Published: 15 December 2024

1. Introduction

According to recent Global Burden of Disease (GBD) estimates, stroke is the second leading cause of death and the third leading cause of disability worldwide, with 12.2 million incident cases of stroke, 143 million disability-adjusted life-years (DALYs) lost, and

6.6 million deaths reported in 2019 [1]. Globally, although life expectancy (LE) increased to 73.2 years in 2021, ageing remains a primary risk factor for stroke events, alongside a ratio of healthy life expectancy (HLE) to LE of 0.83 [2]. On the current trajectory, the average age for a first stroke onset is approximately 70 years, coupled with a reduction in case fatality after stroke [3,4]; the demographic shift is expected to significantly increase the prevalence of stroke by 2030 [5]. Considering the distress caused to patients and families, in addition to the healthcare and social costs [6], the implementation of public health action plans seeking to redress the imbalance of healthcare expenses concentrated towards the last stages of life represents a research priority.

Traditional strategies to curb healthcare costs associated with stroke have predominantly focused on compensatory approaches aiming to alleviate the consequences of impairments instead of tackling their causal factors [7]. Nevertheless, with an enhanced understanding of the pathophysiology and aetiology of the disease, there is robust evidence indicating that modifiable risk factors account for 90% of the risk of stroke [8–11] and can be grouped into specific categories such as diseases (e.g., atrial fibrillation, carotid stenosis, sickle cell disease), physiological factors (e.g., hypertension, high fasting glucose, high body mass index (BMI), high cholesterol, low glomerular filtration rate, chronic inflammation), environmental factors (e.g., air pollution), psychosocial factors (e.g., depression and anxiety, psychosocial stress, job strain, long working hours), and poor lifestyle habits (e.g., dietary items at risk, tobacco, alcohol, and illicit drug abuse, and low physical activity) [12,13]. As the risk of stroke recurrence is highly dependent on the control of these risk factors, the aetiological examination and management of stroke patients should, thus, aim at identifying all potentially modifiable risk factors, as well as their determinants, to provide individualised recommendations for optimal secondary stroke prevention, as promoted in the Stroke Action Plan for Europe (SAP-E) 2018–2020 [12,14].

Of note, whilst dietary risks accounted for 11 million diet-related deaths in 2017, of which cardiovascular diseases were the leading cause worldwide [15], the extant literature has primarily focused on dietary patterns such as the Mediterranean diet, which has been heralded as one of the healthiest patterns exhibiting cardioprotective properties [16–19]. However, amidst the coincidental prominence of obesogenic environments promoting the intake of palatable foods rich in fat, salt, and sugar with high intrinsic addictive properties, there is emerging evidence to now recognise addictive-like eating behaviours as a potentially major, yet understudied, concerns in patients with stroke [20,21].

In a retrospective World Health Organisation (WHO) study examining the impact of mental disorders (based on the Diagnostic and Statistical Manual of Mental Disorders (DSM) IV-TR) on the risk of stroke that included general population surveys in 17 countries (n = 87,250 adults), bulimia nervosa was the mental disorder associated with the highest Odds Ratio (OR) among all disorders evaluated (OR = 3.8; 95% CI: 1.6–9.1), including the abuse or dependence on alcohol or drugs (OR = 2.4; 95% CI [1.5; 3.8] and OR = 2.4; 95% CI [1.1; 5.1], respectively), independently of sociodemographic variables and smoking status [22]. While bulimia nervosa and binge eating disorder are syndromic entities characterised by severe and enduring compulsive overeating that are recognised in the classifications of mental disorders, more recently, the concept of food addiction (FA), defined as an "addiction-like behaviour that develops in association with an excessive, compulsive and dysregulated consumption of energy-dense foods", has emerged as a relatively new approach to understanding problematic eating behaviours [23,24]. Although controversy persists in how to clearly distinguish the diagnosis of FA from other syndromes, such as eating disorders [25], fixed criteria to assess FA have been established to ensure the homogeneity of results between and across studies worldwide [26]. In this context, most of the current research studies focusing on FA use the Yale Food Addiction Scales (YFASs), which have specifically been designed to measure FA by applying the substance-related and addictive disorders criteria of the DSM to the intake of energy-dense food items (DSM-IV-TR: seven criteria assessed by the YFAS; DSM 5: nine criteria assessed by the YFAS 2.0) [25–27]. In effect, similar to addictive drugs, increasing evidence suggests that foods rich in saturated and trans fats, salt and added sugars, which are typical of Western diets, appear to overstimulate neurobiological reward pathways and increase the release of dopamine, thereby triggering FA [28–31].

Importantly, although previous studies have highlighted high YFAS scores in patients with eating disorders (ED), obesity and/or major depressive disorders (MDD) [32–34], the concept of FA in cardiovascular diseases remains largely overlooked. Notably, we were unable to find any prospective studies reporting information on the potential influence of disordered eating behaviours or ED on stroke outcomes. Yet, considering the reported pooled prevalence of FA in the adult population (24%, 95% CI {20; 29}) [35] as well as the negative impact of addictive-like eating behaviours on several markers of metabolic disturbance [36], this research proves important given that the presence of metabolic disturbances has been consistently associated with an increased odds of stroke in the extant literature [37].

Therefore, the aims of this retrospective hospital-based study were to explore the prevalence and severity of FA among stroke survivors and to assess the associations between FA and four critical vascular risk factors for stroke, including hypertension, diabetes, obesity, and dyslipidaemia [38].

2. Materials and Methods

2.1. Study Procedure and Population

This study was a retrospective analysis of patients consecutively hospitalised for a first stroke event at the Neurovascular Unit of the Bordeaux University Hospital between March and July 2019 and discharged to home. Upon admission to the neurovascular unit, all patients are informed about the potential use of their anonymised clinical, imaging, and biological data for teaching and research purposes, and a non-opposition procedure is applied. In acute care, routine evaluations include neuropsychological assessments and a set of self-reported questionnaires. They are administered to patients who understand French well enough, with no and/or medical history or current medical condition preventing their completion according to the referent neurologist (with a visual disability, severe stroke, a disease affecting the nervous system such as epilepsy or dementia, a severe cognitive impairment, psychiatric diagnosis such as neurodevelopmental or schizophrenia spectrum disorders, and/or severe aphasia) and after obtaining an informed verbal consent. For the present study, the authorisation to use retrospective data from medical electronic records for publication was approved by the Research Ethics Committee of Bordeaux University Hospital (CER-BDX-2022-04) in January 2022 and conducted in accordance with the latest version of the Declaration of Helsinki.

2.2. Determination of Food Addiction (FA) in Stroke Patients

In this study, addictive-like eating patterns were only determined using the YFAS 2.0 questionnaire that has been developed by Gearhardt and colleagues [26,39] and validated for French-speaking individuals [27]. Briefly, the YFAS 2.0 is a self-reported questionnaire that is assumed to assess each of the 11 DSM-5 substance use disorders criteria applied to the intake of food items high in saturated fats, refined carbohydrates, and/or sugar and salt (See Supplementary Materials for the YFAS2.0 instruction) plus the associated clinically significant impairment or distress [40]. Although the wider body of the literature focuses primarily on the FA diagnostic scoring option of the scale (i.e., when the participant endorses 2 or more symptoms plus clinically significant impairment or distress), this study also assessed the symptom count scoring option (number of FA symptoms endorsed, without the presence of clinically significant impairment or distress), as well as their proportion across the four domains of addiction symptoms: (1) impaired control; (2) risky use; (3) pharmacological criteria; and (4) social impairment. For individuals endorsing a diagnosis of FA, severity thresholds were also specified (mild: 2–3 symptoms plus impairment or distress; moderate: 4–5 symptoms plus impairment or distress; severe: 6 or more symptoms plus impairment or distress). We complemented our approach to the severity of the phenotype by using a Global Addictive-like eating Profile Severity Index (GAPSI), as explained in statistical analyses Section 2.5.2.

2.3. *Assessment of Stroke Severity*

To evaluate the baseline neurologic outcome and stroke severity in patients, the National Institutes of Health Stroke Scale (NIHSS) was used. The NIHSS is a valid, reliable, and responsive tool assessing domains of (1) consciousness, (2) eye movement, (3) visual fields, (4) facial palsy, (5) motor arm, (6) motor leg, (7) limb ataxia, (8) sensory, (9) language aphasia, (10) speech (dysarthria), and (11) hemi-inattention (neglect). Individual scores from each item are summed, with a minimum and maximum score of 0 and 42, respectively [41].

2.4. *Key Outcome*

This study assessed the association of FA with four of the main vascular risk factors of stroke: obesity; diabetes; hypertension; and dyslipidaemia as independent and cumulative values. BMI was measured using the standard formula (weight (kg)/(height (m^2)) and categorised patients as underweight (BMI < 18.5 kg/m^2), healthy (18.5–24.9 kg/m^2), overweight (25–29.9 kg/m^2), and obese ($\geq$30 kg/m^2), according to the World Health Organisation's criteria for Caucasian populations. Diabetes was diagnosed if the level of haemoglobin A1c (HbA1c) exceeded the cut-point of 48 mmol/mol (6.5%) or if there was a previous medical history of the disease. Patients were considered hypertensive if they presented a medical history of hypertension or if blood pressure exceeded 140/90 mm of mercury (mm Hg). Dyslipidaemia was defined based on fasting serum lipid profile values according to the National Cholesterol Education Program (NCEP) Expert Panel on Detection, Evaluation, and Treatment of High Blood Cholesterol in Adults (ATP III) [42].

2.5. *Statistical Analyses*

2.5.1. Participant Characteristics

Descriptive data were summarised using means (standard deviation (SD)) for continuous variables and frequency for categorical variables. We checked the normality of the key variables of interest by performing the Kolmogorov–Smirnov test and probability plots, and all were not normally distributed. Two-group comparisons for each vascular risk factor (coded as binary indicators), demographic and clinical variables, were performed using univariate analyses for non-normally distributed variables (Mann–Whitney *U* test, Pearson chi-square (χ^2), or Fisher's test for independent sample, as appropriate).

2.5.2. Severity of FA

The YFAS2.0 assesses how frequently (from "Never" to "Every day") in the past year people experienced symptoms related to the difficulties of controlling the intake of energy-dense foods. Gearhardt and colleagues elaborated on a combination of frequency and dichotomous scoring options, where frequency scoring aimed at assessing disordered eating behaviours such as excess consumption or emotional eating, and dichotomous scoring aimed at identifying more severe and problematic eating problems [26]. To determine the severity of the overall addictive-like eating phenotype and take into account the frequency scoring of all the symptom criteria, we computed a Global Addictive-like Eating Profile Index (GAPSI). The items were scored on a four-category ordered scale: 1 = from "Never" to "Less than once a month"; 2 = from "Once a month" to "Two to three times a month"; 3 = from "Once a week" to "Two to three times a week"; and 4 = from "Four to six times a week" to "Every day". As the evaluation of each symptom encompassed several items, the categorisation was based on the one item endorsing the highest frequency score.

A principal component analysis (PCA) was then applied to all the 11 addiction-related symptoms plus 1 item summarising the associated clinically significant impact (distress and/or impairment), scored on the four-category-ordered scale. The first component was used to build a weighted summary or global severity index for the addictive profile (see Supplementary Table S1). PCA scores reflect the combination of the symptoms weighted according to their contribution to the factor. Higher PCA scores reflect higher individual frequency scores on most of the symptom criteria. Restricted cubic splines (three knots) were used to take into account possible departure from linearity in the case of continuous predictors (age and BMI). The number of predictors was deliberately limited to those known from the literature review and univariate testing in order to conform to the 10–15 events per variable rule of thumb (even if the lowest minority class was 20 positive cases out of 98 in the case of diabetes). The parameters of those models were estimated using ridge (L2) penalisation, whereby the tuning of model hyper-parameters (penalty) was performed using repeated 10-fold cross-validations (25 repetitions). The final solution chosen was the one that minimised the cross-validated log likelihood on the optimal penalty parameter the most.

Parameter estimates corrected for overfitting were obtained using bootstrap resampling (B = 200): for each bootstrap sample, the same regression model was used, and the accuracy measure of each parameter was compared to that found in the original sample, and a final optimism corrected estimate was computed by averaging those apparent biases over all bootstrap iterations. The calibration of each regression model was assessed by comparing predicted probabilities with observed frequencies for the corresponding outcome. The pseudo-R-squared value and Somer's D index were used to assess the goodness of fit of each model.

2.5.3. Associations Between Cumulative Vascular Risk Factors and Individual Food Addiction (FA) Symptom

Each vascular risk factor was scored, and the sum of vascular risk factors was treated as ordered categorical variables, ranging from 0 to 4 (i.e., the presence of hypertension (score 1), obesity (score 1), diabetes (score 1), and dyslipidaemia (score 1)). Associations between the number of vascular risk factors, the severity of FA symptoms, and symptom counts were then analysed using Spearman's rank correlation coefficient, which did not assume a normal distribution of the variables. The null hypothesis (H0) was tested, with Spearman's rank correlation coefficient equal to 0. The alternative hypothesis was that the correlation coefficient was different from 0. The null hypothesis (H0) was rejected at $p < 0.05$ ($\alpha = 0.05$). To control for age and sex as potential confounders based on our univariate analyses, partial correlations were also performed. In these analyses, given that multicollinearity between age and sex might obscure the computation because of the overlapping correlation, each confounder was analysed separately.

2.5.4. Statistical Software and Thresholds

All statistical tests were performed using R statistical software version 4.1.0 and R package Regression Modeling Strategies (rms) version 6.1-0 (https://CRAN.R-project.org/package=rms, accessed on 24 October 2024) and by considering a fixed type I error rate of 5%.

3. Results

3.1. Description of the Study Population

Complete data from 101 participants were retrieved from electronic medical records, except for one participant with a missing BMI value. Participant characteristics, captured at baseline and classified according to the presence of vascular risk factors (diabetes, obesity, hypertension, dyslipidaemia), are presented in Table 1. The study sample was predominantly males (60.4%), on average, overweight (BMI: mean (SD), 27.6 (5.77) kg/m^2), with a mean (SD) age of 62.8 (13.7) years. Among all stroke cases, 86.1% were identified as ischemic stroke patients, 5% as haemorrhagic stroke patients, and 8.9% were diagnosed with transient ischaemic attack (TIA). The mean (SD) NIHSS score was at 2.31 (3.13) points for the overall sample, representing a minor stroke severity as per the stroke scale [43].

Table 1. Characteristics of all study participants (n = 101) and univariate between-group comparisons.

Characteristics	Overall	Hypertension			Diabetes			Dyslipidaemia			Obesity		
		HTN− (n = 49)	HTN+ (n = 52)	p-Value, (ES)	DIA− (n = 80)	DIA+ (n = 21)	p-Value, (ES)	DYS− (n = 67)	DYS+ (n = 34)	p-Value, (ES)	OB− (n = 71)	OB+ (n = 29)	p-Value, (ES)
Sex, % men (n)	60.40 (61)	61.20 (30)	59.60 (31)	0.870 (0.387)	56.30 (45)	76.20 (16)	0.096 (0.165)	56.70 (38)	67.60 (23)	0.288 (0.106)	63.40 (45)	51.70 (15)	0.320 (−0.099)
Age, years (mean (SD))	62.80 (13.7)	56.30 (14.0)	68.90 (10.1)	**<0.001 (−0.461)**	61.70 (14.7)	66.80 (7.80)	0.215 (−0.124)	60. 60 (14.6)	67.10 (10.6)	**0.032 (−0.214)**	61.40 (14.8)	66.40 (9.87)	0.305 (−0.102)
NIHSS (mean (SD))	2.31 (3.13)	1.84 (2.94)	2.75 (3.30)	**0.014 (0.370)**	2.34 (3.42)	2.19 (1.66)	0.151 (0.253)	2.06 (2.48)	2.79 (4.13)	0.470 (0.403)	2.13 (3.08)	2.83 (3.29)	0.063 (0.381)
BMI*, kg/m^2 (mean (SD)) (n = 100)	27.60 (5.77)	26.00 (5.02)	28.90 (6.22)	**0.009 (−0.260)**	27.10 (5.52)	29.00 (6.75)	**0.034 (−0.212)**	26.60 (5.07)	29.20 (6.86)	**<0.001 (0.807)**	24.60 (2.96)	34.50 (5.01)	**<0.001 (−0.777)**
Comorbidities													
Obesity, % (n) (n = 100)	29.00 (29)	18.40 (9)	39.20 (20)	**0.022 (0.629)**	26.60 (21)	38.10 (8)	0.310 (0.572)	23.90 (16)	39.40 (13)	0.110 (0.886)	-	-	-
Dyslipidaemia, % (n)	33.70 (34)	14.30 (7)	51.90 (27)	**<0.001 (0.452)**	26.30 (21)	61.90 (13)	**0.002 (0.750)**	-	-	-	28.20 (20)	44.80 (13)	0.110 (0.773)
Diabetes, % (n)	20.80 (21)	6.10 (3)	34.60 (18)	**<0.001 (0.376)**	-	-	-	11.90 (8)	38.20 (13)	**0.002 (0.763)**	18.30 (13)	27.60 (8)	0.301 (0.763)
Hypertension, % (n)	51.50 (52)	-	-	-	42.50 (34)	85.70 (18)	**<0.001 (0.654)**	37.30 (25)	79.40 (27)	**<0.001 (0.950)**	43.70 (31)	69.0 (20)	**0.022 (0.747)**

HTN, DIA, DYS, OB−: patients without hypertension, diabetes, dyslipidemia, obesity; HTN, DIA, DYS, OB+: patients with hypertension, diabetes, dyslipidemia, obesity; ES: effect size; BMI: body mass index; BMI* n = 100; NIHSS: National Institute of Health Stroke Scale; SD: Standard deviation. Bold figures indicate significance at $p < 0.05$.

3.2. Prevalence of Food Addiction (FA) Diagnosis and Symptoms

Table 2 shows the prevalence of patients with a diagnosis of FA and the detailed prevalence of addictive-like eating behaviours by symptoms endorsed. In this study, 5% (n = 5) of participants, all with ischemic stroke, endorsed a diagnosis of FA. Interestingly, whereas the endorsement of either clinical distress or impairment is necessary to establish an FA diagnosis, these factors were only experienced by 3.0% and 7.9% of patients, respectively, thereby corresponding with the overall low prevalence of FA in this sample. However, 23.8% of patients screened positive for at least two of the symptom criteria, and 9.0% of patients endorsed at least four symptoms. The most prevalent symptoms (i.e., >10%) were "Inability to cut down" (16.8%), "Use in physically hazardous situations" (15.8%), "Use despite social/interpersonal problems" (12.9%), "Feelings of withdrawal symptoms" (11.9%), and "Tolerance" (10.9%). When combined under specific domains, "Impaired control" was the most prevalent domain, with 25.7% of patients experiencing at least one symptom of this domain.

Table 2. Prevalence of Food Addiction (FA) diagnosis and detailed symptom count (n = 101).

	Prevalence, % (n)
FA diagnosis	
Two or more symptoms plus clinically significant distress or impairment	5.0 (5)
Symptom criteria	
(1) Inability to cut down	16.8 (17)
(2) Physically hazardous situations	15.8 (16)
(3) Interpersonal problems	12.9 (13)
(4) Withdrawal	11.9 (12)
(5) Time spent	10.9 (11)
(6) Tolerance	8.9 (9)
(7) Loss of control	6.9 (7)
(8) Adverse consequences	5.9 (6)
(9) Craving	5.9 (6)
(10) Impaired daily functioning	5.0 (5)
(11) Activities given up	4.0 (4)
Clinical significance	
Distress	3.0 (3)
Impairment	7.9 (8)
Domains (symptom criteria)	
Impaired control (symptoms 1, 5, 7, 9)	25.7 (26)
Risky use (symptoms 2, 8)	18.8 (19)
Pharmacological criteria (symptoms 4, 6)	16.8 (17)
Social impairment (symptoms 3, 10, 11)	16.8 (17)
Symptom count	
No symptom	61.4 (62)
One symptom endorsed	14.9 (15)
Two symptoms endorsed	5.9 (6)
Three symptoms endorsed	8.9 (9)
Four symptoms endorsed	2.0 (2)
Five symptoms endorsed	2.0 (2)
Six symptoms endorsed	2.0 (2)
Seven symptoms endorsed	2.0 (2)

3.3. Food Addiction (FA) Diagnosis, Its Severity, and the Association with Vascular Risk Factors

Table 3 shows the characteristics of patients who met the diagnosis of FA. The mean (SD) age of the patients with FA was 57.0 (13.7) years, with three individuals out of five living with obesity and being females. Four out of five of the patients experienced severe FA, with only one patient suffering from mild FA but living with multi-morbidities, including obesity, hypertension, dyslipidemia and diabetes (Patient 1). The GAPSI score was 2.7 in the patients with mild FA and ranged from 5.2 to 7.2 in those experiencing severe FA.

Table 3. Characteristics of patients with a Food Addiction (FA) diagnosis.

Characteristics	Patient 1	Patient 2	Patient 3	Patient 4	Patient 5
Sex	Male	Female	Male	Female	Female
Age, y	63	38	64	48	72
NIHSS	3	7	11	1	2
Weight status	Obese	Healthy	Obese	Healthy	Obese
BMI, kg/m^2	31.6	24.4	40.8	21.3	37.2
Hypertension	Yes	No	No	No	Yes
Diabetes	Yes	No	No	No	No
Dyslipidaemia	Yes	Yes	Yes	No	Yes
FA severity	Mild	Severe	Severe	Severe	Severe
GAPSI	2.7	7.2	6.7	5.2	11.2
YFAS symptom criteria:					
1. Substance taken in larger amounts and for longer periods than intended		x		x	
2. Persistent desire or repeated unsuccessful attempts to quit		x	x	x	
3. Much time/activity to obtain, use, recover	x		x	x	x
4. Important social, occupational, or recreational activities given up or reduced	x		x		x
5. Use continues despite knowledge of adverse consequences			x		x
6. Tolerance		x	x	x	
7. Characteristic withdrawal symptoms; substance taken to relieve withdrawal	x	x	x		x
8. Continued use despite social or interpersonal problems		x		x	x
9. Failure to fulfil major role obligations (e.g., work, school, home)			x		x
10. Use in physically hazardous situations		x			x
11. Craving or a strong desire or urge to use		x		x	x
12. Use causes clinically significant impairment or distress	x	x	x	x	x

NIHSS: National Institute of Health Stroke Scale; BMI: Body mass index; GAPSI: Global Addictive-like Eating Profile Severity Index.

As shown in Table 4, dyslipidemia was the only vascular risk factor significantly associated with the FA diagnosis (p = 0.043, 95% CI [−0.21; 0.01]), with four out of five patients with an FA diagnosis having dyslipidemia, whereas diabetes was present in only one patient. Higher GAPSI scores were also associated with dyslipidemia (p = 0.016, 95% CI [−2.16; −0.21]) and diabetes (p = 0.038, 95% CI [−1.77; 0.25]) in univariate comparisons. However, GAPSI scores were independently associated with dyslipidemia only (p = 0.05; OR = 1.25; 95% CI = 1.00–1.56) (See Supplementary Materials for the detailed regression models with each vascular risk factor).

Table 4. Associations between Food Addiction diagnosis by vascular stroke risk factor and the Global Addictive-like Eating Profile Severity Index (GAPSI).

		Vascular Risk Factors															
		Hypertension				Diabetes				Dyslipidaemia				Obesity			
Characteristics	**Overall**	**HTN−** **($n = 49$)**	**HTN+** **($n = 52$)**	***p*-Value**	**95% CI**	**DIA−** **($n = 80$)**	**DIA+** **($n = 21$)**	***p*-Value**	**95% CI**	**DYS−** **($n = 67$)**	**DYS+** **($n = 34$)**	***p*-Value**	**95% CI**	**OB−** **($n = 71$)**	**OB+** **($n = 29$)**	***p*-Value**	**95% CI**
FA diagnosis, % (*n*)	5 (5)	40 (2)	60 (3)	0.671	[−0.10; 0.07]	80 (4)	20 (1)	0.964	[−0.10; 0.11]	20 (1)	80 (4)	**0.043**	[−0.21; 0.01]	40 (2)	60 (3)	0.151	[−0.19; 0.04]
GAPSI, Mean (SD)	-3.05^{-15} (2.23)	−0.18 −2.25	0.17 −2.23	0.150	[−1.23; 0.53]	−0.16 −2.28	0.6 −1.96	**0.038**	[−1.77; 0.25]	−0.37 −1.77	0.72 −2.83	**0.016**	[−2.16; −0.21]	−0.31 −1.81	0.7 −2.96	0.090	[−2.21; 0.19]

GAPSI: Global Addictive-like Eating Profile Severity Index; 95% CI: 95% confidence interval. Bold figures indicate significance at $p < 0.05$.

3.4. Associations Between the Food Addiction (FA) Symptom Criteria and Vascular Risk Factor Scores

The correlation coefficients, as well as *p*-values, are presented in Table 5. The relationship between the total number of symptoms endorsed and the number of vascular risk factors was significant only in univariate analyses. When analysing the severity of each specific symptom criterion, there were no significant associations observed with the number of vascular risk factors and most of the FA symptoms, except for (i) Time spent, (ii) Tolerance, and (iii) Use despite adverse emotional or physical consequences. These correlations remained significant after controlling for age and sex.

Table 5. Correlations between the number of vascular risk factors (0–4), the symptom count, and the severity of each symptom criterion. Values presented are correlation coefficients, ρ (rho), and *p*-value.

	Association with Number of Vascular Risk Factors		
	Unadjusted, ρ (*p*-Value)	**Adjusted for Age, ρ (*p*-Value)**	**Adjusted for Sex, ρ (*p*-Value)**
Number of symptoms endorsed	**0.265 (0.007)**	0.194 (0.055)	0.174 (0.083)
Severity of symptoms criteria			
(1) Inability to cut down	0.028 (0.782)	−0.009 (0.928)	0.023 (0.817)
(2) Physically hazardous situations	−0.042 (0.680)	−0.004 (0.968)	−0054 (0.597)
(3) Interpersonal problems	−0.113 (0.261)	−0.057 (0.575)	−0.116 (0.249)
(4) Withdrawal	0.087 (0.387)	0.021 (0.833)	0.051 (0.616)
(5) Time spent	**0.219 (0.028)**	**0.212 (0.035)**	**0.236 (0.018)**
(6) Tolerance	**0.260 (0.009)**	**0.343 (<0.001)**	**0.319 (0.001)**
(7) Loss of control	0.132 (0.189)	0.041 (0.684)	0.021 (0.837)
(8) Use despite adverse consequences	**0.230 (0.020)**	**0.251 (0.012)**	**0.214 (0.033)**
(9) Craving	0.072 (0.472)	0.094 (0.357)	0.059 (0.558)
(10) Impaired daily functioning	−0.065 (0.518)	0.010 (0.922)	−0.024 (0.813)
(11) Activities given up	0.081 (0.419)	0.108 (0.287)	0.103 (0.307)

4. Discussion

4.1. Principal Findings

To the best of our knowledge, this was the first study to investigate the prevalence of FA and the association of addictive-like eating patterns in the presence of vascular risk factors in a sample of adults with a first-ever mild stroke event. The diagnostic threshold for FA (i.e., two or more symptoms plus clinically significant impairment or distress) was only met by 5% of participants. From this sub-sample group, dyslipidaemia was the only vascular risk factor, which was significantly associated with a diagnosis of FA, and the severity of the addictive profile was independently associated with dyslipidemia only. Concerning the relationship between vascular risk factors and the severity of FA symptoms in the overall sample, significant associations were noted between the number of vascular risk factors and the severity of Time spent, Tolerance, and Use despite adverse consequences symptom criteria, both in univariate and multivariate analyses. However, the number of vascular risk factors and total number of symptoms endorsed were significantly correlated in univariate analyses only.

4.2. Prevalence of Food Addiction (FA) Diagnosis and Comparison with Other Studies

Compared with the average prevalence of FA reported in the general French-speaking population at 8.2% [27], our study reported a slightly lower percentage of participants who met the diagnostic threshold for FA at 5%. One potential explanation could pertain to the low endorsement of both clinical distress and impairment (clinical distress: 3%; clinical impairment: 7.9%), either of which is required to establish an FA diagnosis. Based on the YFAS 2.0 scoring instructions, given that clinically significant impairment or distress should be experienced at least twice a week to meet the diagnostic criterion, it is possible that the pre-defined thresholds were too high for some patients, thereby precluding the diagnosis of FA. In addition, whereas clinical impairment or distress has more often been reported among young females [44,45] and people living with obesity [46,47], our overall study sample was predominantly males (60.4%), in their later adulthood stages at the mean (SD) age of 62.8 (13.7) years, and with a mean (SD) BMI representing overweight at 27.6 (5.77) kg/m^2. In this context, the demographics of our overall study sample may have also precluded a diagnosis of FA in many participants. This finding could, in effect, be substantiated by the fact that our subsample of patients with an FA diagnosis was, on average, 5 years younger than the overall sample, of whom two were females with severe FA (Table 3). However, given that 23.8% of participants screened positive for at least two FA symptoms, the use of the YFAS 2.0 questionnaire solely as a diagnostic scoring option appears reductive in the context of stroke, considering that the types and number of symptoms with and without the endorsement of clinical distress or impairment criterion could be informative for research and treatment [48], as discussed in Section 4.3.

4.3. Endorsement Rates for Food Addiction (FA) Symptom Criteria in the Overall Sample

Overall, 38.6% of the patients screened positive for at least one of the 11 FA symptom criteria (i.e., without clinical impairment or distress). Consistent with other studies [45,49,50], the most frequent symptom endorsed by the current sample was "Inability to cut down". One potential explanation underpinning this common finding across cohorts may pertain to the acquired benefits from the ubiquity of low-cost, energy-dense, and palatable ultra-processed foods (UPFs) and the abundance of external cues recalling triggers of snacking behaviours [51]. Although UPFs form a highly heterogeneous food category and also include low-calorie products, products "fortified" with beneficial nutrients or frozen meals [52], the majority of UPFs are high in energy density, salts, added sugars, saturated and trans fats, as well as additives [53]. Mechanistically, preclinical and human studies have demonstrated that a repeated intake of UPFs triggers addiction-like biological (e.g., dopaminergic sensitisation) and behavioural responses (e.g., tolerance, withdrawal, use despite consequences) through the pharmacokinetic properties of rewarding ingredients (e.g., fatty–salty and fatty–sugary) that are rapidly absorbed by the system [54]. However, a complementary assessment of dietary intake, allowing for a detailed analysis regarding the amount of high-fat or high-sugar foods consumed, would be needed to confirm these explanations.

4.4. Association Between Food Addiction (FA) Diagnosis and Vascular Risk Factors

In this case series (n = 5 with an FA diagnosis), there were no robust associations between FA diagnosis and diabetes, obesity, and/or hypertension. Clinically, given that it has been shown that type 2 diabetic patients with an FA diagnosis are mostly in the age range of 20–29 years [55], it is possible that associations between an FA diagnosis and vascular risk factors may be stronger in younger stroke survivors. However, more needs to be understood about developmental changes in healthy and unhealthy food preferences [56], as several studies have shown age-related effects on central regulation [57,58]. Compared to older adults, younger individuals have been shown to be more motivated by food preferences, to experience greater food cravings for unhealthy foods, and to have increased striatal sensitivity to food stimuli, all of which corresponded with an imbalanced development of the prefrontal cortex and limbic system [59]. Importantly, besides the potential long-term neurological repercussions in younger individuals [60], these connections between brain health and dietary intake also parallel the premature onset of vascular risk factors for cardiovascular diseases [61–63]. To this end, the lack of significant relationship in our study sample could be due to the fact that the patients of this study belonged primarily to Generation X and Boomers II cohorts and, therefore, might have been less exposed to calorie-dense environments in their earlier stages of life.

Nevertheless, whilst the possibility of a type I error cannot be negated with regard to the limited sample size, FA and dyslipidaemia were significantly associated in this study sample. Moreover, if dyslipidaemia was the only vascular risk factor significantly associated with FA in this study sample, there were more patients who suffered from dyslipidaemia (n = 34) compared with diabetes (n = 21). From a cultural perspective, considering that older French adults are more likely to regularly consume higher quantities of high-fat foods (e.g., butter, cheeses, sausages, and other charcuterie) than high-sugar foods as part of their daily diets [64,65], it may be possible that the association between FA and dyslipidaemia is, thus, more significant in this study sample. However, despite not meeting the criteria for an FA diagnosis, similar results were reported by Nelder and colleagues in the general Newfoundland population, whereby YFAS symptoms were significantly associated with triglyceride levels and inversely associated with high-density lipoproteins (HDL) levels in a larger study sample of healthy adults [36]. Mechanistically, the associations between FA and dyslipidaemia could be supported by preclinical studies, whereby prolonged high-fat intake in rodents has been shown to reduce mesolimbic dopamine (DA) function and nucleus accumbens (NAc) DA overflow, besides modulating striatal neuroadaptive responses and blunting DA reuptake in the NAc [66–69]. Importantly, although evidence for causality remains enigmatic, these observations could be potentially problematic considering the co-existence of diabetes, obesity, and hypertension with dyslipidaemia [70–72]. However, given that our own results indicated no significant correlation between the number of vascular risk factors and symptom counts in controlled analyses and no significant association between the number of vascular risk factors and most FA symptoms in multivariate analyses (except for Time spent, Tolerance, and Use despite adverse consequences), larger and longer-term studies are warranted to improve understanding of the impact of such eating behaviours on health, as well as the direction of association between FA and vascular risk factors.

4.5. Strengths and Limitations of This Study

The sample size analysed was rather small, thereby reducing the statistical power to detect potential significant associations, and even with multivariable adjustments, measurement error-related or residual confounding cannot be excluded in our exploratory observational study design. Moreover, due to the cross-sectional design of this study, our statistical results inherently possess limitations that preclude causal interpretations.

The final sample lacked age and sex diversity. As previously discussed, these demographic factors are of special interest given that the prevalence of FA is not only higher in young than older population but also more elevated among females than males. In the present study, the age distribution is as expected for a stroke population, especially of minor or moderate severity. While the men-to-women distribution was not representative of the typical sex ratio of stroke patients, it corresponded to that of a non-severe stroke population. In addition, whereas stroke and FA association may differ by race, ethnicity, genetic composition and physical activity level [9,73,74], our study did not measure these potential key confounders, thereby impacting the generalisability of the findings. Indeed, beyond the numerous studies that highlighted a significant genetic component in the occurrence of stroke, a dopamine genetic risk has been associated with FA [75–78]. Blacks, Hispanics, and those with sedentary behaviours have also been shown to have an increased risk of both stroke and FA [79–81].

Regarding the evaluation of at-risk lifestyle behaviours among the stroke population, the possibility of recall and social desirability biases from the self-reported YFAS 2.0 questionnaire cannot be excluded. Therefore, future studies with larger and more diverse samples, including a complimentary assessment of dietary intake that would ensure a detailed analysis regarding the amount of high-fat or high-sugar foods consumed, are needed to draw firm conclusions.

5. Conclusions

From the evaluation of the extant literature, our study findings emphasise a research gap pertaining to disordered eating patterns in people with stroke. Our study highlighted the potential importance of considering addictive-like eating behaviours as part of the management of stroke patients. Whereas there is still some uncertainty from the substantive Cochrane Review regarding the benefits of adopting healthy dietary patterns such as a Mediterranean-style diet for stroke secondary prevention [19], we believe that administering the YFAS 2.0 questionnaire as part of routine evaluations could be used to identify patients with specific unmet needs and unhealthy eating patterns in their care pathways. In this context, to optimise the secondary prevention of stroke, it is important to recognise addictive-like eating behaviours as complex and multifaceted, thus requiring a multidisciplinary team approach. For example, the collaboration between not only neurologists and dietitians but also with addictologists/psychiatrists and psychologists specialised in disordered eating and associated disorders may be conducive to reducing the determinants of such compulsive overeating behaviours. Through a multidisciplinary lens, future prospective studies should prioritise the investigation of FA and its symptoms in larger and more diverse samples of stroke patients so as to better guide clinical practice and achieve precision medicine.

Supplementary Materials: The following supporting information can be downloaded at: https://www.mdpi.com/article/10.3390/nu16244327/s1, Table S1. Principal component analysis on the YFAS2.0 items used to compute the Global Addictive-like eating Profile Severity Index (GAPSI). Figure S1. Predicted values of Pr(Dyslipidemia).

Author Contributions: Conceptualisation, I.S. and S.B.; methodology, I.S., S.B. and C.L.; formal analysis, B.A.S., Y.R., C.L. and S.B.; investigation, Y.R. and S.B.; data curation, B.A.S., Y.R. and S.B.; writing—original draft preparation, B.A.S., I.S. and S.B.; writing—review and editing, B.A.S., Y.R., C.L., I.S. and S.B.; supervision, I.S. and S.B.; project administration, I.S. and S.B. All authors have read and agreed to the published version of the manuscript.

Funding: This research received no external funding. Yolaine Rabat was a PhD fellow funded by the Ministry of Research and Higher Education. Bibi Aliya Seelarbokus is a PhD student funded by the Neurocampus International Graduate Program managed by the Agency Nationale de la Recherche (French National Research Agency) under reference ANR-17-EURE-0028.

Institutional Review Board Statement: This study was conducted in accordance with the Declaration of Helsinki and received local ethical board approval (protocol code CER-BDX-2022-04 and date 26 January 2022).

Informed Consent Statement: Informed verbal consent was obtained from all subjects involved in this study. In this study, upon admission to the neurovascular unit of Bordeaux University Hospital, all patients were orally informed about the potential use of their anonymised clinical, imaging, and biological data for teaching and research purposes, and a non-opposition procedure was applied. All data remained strictly confidential.

Data Availability Statement: The data presented in this study are available upon reasonable request from the corresponding author. The data are not publicly available due to specifications from the study's sponsor.

Acknowledgments: The authors would like to thank all patients and the staff from Bordeaux University Hospital Neurovascular Unit for their kind contribution to this research.

Conflicts of Interest: The authors declare no conflicts of interest. Igor Sibon has served as an advisor for Servier and Boehringer Ingelheim and has received teaching honoraria from Medtronic and Bayer. The French Ministry of Research and Higher Education had no role in the design, execution, interpretation, or writing of this study.

References

1. eClinicalMedicine. The rising global burden of stroke. *eClinicalMedicine* **2023**, *59*, 102028. [CrossRef] [PubMed]
2. Dattani, S.; Rodés-Guirao, L.; Ritchie, H.; Ortiz-Ospina, E.; Roser, M. Life Expectancy. Available online: https://ourworldindata.org/life-expectancy (accessed on 14 October 2024).

3. Haute-Autorité-de-Santé. Stroke: Early management (alert, prehospital phase, initial hospital phase, indications for thrombolysis). *Clin. Pract. Guidel.* **2009**. Available online: https://www.has-sante.fr/upload/docs/application/pdf/2010-03/stroke_early_management_-_guidelines_-_english_version.pdf (accessed on 14 October 2024).
4. Li, C.; Baek, J.; Sanchez, B.N.; Morgenstern, L.B.; Lisabeth, L.D. Temporal trends in age at ischemic stroke onset by ethnicity. *Ann. Epidemiol.* **2018**, *28*, 686–690.e682. [CrossRef] [PubMed]
5. Pu, L.; Wang, L.; Zhang, R.; Zhao, T.; Jiang, Y.; Han, L. Projected Global Trends in Ischemic Stroke Incidence, Deaths and Disability-Adjusted Life Years From 2020 to 2030. *Stroke* **2023**, *54*, 1330–1339. [CrossRef]
6. Chevreul, K.; Durand-Zaleski, I.; Gouépo, A.; Fery-Lemonnier, E.; Hommel, M.; Woimant, F. Cost of stroke in France. *Eur. J. Neurol.* **2013**, *20*, 1094–1100. [CrossRef]
7. Grefkes, C.; Fink, G.R. Recovery from stroke: Current concepts and future perspectives. *Neurol. Res. Pract.* **2020**, *2*, 17. [CrossRef]
8. Feigin, V.L.; Roth, G.A.; Naghavi, M.; Parmar, P.; Krishnamurthi, R.; Chugh, S.; Mensah, G.A.; Norrving, B.; Shiue, I.; Ng, M.; et al. Global burden of stroke and risk factors in 188 countries, during 1990–2013: A systematic analysis for the Global Burden of Disease Study 2013. *Lancet Neurol.* **2016**, *15*, 913–924. [CrossRef]
9. Boehme, A.K.; Esenwa, C.; Elkind, M.S. Stroke Risk Factors, Genetics, and Prevention. *Circ. Res.* **2017**, *120*, 472–495. [CrossRef]
10. Hankey, G.J. Population Impact of Potentially Modifiable Risk Factors for Stroke. *Stroke* **2020**, *51*, 719–728. [CrossRef]
11. Zeng, X.; Deng, A.; Ding, Y. The INTERSTROKE study on risk factors for stroke. *Lancet* **2017**, *389*, 35. [CrossRef]
12. Hankey, G.J. Stroke. *Lancet* **2017**, *389*, 641–654. [CrossRef] [PubMed]
13. O'Donnell, M.J.; Chin, S.L.; Rangarajan, S.; Xavier, D.; Liu, L.; Zhang, H.; Rao-Melacini, P.; Zhang, X.; Pais, P.; Agapay, S.; et al. Global and regional effects of potentially modifiable risk factors associated with acute stroke in 32 countries (INTERSTROKE): A case-control study. *Lancet* **2016**, *388*, 761–775. [CrossRef] [PubMed]
14. ESO. Stroke-Action-Plan-For-Europe. Available online: https://eso-stroke.org/projects/stroke-action-plan/ (accessed on 14 October 2024).
15. Afshin, A.; Sur, P.J.; Fay, K.A.; Cornaby, L.; Ferrara, G.; Salama, J.S.; Mullany, E.C.; Abate, K.H.; Abbafati, C.; Abebe, Z.; et al. Health effects of dietary risks in 195 countries, 1990–2017: A systematic analysis for the Global Burden of Disease Study 2017. *Lancet* **2019**, *393*, 1958–1972. [CrossRef]
16. Martínez-González, M.A.; Gea, A.; Ruiz-Canela, M. The Mediterranean Diet and Cardiovascular Health. *Circ. Res.* **2019**, *124*, 779–798. [CrossRef]
17. Estruch, R.; Ros, E.; Salas-Salvadó, J.; Covas, M.-I.; Corella, D.; Arós, F.; Gómez-Gracia, E.; Ruiz-Gutiérrez, V.; Fiol, M.; Lapetra, J.; et al. Primary Prevention of Cardiovascular Disease with a Mediterranean Diet Supplemented with Extra-Virgin Olive Oil or Nuts. *N. Engl. J. Med.* **2018**, *378*, e34. [CrossRef]
18. Widmer, R.J.; Flammer, A.J.; Lerman, L.O.; Lerman, A. The Mediterranean diet, its components, and cardiovascular disease. *Am. J. Med.* **2015**, *128*, 229–238. [CrossRef]
19. Rees, K.; Takeda, A.; Martin, N.; Ellis, L.; Wijesekara, D.; Vepa, A.; Das, A.; Hartley, L.; Stranges, S. Mediterranean-style diet for the primary and secondary prevention of cardiovascular disease. *Cochrane Database Syst. Rev.* **2019**, *2019*, CD009825. [CrossRef]
20. Davis, C. From Passive Overeating to "Food Addiction": A Spectrum of Compulsion and Severity. *Int. Sch. Res. Not.* **2013**, *2013*, 435027. [CrossRef]
21. Rabat, Y.; Berthoz, S.; Sibon, I. Is addictive-like eating an overlooked stroke risk factor? A study case. *Eat. Weight. Disord.* **2021**, *26*, 2801–2806. [CrossRef]
22. Swain, N.R.; Lim, C.C.W.; Levinson, D.; Fiestas, F.; de Girolamo, G.; Moskalewicz, J.; Lepine, J.-P.; Posada-Villa, J.; Haro, J.M.; Medina-Mora, M.E.; et al. Associations between DSM-IV mental disorders and subsequent non-fatal, self-reported stroke. *J. Psychosom. Res.* **2015**, *79*, 130–136. [CrossRef]
23. Piccinni, A.; Marazziti, D.; Vanelli, F.; Franceschini, C.; Baroni, S.; Costanzo, D.; Cremone, I.M.; Veltri, A.; Dell'Osso, L. Food addiction spectrum: A theoretical model from normality to eating and overeating disorders. *Curr. Med. Chem.* **2015**, *22*, 1631–1638. [CrossRef] [PubMed]
24. Imperatori, C.; Fabbricatore, M.; Vumbaca, V.; Innamorati, M.; Contardi, A.; Farina, B. Food Addiction: Definition, measurement and prevalence in healthy subjects and in patients with eating disorders. *Riv. Di Psichiatr.* **2016**, *51*, 60–65. [CrossRef]
25. Hauck, C.; Cook, B.; Ellrott, T. Food addiction, eating addiction and eating disorders. *Proc. Nutr. Soc.* **2020**, *79*, 103–112. [CrossRef]
26. Gearhardt, A.N.; Corbin, W.R.; Brownell, K.D. Preliminary validation of the Yale Food Addiction Scale. *Appetite* **2009**, *52*, 430–436. [CrossRef]
27. Brunault, P.; Courtois, R.; Gearhardt, A.N.; Gaillard, P.; Journiac, K.; Cathelain, S.; Réveillère, C.; Ballon, N. Validation of the French Version of the DSM-5 Yale Food Addiction Scale in a Nonclinical Sample. *Can. J. Psychiatry* **2017**, *62*, 199–210. [CrossRef]
28. Gearhardt, A.N.; Davis, C.; Kuschner, R.; Brownell, K.D. The addiction potential of hyperpalatable foods. *Curr. Drug Abus. Rev.* **2011**, *4*, 140–145. [CrossRef]
29. Gordon, E.L.; Ariel-Donges, A.H.; Bauman, V.; Merlo, L.J. What Is the Evidence for "Food Addiction?" A Systematic Review. *Nutrients* **2018**, *10*, 477. [CrossRef]
30. Wang, G.J.; Volkow, N.D.; Thanos, P.K.; Fowler, J.S. Imaging of brain dopamine pathways: Implications for understanding obesity. *J. Addict. Med.* **2009**, *3*, 8–18. [CrossRef]
31. Pelchat, M.L.; Johnson, A.; Chan, R.; Valdez, J.; Ragland, J.D. Images of desire: Food-craving activation during fMRI. *Neuroimage* **2004**, *23*, 1486–1493. [CrossRef]

32. Lerma-Cabrera, J.M.; Carvajal, F.; Lopez-Legarrea, P. Food addiction as a new piece of the obesity framework. *Nutr. J.* **2016**, *15*, 5. [CrossRef]
33. Gearhardt, A.N.; Boswell, R.G.; White, M.A. The association of "food addiction" with disordered eating and body mass index. *Eat. Behav.* **2014**, *15*, 427–433. [CrossRef]
34. Pedram, P.; Wadden, D.; Amini, P.; Gulliver, W.; Randell, E.; Cahill, F.; Vasdev, S.; Goodridge, A.; Carter, J.C.; Zhai, G.; et al. Food Addiction: Its Prevalence and Significant Association with Obesity in the General Population. *PLoS ONE* **2013**, *8*, e74832. [CrossRef] [PubMed]
35. Praxedes, D.R.S.; Silva-Júnior, A.E.; Macena, M.L.; Oliveira, A.D.; Cardoso, K.S.; Nunes, L.O.; Monteiro, M.B.; Melo, I.S.V.; Gearhardt, A.N.; Bueno, N.B. Prevalence of food addiction determined by the Yale Food Addiction Scale and associated factors: A systematic review with meta-analysis. *Eur. Eat. Disord. Rev.* **2022**, *30*, 85–95. [CrossRef] [PubMed]
36. Nelder, M.; Cahill, F.; Zhang, H.; Zhai, G.; Gulliver, W.; Teng, W.; Shan, Z.; Sun, G. The Association Between an Addictive Tendency Toward Food and Metabolic Characteristics in the General Newfoundland Population. *Front. Endocrinol.* **2018**, *9*, 661. [CrossRef] [PubMed]
37. Moghadam-Ahmadi, A.; Soltani, N.; Ayoobi, F.; Jamali, Z.; Sadeghi, T.; Jalali, N.; Vakilian, A.; Lotfi, M.A.; Khalili, P. Association between metabolic syndrome and stroke: A population based cohort study. *BMC Endocr. Disord.* **2023**, *23*, 131. [CrossRef]
38. Arboix, A. Cardiovascular risk factors for acute stroke: Risk profiles in the different subtypes of ischemic stroke. *World J. Clin. Cases* **2015**, *3*, 418–429. [CrossRef]
39. Gearhardt, A.N.; Corbin, W.R.; Brownell, K.D. Development of the Yale Food Addiction Scale Version 2.0. *Psychol. Addict. Behav.* **2016**, *30*, 113–121. [CrossRef]
40. American Psychiatric Association. *Diagnostic and Statistical Manual of Mental Disorders: DSM-5™*, 5th ed.; American Psychiatric Publishing, Inc.: Arlington, VA, USA, 2013; p. 947.
41. Kwah, L.K.; Diong, J. National Institutes of Health Stroke Scale (NIHSS). *J. Physiother.* **2014**, *60*, 61. [CrossRef]
42. Third Report of the National Cholesterol Education Program (NCEP) Expert Panel on Detection, Evaluation, and Treatment of High Blood Cholesterol in Adults (Adult Treatment Panel III) final report. *Circulation* **2002**, *106*, 3143–3421. [CrossRef]
43. Hage, V. The NIH Stroke Scale: A Window into Neurological Status. *Nurs. Spectr.* **2011**, *24*, 44–49.
44. Pilgrim, A.L.; Robinson, S.M.; Sayer, A.A.; Roberts, H.C. An overview of appetite decline in older people. *Nurs. Older People* **2015**, *27*, 29–35. [CrossRef] [PubMed]
45. Flint, A.J.; Gearhardt, A.N.; Corbin, W.R.; Brownell, K.D.; Field, A.E.; Rimm, E.B. Food-addiction scale measurement in 2 cohorts of middle-aged and older women. *Am. J. Clin. Nutr.* **2014**, *99*, 578–586. [CrossRef] [PubMed]
46. Carr, M.M.; Lawson, J.L.; Wiedemann, A.A.; Barnes, R.D. Examining impairment and distress from food addiction across demographic and weight groups. *Eat. Behav.* **2021**, *43*, 101574. [CrossRef]
47. Oliveira, J.; Colombarolli, M.S.; Cordás, T.A. Prevalence and correlates of food addiction: Systematic review of studies with the YFAS 2.0. *Obes. Res. Clin. Pract.* **2021**, *15*, 191–204. [CrossRef]
48. Whatnall, M.; Skinner, J.A.; Leary, M.; Burrows, T.L. Food Addiction: A Deep Dive into 'Loss of Control' and 'Craving'. *Curr. Addict. Rep.* **2022**, *9*, 318–325. [CrossRef]
49. Meule, A.; Gearhardt, A.N. Five years of the Yale Food Addiction Scale: Taking stock and moving forward. *Curr. Addict. Rep.* **2014**, *1*, 193–205. [CrossRef]
50. Albayrak, Ö.; Föcker, M.; Kliewer, J.; Esber, S.; Peters, T.; de Zwaan, M.; Hebebrand, J. Eating-related Psychopathology and Food Addiction in Adolescent Psychiatric Inpatients. *Eur. Eat. Disord. Rev.* **2017**, *25*, 214–220. [CrossRef]
51. Leung, C.W.; Parnarouskis, L.; Slotnick, M.J.; Gearhardt, A.N. Food Insecurity and Food Addiction in a Large, National Sample of Lower-Income Adults. *Curr. Dev. Nutr.* **2023**, *7*, 102036. [CrossRef]
52. Monteiro, C.A.; Cannon, G.; Levy, R.B.; Moubarac, J.C.; Louzada, M.L.; Rauber, F.; Khandpur, N.; Cediel, G.; Neri, D.; Martinez-Steele, E.; et al. Ultra-processed foods: What they are and how to identify them. *Public Health Nutr.* **2019**, *22*, 936–941. [CrossRef]
53. Schulte, E.M.; Gearhardt, A.N. Development of the Modified Yale Food Addiction Scale Version 2.0. *Eur. Eat. Disord. Rev.* **2017**, *25*, 302–308. [CrossRef]
54. Schulte, E.M.; Avena, N.M.; Gearhardt, A.N. Which Foods May Be Addictive? The Roles of Processing, Fat Content, and Glycemic Load. *PLoS ONE* **2015**, *10*, e0117959. [CrossRef] [PubMed]
55. Yang, F.; Liu, A.; Li, Y.; Lai, Y.; Wang, G.; Sun, C.; Sun, G.; Shan, Z.; Teng, W. Food Addiction in Patients with Newly Diagnosed Type 2 Diabetes in Northeast China. *Front. Endocrinol.* **2017**, *8*, 218. [CrossRef] [PubMed]
56. Serrano-Gonzalez, M.; Herting, M.M.; Lim, S.L.; Sullivan, N.J.; Kim, R.; Espinoza, J.; Koppin, C.M.; Javier, J.R.; Kim, M.S.; Luo, S. Developmental Changes in Food Perception and Preference. *Front. Psychol.* **2021**, *12*, 654200. [CrossRef] [PubMed]
57. Giuliani, N.R.; Pfeifer, J.H. Age-related changes in reappraisal of appetitive cravings during adolescence. *Neuroimage* **2015**, *108*, 173–181. [CrossRef] [PubMed]
58. Silvers, J.A.; Shu, J.; Hubbard, A.D.; Weber, J.; Ochsner, K.N. Concurrent and lasting effects of emotion regulation on amygdala response in adolescence and young adulthood. *Dev. Sci.* **2015**, *18*, 771–784. [CrossRef]
59. Galván, A.; McGlennen, K.M. Enhanced striatal sensitivity to aversive reinforcement in adolescents versus adults. *J. Cogn. Neurosci.* **2013**, *25*, 284–296. [CrossRef]
60. Lowe, C.J.; Morton, J.B.; Reichelt, A.C. Adolescent obesity and dietary decision making-a brain-health perspective. *Lancet Child Adolesc. Health* **2020**, *4*, 388–396. [CrossRef]

61. Victor, A.; Silva, R.d.C.R.; Silva, N.d.J.; Ferreira, A.; Barreto, M.L.; Campello, T. Influence of Unhealthy Food Environment on Premature Cardiovascular Disease Mortality in Brazil: An Ecologic Approach. *Am. J. Prev. Med.* **2023**, *64*, 285–292. [CrossRef]
62. Bigna, J.J.; Noubiap, J.J. The rising burden of non-communicable diseases in sub-Saharan Africa. *Lancet Glob. Health* **2019**, *7*, e1295–e1296. [CrossRef]
63. Ryder, J.R.; Northrop, E.; Rudser, K.D.; Kelly, A.S.; Gao, Z.; Khoury, P.R.; Kimball, T.R.; Dolan, L.M.; Urbina, E.M. Accelerated Early Vascular Aging Among Adolescents With Obesity and/or Type 2 Diabetes Mellitus. *J. Am. Heart Assoc.* **2020**, *9*, e014891. [CrossRef]
64. Razanamahefa, L.; Lafay, L.; Oseredczuk, M.; Thiébaut, A.; Laloux, L.; Gerber, M.; Astorg, P.; Berta, J.L. Dietary fat consumption of the French population and quality of the data on the composition of the major food groups. *Bull. Cancer* **2005**, *92*, 647–657. [PubMed]
65. Ferrières, J. The French paradox: Lessons for other countries. *Heart* **2004**, *90*, 107–111. [CrossRef] [PubMed]
66. Davis, J.F.; Tracy, A.L.; Schurdak, J.D.; Tschöp, M.H.; Lipton, J.W.; Clegg, D.J.; Benoit, S.C. Exposure to elevated levels of dietary fat attenuates psychostimulant reward and mesolimbic dopamine turnover in the rat. *Behav. Neurosci.* **2008**, *122*, 1257–1263. [CrossRef]
67. Sharma, S.; Fulton, S. Diet-induced obesity promotes depressive-like behaviour that is associated with neural adaptations in brain reward circuitry. *Int. J. Obes. (Lond.)* **2013**, *37*, 382–389. [CrossRef]
68. Cone, J.J.; Chartoff, E.H.; Potter, D.N.; Ebner, S.R.; Roitman, M.F. Prolonged high fat diet reduces dopamine reuptake without altering DAT gene expression. *PLoS ONE* **2013**, *8*, e58251. [CrossRef]
69. Hryhorczuk, C.; Florea, M.; Rodaros, D.; Poirier, I.; Daneault, C.; Des Rosiers, C.; Arvanitogiannis, A.; Alquier, T.; Fulton, S. Dampened Mesolimbic Dopamine Function and Signaling by Saturated but not Monounsaturated Dietary Lipids. *Neuropsychopharmacology* **2016**, *41*, 811–821. [CrossRef]
70. Dalal, J.J.; Padmanabhan, T.N.; Jain, P.; Patil, S.; Vasnawala, H.; Gulati, A. LIPITENSION: Interplay between dyslipidemia and hypertension. *Indian J. Endocrinol. Metab.* **2012**, *16*, 240–245. [CrossRef]
71. Wu, L.; Parhofer, K.G. Diabetic dyslipidemia. *Metabolism* **2014**, *63*, 1469–1479. [CrossRef]
72. Vekic, J.; Zeljkovic, A.; Stefanovic, A.; Jelic-Ivanovic, Z.; Spasojevic-Kalimanovska, V. Obesity and dyslipidemia. *Metabolism* **2019**, *92*, 71–81. [CrossRef]
73. Kuriakose, D.; Xiao, Z. Pathophysiology and Treatment of Stroke: Present Status and Future Perspectives. *Int. J. Mol. Sci.* **2020**, *21*, 7609. [CrossRef]
74. Gallanagh, S.; Quinn, T.J.; Alexander, J.; Walters, M.R. Physical activity in the prevention and treatment of stroke. *ISRN Neurol.* **2011**, *2011*, 953818. [CrossRef] [PubMed]
75. Guo, J.M.; Liu, A.J.; Su, D.F. Genetics of stroke. *Acta Pharmacol. Sin.* **2010**, *31*, 1055–1064. [CrossRef] [PubMed]
76. Cornelis, M.C.; Flint, A.; Field, A.E.; Kraft, P.; Han, J.; Rimm, E.B.; van Dam, R.M. A genome-wide investigation of food addiction. *Obesity* **2016**, *24*, 1336–1341. [CrossRef]
77. Carlier, N.; Marshe, V.S.; Cmorejova, J.; Davis, C.; Müller, D.J. Genetic Similarities between Compulsive Overeating and Addiction Phenotypes: A Case for "Food Addiction"? *Curr. Psychiatry Rep.* **2015**, *17*, 96. [CrossRef]
78. Romer, A.L.; Su Kang, M.; Nikolova, Y.S.; Gearhardt, A.N.; Hariri, A.R. Dopamine genetic risk is related to food addiction and body mass through reduced reward-related ventral striatum activity. *Appetite* **2019**, *133*, 24–31. [CrossRef]
79. Gardener, H.; Sacco, R.L.; Rundek, T.; Battistella, V.; Cheung, Y.K.; Elkind, M.S.V. Race and Ethnic Disparities in Stroke Incidence in the Northern Manhattan Study. *Stroke* **2020**, *51*, 1064–1069. [CrossRef]
80. Wang, Z.; Jin, X.; Liu, Y.; Wang, C.; Li, J.; Tian, L.; Teng, W. Sedentary behavior and the risk of stroke: A systematic review and dose-response meta-analysis. *Nutr. Metab. Cardiovasc. Dis.* **2022**, *32*, 2705–2713. [CrossRef]
81. Carr, M.M.; Schulte, E.M.; Saules, K.K.; Gearhardt, A.N. Measurement Invariance of the Modified Yale Food Addiction Scale 2.0 Across Gender and Racial Groups. *Assessment* **2020**, *27*, 356–364. [CrossRef]

nutrients

MDPI

Article

Psychoneurological Links Contributing to Body Mass Index and Eating Disorder Severity

Geovanny Genaro Reivan Ortiz [1,*], Braulio Elizalde [2], Cristhian Tapia [2] and Roser Granero [3]

1 Catholic University of Cuenca, Cuenca 010107, Ecuador
2 Ministry of Public Health, Mental Health Area Zonal 6, Cuenca 010107, Ecuador
3 Department of Psychobiology and Methodology, Universitat Autònoma de Barcelona, 08193 Barcelona, Spain; roser.granero@uab.cat
* Correspondence: greivano@ucacue.edu.ec

Abstract: Background-objectives: Multiple dynamic interacting factors contribute to the presence and progression of eating disorders (ED). Empirical research has provided mixed findings regarding the mechanisms explaining the contribution of body mass index (BMI) to the diverse ED endophenotypes. The present study aims to evaluate the underlying processes (direct and indirect effects) contributing to BMI and ED severity, considering the contribution of multiple neuropsychological constructs. Method: Path analysis, implemented through structural equation models (SEM), was applied to a sample of N = 193 ED patients, men and women, aged 17 to 50 years old, and diagnosed with bulimia nervosa, night eating syndrome, binge eating disorder, and other specified feeding. Results: BMI was directly associated with ED severity level. The ED symptom level was also a mediational link into the relationship between BMI with emotion regulation strategies, decision-making capacity, stress levels, and impulsiveness. Multigroup SEM revealed invariance of the structural coefficients by sex, but differences according to the ED subtype. Conclusions: This study provides new empirical evidence on predictors of ED severity, focusing on the role of impaired decision-making and BMI. Our results could contribute to new intervention plans with techniques specifically aimed at improving emotional regulation capacity, decreasing impulsivity levels, and improving reasoning skills. Nutrition education plans may also play a key role for preventing the onset and progression of ED, helping patients understand how food affects their physical and emotional health and how to manage anxiety and fears related to food.

Keywords: emotion regulation; decision-making; impulsivity; anxiety; stress; eating disorders; body mass index

Academic Editor: Mauro Cataldi

Received: 25 November 2024
Revised: 6 January 2025
Accepted: 13 January 2025
Published: 15 January 2025

Citation: Reivan Ortiz, G.G.; Elizalde, B.; Tapia, C.; Granero, R. Psychoneurological Links Contributing to Body Mass Index and Eating Disorder Severity. *Nutrients* **2025**, *17*, 296. https://doi.org/10.3390/nu17020296

1. Introduction

Nutrition and diet are crucial elements of health. Studies have demonstrated that a balanced diet containing all essential nutrients is vital for optimal brain performance and cognitive function. Conversely, diets lacking in nutritional quality or are excessively abundant in calories have been linked to various negative health outcomes [1], including overweightness/obesity and even brain damage. Persistent alterations in nutritional habits affect brain chemistry and psychological processes, contributing to the onset and progression of eating disorders.

Malnutrition affects metabolic health through diverse biological pathways and determines the obesogenic effects of food, contributing to reduced body mass index (BMI) but also obesity [2]. BMI is a measure that relates body weight to height, and it is typically interpreted as an index of body fat and of healthy weight. Low BMI, which is categorized as underweight (less than 18.5 kg/m^2 among adulthood population), suggests that the body may not be receiving the nutrients required for a healthy state and can lead to physical illness (such as osteoporosis, skin-hair-teeth problems, anemia, or irregular periods) and mental disease (such as depression, anxiety, or anorexia). On the other end of the scale, a high BMI is categorized as overweight (BMI higher than 25 and lower than 30) or obesity (BMI of 30 or greater), indicates excessive body fat deposits that can also impair health, increasing the likelihood of multiple health issues and severe comorbidities (such as heart disease, diabetes, hypertension, metabolic syndrome, substance abuse, depression, anxiety, and eating behavior related problems) [3–6].

Overweightness and obesity are complex multifactorial diseases, primarily stemming from an imbalance between energy intake (diet) and energy expenditure (physical activity). The eating disorders (ED) defined in the current version of the Diagnostic and Statistical Manual of Mental Disorders DSM-5 [7] more frequently associated with overweightness and obesity are bulimia nervosa (BN, characterized by episodes of overeating followed by regret and purging behaviors), night eating syndrome (NES, where individuals consume large amounts of food after dinner and may wake up at night to eat), binge eating disorder (BED, in which individuals eat an excessively large amount of food in a short period while feeling a loss of control), and other specific feeding and eating disorders (OSFED, which present incomplete or atypical symptoms of eating disorders). The global prevalence of ED is increasing for all subtypes and more affected people have sought professional help in recent decades [6].

The links between ED with BMI are complex, and it has been suggested that there are diverse mediational links that contribute, including emotional regulation strategies [2,8–11], impairing eating attitudes [12], negative mood states [6,10], and different neuropsychological processes (such as impaired decision-making [13–19]). Impulsivity has also been observed within some pathways, and the transdiagnostic role of this construct has been suggested [20].

Firstly, the difficulties in managing and responding to emotional experiences have been widely linked with overeating (for example, binge episodes) and purging behaviors (aimed at weight control/reduction). Interestingly, the emotion-driven model addresses overeating because of the dysfunction in emotional and cognitive processing [2]. This view holds that decision-making inherently relies on emotional processes that provide important implicit and explicit knowledge by which the individual can make fast and adaptive decisions [14]. Concretely, homeostatic control of food intake seems strongly influenced by the brain reward system [15]. Since dopamine and serotonin participate in the regulation of appetite, in dietary balance, and in food reward [16], it may be the case that impairing the functioning of these two neurotransmitters is related to decision-making, emotional eating, and addictive behavior. In addition, impaired decision-making under conditions of uncertainty has been associated with the concrete expression and maintenance of ED [14], and it has been suggested that both ED and obese individuals may share a similar incapacity to modulate reward and punishment using a long-term perspective, with their behavior guided by immediate rewards (restrictive eating, binges, and compensatory behaviors such as purges or laxatives), despite the severe long-term effects on their bodies and weight. This process could also explain the high resistance to change among ED patients.

Secondly, emotional dysregulation has been found to be associated with impulse control difficulties and decision-making deficits, two critical mechanisms in the basis of the onset and the chronic course of ED [13,17]. Concretely, high impulsivity and impaired emotion regulation capacities at a younger age have been related to the emergence of eating behavior symptoms later via suboptimal decision-making [18]. Reduced functionality of the ventromedial prefrontal cortex has been associated with worse decision-making performance among patients with ED [16].

Regarding mood states, perceived levels of anxiety and stress are powerful risk factors for overweightness/obesity and ED [6,10,11]. Epidemiological research shows that social anxiety and generalized anxiety are the most common psychiatric comorbidities in patients with ED, with rates around 50% in AN, BN, and BED. Studies have observed a relationship between neuropsychological performance and anxiety levels within samples of patients with ED [19], suggesting that: (a) executive functions could achieve a transdiagnostic process in ED and obesity, and (b) this process could provide explanations for the inability to regulate food intake and other dysfunctional eating behaviors among these patients.

But despite recognizing the associations between the multiple neuropsychological processes on the profiles of ED, few studies have analyzed the effect of these underlying mechanisms and the mediational links between these variables on the patients' BMI and symptoms of the ED, over a broad spectrum of ED and weight. The aim of this study is to explore the pathways between emotional regulation, eating behavior style, decision-making, impulsiveness, anxiety, and perceived stress on the BMI and severity of the ED, among a sample of patients diagnosed with OSFED, BED, NES, and BN.

2. Materials and Methods

2.1. Participants

The study included a sample of patients diagnosed with BN ($n = 42$), NES ($n = 31$), BED ($n = 37$), and OSFED ($n = 83$) who consecutively attended to the psychiatry outpatient area of the Customer Care Program, Citizen "Mental Health" of the Ministry of Public Health of Ecuador. The diagnosis of the patients was made by the experienced psychiatrists in charge of the program. The inclusion criteria for this study were ages 17 to 50 years and met clinical criteria for BN, NES, BED, and OSFED according to DSM-5 criteria. Exclusion criteria were psychoactive substance dependence, significant medical or neurological disease, and severe cognitive impairment (such as Alzheimer's disease).

The included patients met the criteria established by the DSM-5 for diagnosis at least 2 months before entering the study. Likewise, they did not report being under the effect of any medication or psychotropic drug at the arrival to the therapy unit.

2.2. Measures

BMI was calculated by dividing the weight (in kilograms) by the height (in meters squared). The weight was measured with a 500 KL eye-level digital Healthometer medical scale, 500 pound/485.0 kg capacity, manufactured in the USA, used to calculate BMI (BMI = weight (kg)/[height (m)]^2.

The symptom level was measured with the Eating Disorder Inventory level (EDI-3) [20]. This is a self-report instrument used to assess psychological traits and constructs clinically related to ED. The questionnaire consists of 91 items registered in a Likert-type scale (from 0 to 5), organized in the following primary scales: drive for thinness, bulimia, body dissatisfaction, low self-esteem, personal alienation, interpersonal insecurity, interpersonal distrust, interoceptive deficits, emotional dysregulation, perfectionism, asceticism, and maturity fears. A total score in the whole questionnaire is interpreted as the ED severity level. In this work, the Cronbach's alpha ranged between 0.83 and 0.91.

The anxiety level was assessed with the Goldberg Anxiety and Depression Scale (GADS) [21]. This self-report tool consists of 18 items (registered with a binary scale yes/no) structured in two primary scales for assessing anxiety and depression symptoms.

The anxiety scale was used in the study with an adequate internal consistency in the sample ($\alpha = 0.75$).

The stress level was assessed with the Perceived Stress Scale (PSS-10) [22]. This is a 10-item tool designed to assess perceived stress over the last month, based on 10 items registered through a Likert-type scale (0 = Never, 1 = Almost Never, 2 = Sometimes, 3 = Often and 4 = Very often). The Cronbach's alpha coefficient of in the study was adequate ($\alpha = 0.79$).

Emotional regulation capacities were assessed with the Emotional Regulation Questionnaire (ERQ) [23]. This is a self-report tool containing two first-order scales: cognitive reappraisal and expressive suppression. A total score is also available based on the sum of all the items. The responses are registered through a seven-point Likert scale (from 1 "totally disagree" to 7 "totally agree"). In this work the Cronbach's alpha coefficient was $\alpha = 0.70$ for the cognitive reappraisal subscale and $\alpha = 0.78$ on the expressive suppression subscale.

Impulsivity level was assessed with the Plutchick Impulsivity Scale (PIS) [24,25]. This self-report scale consists of 15 Likert type items scored from 0 to 3 (never, sometimes, often, almost, and always). The aim is to obtain a measure of the control capacity for self-control, planning and action in the future, physiological behaviors, and spontaneous action. A total score calculated as the sum of the items is usually employed as a global measure of the impulsiveness levels. In this work, the Cronbach's alpha coefficient was $\alpha = 0.70$.

The decision-making capacity was assessed with the General Decision-Making Style (GDMS) [26]. This is a 25 items questionnaire (registered with a Likert scale scored from 1 = "Strongly disagree" to 5 = "Strongly agree") developed to assess an individuals' decision-making styles in five approaches: rational (logical approach to decisions by searching information and alternatives, and carefully thought out), intuitive (decisions based on people's hunches or feelings), dependent (decision process based on searching advice and guidance from others), avoidant (procrastinating and avoidant decision rules), and spontaneous (quick decision process). This study analyzed a total score, calculated by summing the responses to the items. Higher values indicate a greater level of deterioration. In this work, Cronbach's alpha coefficient in the study was $\alpha = 0.81$.

2.3. Procedure

The study was carried out in accordance with the latest version of the Declaration of Helsinki. The Research Ethics Committee of the Catholic University of Cuenca and the Clinical Research Ethics Committee of the Ecuadorian Ministry of Public Health approved the study. Signed consent was also obtained from the participants.

Physicians and psychiatrists with high experience in the treatment of ED carried out the assessment of the patients at the baseline (at the arrival to the therapy unit). Data collection was 8 months (from February 2023 to September 2023). Clinicians helped participants complete the measurement tools to avoid the presence of missing data.

2.4. Statistical Analysis

Statistical analysis was performed with Stata18 for Windows (Stata-Corp, College Station, TX, USA) [27]. Firstly, the correlation matrix between the variables analyzed in the study was obtained. The clinical relevance of the correlation coefficients (R) was not based on the results of the significance tests using Pearson's correlation model since this test provides results that are directly based on the sample size: very weak correlation coefficients (close to zero) achieve significant results ($p < 0.05$) with large samples, while correlation coefficients very far from zero achieve non-significant results ($p > 0.05$) with low samples. In this work, relevant correlations were considered for R-coefficients with effect size within the ranges moderate (|R| > 0.24) to large (|R| > 0.37) (these two thresholds are equivalent to the classical Cohen's-*d* 0.50 and 0.80) [28].

The study of the underlying processes associated with BMI was conducted with path analysis procedure, which constitutes a straightforward extension of classical multiple regression modeling. The aim of this statistical method is to estimate the significance and magnitude of the relationships among a set of variables, including mediational links (direct and indirect effects) [29]. Path analysis in this work was developed as a case of structural equation modeling (SEM). In psychology, this method has been used for the study of the etiopathogenesis of several processes, allowing for the estimation of the magnitude and significance of the hypothesized associations into a set of variables and facilitating testing mediational links. While path analysis has been historically used to disprove a "model" that postulates potential causal relations among variables, currently this method is also employed for both exploratory and confirmatory modeling (it allows both theory testing and theory development). The rationale for the model specification (synopsized in the path-diagram) was based on the theoretical background provided by the cumulated empirical evidence. All parameters were free estimated (no values were assumed, and coefficients were directly estimated by the SEM). In this work, the maximum-likelihood estimation method was used, and multi-group processes were tested to assess invariance by participants' sex and diagnostic subtype. Goodness-of-fit was considered based on the usual statistical measures [30,31]: non-significant result in the chi-square (χ^2) test, Root Mean Square Error of Approximation RMSEA < 0.08, Tucker–Lewis Index TLI > 0.90, Bentler's Comparative Fit Index CFI > 0.90, and Standardized Root Mean Square Residual SRMR < 0.10.

3. Results

3.1. Descriptive Statistics for the Sample

The frequency distribution of the variables analyzed in the study and the comparison between the diagnostic subtypes are displayed in Table 1. Most participants in the complete sample were women (64.2%), and the mean age was 32.1 years (SD = 6.26). No differences between the diagnostic groups were found.

Table 1. Descriptive statistics for the variables of the study by diagnostic subtype group.

	OSFED (n = 83)		**BED (n = 37)**		**NES (n = 31)**		**BN (n = 42)**			
	n	%	n	%	n	%	n	%	χ^2	p
Sex										
Women	52	62.7%	23	62.2%	22	71.0%	27	64.3%	0.77	0.856
Men	31	37.3%	14	37.8%	9	29.0%	15	35.7%		
	Mean	SD	Mean	SD	Mean	SD	Mean	SD	F-stat	p
Age	32.20	6.21	32.38	6.61	32.16	6.21	31.76	6.31	0.071	0.975
Emotion dysregulation	12.47	4.35	12.95	4.48	13.55	5.62	12.95	4.04	0.452	0.716
Decision-making	12.93	5.96	14.32	6.58	14.00	5.68	14.60	6.12	0.905	0.440
Impulsivity	14.45	4.28	14.81	4.91	14.65	4.82	14.79	5.01	0.077	0.972
Anxiety	14.39	4.90	15.16	5.75	15.77	6.06	15.52	5.52	0.713	0.545
Stress	22.70	7.19	24.70	9.05	24.74	9.67	24.00	8.47	0.769	0.513
Eating symptom level	4.93	2.13	4.95	2.20	5.68	3.32	5.31	2.73	0.815	0.487
BMI (kg/m^2)	29.35	10.73	27.84	7.37	30.65	13.81	30.93	13.27	0.590	0.622

Note. SD: standard deviation. OSFED: other specified feed and eating disorder. BED: binge eating disorder. NES: night eating syndrome. BN: bulimia nervosa. Comparison between the groups through chi-square (χ^2) for categorical variables and analysis of variance (ANOVA) for quantitative variables.

The correlation matrix between the variables considered in the study is displayed in Table 2. Positive coefficients were obtained (R values within the ranges mild-moderate to large-high), suggesting the relationships between difficulties with emotion regulation, higher impairment in cognitive decision-making, higher impulsivity, higher anxiety, higher stress, higher eating symptom level, and higher BMI.

Table 2. Correlation matrix.

		2	3	4	5	6	7	8	9
1	Age	0.030	0.110	0.111	0.029	0.026	0.017	0.052	−0.080
2	Emotion dysregulation		**0.607** †	**0.262** †	**0.803** †	**0.467** †	**0.356** †	**0.245** †	−0.105
3	Decision-making			**0.333** †	**0.632** †	**0.525** †	0.234	**0.277** †	−0.133
4	Impulsivity				0.221	**0.586** †	**0.366** †	0.187	0.031
5	Anxiety					**0.445** †	**0.321** †	**0.284** †	−0.117
6	Stress						**0.467** †	**0.345** †	−0.114
7	Eating symptom level							**0.468** †	−0.010
8	BMI (kg/m^2)								0.010
9	Sex								---

Note. † Bold: effect size within the ranges mild–moderate to large–high.

3.2. Path Analysis

Figure 1 shows the path diagram with the standardized coefficients obtained in the whole sample. Adequate goodness-of-fit was obtained for the SEM (see fit-indexes reported in the first line of Table 3). The results obtained in this model showed a direct effect of the EDI-3 total score on the BMI (the higher the ED symptom level, the higher the BMI). Severity of the ED was also a mediational variable within different paths: (a) difficulties with emotion regulation, higher impaired decision-making, higher impulsivity levels, increased stress levels, and higher stress levels contributed to ED with higher severity levels, which then contributed to an increased BMI; (b) higher emotion dysregulation and higher impulsivity also directly impacted severity levels of ED, which then increase BMI values. The path diagram displayed in Figure 1 also indicates that anxiety levels were directly increased for patients with difficulties with emotion regulation and decision-making.

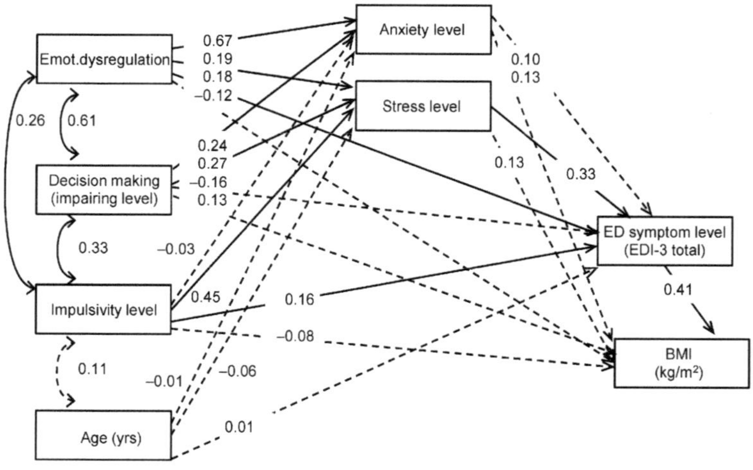

Figure 1. Path diagram: standardized coefficients in the complete sample. Note. Continuous line: significant parameter. Dash line: non-significant parameter.

Table 3. Fit statistics for the SEM.

	χ^2	*p*	RMSEA	CFI	TLI	SRMR
Single	1.220	0.544	0.001	0.999	0.999	0.008
Invariance by sex	0.885	0.927	0.001	0.999	0.999	0.008
Invariance by diagnostic subtype	4.903	0.768	0.001	0.999	0.999	0.019

Note. SD: standard deviation. RMSEA: Root mean squared error of approximation. CFI: Comparative fit index. TLI: Tucker–Lewis index. SRMR: Standardized root mean squared residual.

The multi-group models defined to assess the invariance of the SEM by patients' sex and diagnostic subtype obtained adequate goodness-of-fit (Table 3). Table 4 shows the tests for the unvarying of the structural coefficients, the covariances, and the global fit statistics. In relation to sex, join test showed invariance of the structural coefficients (the only difference was for the coefficient measuring the association between impulsivity and stress) and for the fitting indexes, but differences for the covariances emerged (two coefficients were different between sexes: impulsivity correlated with age and with decision-making only among the women's subsample). Table S1 (Supplementary Materials) shows the structural coefficients obtained in the multi-group model defined to assess invariance by participants' sex.

Table 4. Tests for group invariance.

		Sex				Diagnostic Subtype			
Structural Coeff.			χ^2	*df*	*p*		χ^2	*df*	*p*
Stress	Age		0.022	1	0.881		4.963	3	0.175
	Impulsivity		8.419	1	**0.004** *		2.730	3	0.435
	decision-making		1.949	1	0.163		4.695	3	0.196
	Emotion dysregulation		2.518	1	0.113		8.183	3	**0.042** *
Anxiety	Age		0.002	1	0.968		5.067	3	0.167
	Impulsivity		0.172	1	0.678		3.001	3	0.392
	decision-making		1.263	1	0.261		5.436	3	0.143
	Emotion dysregulation		0.711	1	0.399		1.350	3	0.717
Symptoms of ED	Stress		1.774	1	0.183		0.344	3	0.952
	Anxiety		1.383	1	0.240		5.405	3	0.144
	Age		1.240	1	0.266		5.752	3	0.124
	Impulsivity		0.723	1	0.395		6.920	3	0.075
	decision-making		0.023	1	0.880		5.978	3	0.113
	Emotion dysregulation		1.209	1	0.272		1.485	3	0.686
BMI	Stress		0.744	1	0.388		3.759	3	0.289
	Anxiety		0.008	1	0.929		1.805	3	0.614
	ED symptom level		2.588	1	0.108		12.767	3	**0.005** *
	Impulsivity		0.164	1	0.685		4.717	3	0.194
	decision-making		0.026	1	0.872		8.011	3	**0.046** *
	Emotion dysregulation		0.634	1	0.426		4.119	3	0.249
Join tests	Parameters		χ^2	*df*	*p*		χ^2	*df*	*p*
	Structural coefficients		24.940	20	0.204		108.873	60	**0.001** *
	Covariances		18.610	10	**0.045** *		22.520	30	0.835
	Fit-statistics	Women	0.432	2	0.806	OSFED	0.296	2	0.862
		Men	0.453	2	0.797	BED	1.172	2	0.557
						NES	1.850	2	0.397
						BN	1.584	2	0.453

Note. *df*: degrees of freedom. OSFED: other specified feed and eating disorder. BED: binge eating disorder. NES: night eating syndrome. BN: bulimia nervosa. * Bold: significant test.

The multi-group model defined to assess the invariance of the SEM by diagnostic subtype 4 showed unvarying covariances and global fit statistics but differences in the structural coefficients. Figure 1 shows the path diagrams with the standardized coefficients obtained from each diagnosis. The test of invariance for each structural coefficient reported differences for: (a) the contribution of emotion dysregulation to the stress level (a significant coefficient was found for NES and BN, while no association was identified for OSFED and BED); (b) the effect of ED symptom severity on BMI (the relationship was identified for OSFED, NES, and BN but was not relevant for BED); and (c) the impact of decision-making on BMI (a significant association only found among the OSFED group) (see Table S2, Supplementary, for the structural coefficients obtained in the multi-group model defined, including the diagnostic subtype as a group).

4. Discussion

This study aimed to explore the pathways between eating related symptoms (disordered eating characteristics), emotional dysregulation, impaired decision-making, impulsiveness, anxiety, stress, and BMI, among patients diagnosed with ED (OSFED, BED, NES, and BN).

The results indicated that higher levels of symptoms of ED directly impacted the BMI (direct effect). This observation is consistent with previous studies [32] that observed the pathognomonic nature of disordered/impairing eating behaviors on the body composition (and particularly on BMI) [33]. It is well known that some ED subtypes (such as BN and BED) show symptoms related to the sensation of loss of control, a feature strongly linked with the inability to stop eating. Patients within these ED categories also report eating faster than normal (even being alone) and argue that this eating style may prevent others from realizing how much they eat (a behavior contributing to the chronification) [33,34].

Another relevant result of our study is the identification of levels of symptoms of ED as a mediational link in various pathways. In particular, difficulties with emotional regulation, greater deterioration in decision-making, higher levels of impulsivity, and increased stress levels contributed to higher levels of severe symptoms in the ED, which finally lead to higher BMI. These results are consistent with previous studies that outline the influence of emotional dysregulation [8–11], difficulties in decision-making [13,14,18,19], and impulsivity [35,36], on increased anxiety and perceived stress, which next lead to impairing/disordered eating behaviors. Our results support previous studies that suggest that stress plays an important role in the onset and development of ED [37–39]. Concretely, stress has been associated with an increased likelihood of being overweight/obese [40–42], arguing that exposure to life events may release appetite hormones that increase the desire for foods rich in fats and sugars [40] with weak efforts for healthy activity levels [43]. Studies have also observed that participants who reported a higher perception of stress were more likely to indicate a lower intake of fruits, vegetables, and proteins, but higher consumption of salty and sweet snacks and less participation in physical activities [42]. A meta-analysis of prospective studies has also revealed that psychosocial stressors, including acute stressful events (for example, being fired or losing a loved one) are risk factors for increased BMI [43]. Other forms of psychosocial stressors have also been postulated as potential risk factors for overweight and obesity in adulthood, such as weight discrimination (i.e., unfair treatment of a person based on their weight) [44], childhood trauma (e.g., physical abuse, verbal abuse, witnessed abuse, humiliation, neglect) [45], financial stress (e.g., difficulty paying bills) [46], and conflicts in interpersonal relationships (e.g., adverse exchanges and conflicts) [47].

Our study also evidenced the mediating role of the severity of the symptoms of ED on BMI levels. The pathways showed that difficulties with emotional regulation capacity and higher levels of impulsivity directly impacted the severity levels of ED, and the more impaired they were, the more severe the ED were and the higher the BMI was. This new empirical observation reinforces previous studies that concluded that both emotion regulation and impulsiveness are key features in the genesis and maintenance of disordered eating behaviors [48–52].

Related to the previous result, this work showed that anxiety levels were directly related to the individuals' difficulties regulating their emotions as well as to impaired decision-making. The crucial role of negative mood states and concrete anxiety states on the etiopathogenesis of multiple mental disorders has been systematically reported [53,54]. Existing research also suggests that emotion regulation skills are transdiagnostic factors for the development and course of anxiety discrders [53,54] and also for the different subtypes of ED [54,55]. It could be that individuals with difficulties managing emotional responses and eating experiences accumulate periods of more serious stress, which can evolve into anxiety levels and subsequently to greater severity of their ED [10,33,54]. Studies have also observed that patients with poor emotional awareness reported higher anxiety levels [54,56,57], suggesting that these subjects typically avcid situations of high emotional cost because of the hard time coping with these states. That is, since emotional awareness capacities allow people to acknowledge the type of emotions and the degree to which they are experienced, the difficulties with recognizing negative emotions should increase distress tolerance, capacities for managing conflict, and impairing decision-making. All these features form the basis of the severity of ED, and therefore are mediational links for the BMI. These pathways have been suggested based on the empirical results obtained in previous studies with samples of overweight and/or obese patients [12,38,39,43,50,58] and patients with ED [59,60]. Previous studies identified the direct contribution of emotional regulation on the perceived stress levels among NES [3,61–63], BN [57,64,65], BED [2,4,5,18,36,37,52,58], and OSFED [66–68].

The association between high anxiety and impaired decision-making has also been reported in previous research analyzing the diverse endophenotypes of ED [13,14,18,19,69]. Both features have been identified as triggers for disordered eating (restrictive or compulsive eating, irregular or inflexible eating patterns), and for multiple behaviors present in people with ED (fasting, binges, skipping meals, self-induced vomiting, use of diet pills, use of laxatives-diuretics, etc.). Furthermore, the study of the neurobiology of ED has identified multifaceted interaction systems involving both neural and physical substrates for hunger and satiety, including the diverse processes implicated in eating (hedonic/reward-based homeostatic/appetitive actions) [70]. The reward circuitry includes multiple brain areas (ventral striatum, amygdala, thalamus, and midbrain neuros), as well as neurotransmitters and neuropeptides (dopamine, serotonin, opioids, endocannabinoids, orexigenic peptides, and glutamate) [71]. Studies aimed at investigating the neural correlations of decision-making processes among patients with ED have observed aberrant functioning of these brain areas [72]. For example, poor cognitive flexibility in AN seems characterized by impaired functioning of the frontoparietal control network, and this weakened performance may contribute to dysregulation in gcal-directed cognition and decision-making [73]. The difficulties with cognitive performance in BN patients have been associated with premotor cortex and dorsal striatum [65]. Etiological studies have also associated high anxiety levels and body shape concerns among AN patients with abnormal brain functioning, concretely with prefrontal and cingulate brain response [70,74,75], and with lower caudate or parietal activity [75], which are also strongly related with cognition processes. But these studies should be considered with caution, despite the number of studies aimed at identifying brain structures and structural connectivity contributing to AN, BN, and OB (such as food restriction, binge-eating or purging behaviors, cognitive and emotional factors), empirical research is still low for BED.

Regarding the differences by sex, our study showed invariance for the SEM. This result seems inconsistent with previous studies which observed differences between men and women in most of the variables analyzed in this work (female sex were related to higher impulsivity levels, more perceived stress, more difficulties in decision-making, and higher severity of ED) [59,60,76–78]. Regarding this supposed discrepancy, it should be considered that our study did not analyze mean differences between men and women in these constructs, but rather assessed whether the underlying relationships (the structural coefficients) were similar. For example, our objective was not to identify differences in the symptom levels of ED between the sexes, but to test the contribution of the severity of ED on BMI (measuring the direct and indirect effects).

Similarly, we obtained invariance based on the subtype of the ED. Previous research has also outlined differences within the different groups of ED, even between BED and obese patients [59]. In fact, given the high concurrence between these diseases, both clinical conditions have some shared behaviors and features (overeating and high BMI), and etiology and behaviors were expected to have a similar presentation. However, emerging studies evidence divergent neurobiological [79,80] and psychological processes, implied in impulsivity/compulsivity response, reward processing and emotional reactivity. Our study has evidenced structural invariance related with the subtypes of ED, suggesting that the relationships pattern and the strengths of the associations did not statistically differ between the ED groups. That is, the underlying relationships between the variables analyzed in the study work in the same way across the different types of ED.

There are several limitations in the present study. First, while structural invariance was analyzed by the subtypes of the ED, no differentiation was made within each group of ED (for example, differentiating between BN-restrictive and BN-purgative). Second, comorbidities associated with eating disorders were not considered (such as diseases related to obesity, joint problems, heart disease, type 2 diabetes, gastroesophageal reflux disease, and some sleep-related breathing disorders). Finally, the sample size could be considered too small to achieve statistical power for path-analysis. However, it must be considered that the sample size requirements for these models seem to rely on outdated rules-of-thumb. Some current studies have been analyzed through Monte-Carlo procedures where the sample size requirements for some common types of SEMs is different, including variation by the number of factors, number of indicators, strength of the indicator loadings and the regressive paths and the amount of missing data per indicator [81,82]. For example, the study of Wolf and colleagues, performed with respect to statistical power, bias in the parameter estimates, and overall solution propriety, revealed that the sample requirements were into a very broad range (from 30 to 460), depending on the analysis characteristics [83]. The most interesting finding is that overall, solutions that met fitting at a given sample size were stable relative to the results of the analysis at the next largest sample sizes. Other studies have also observed that the appropriate sample size for a SEM depends on the complexity of the model, such as the following: (a) the number of parameters (at least 10 cases for each free parameter in the model [84]; (b) the complexity of the path diagram (200 to 500 for models without latent variables, and 500–1000 for models with latent variables) [85].

This study has various strengths. First the inclusion of multiple variables contributing to impaired eating behaviors, eating symptom severity, and BMI. While several previous studies analyzed the direct impact of multiple psychological features on the BMI among patients who met different diagnoses of ED, to our knowledge, this is the first study to include a broad set of indicators in a mediational model (path analysis) that allows measurement of both direct and indirect effects. This work has modeled the underlying processes between emotion regulation, impulsiveness, negative emotions (anxiety and stress), performance on decision-making, symptom severity of ED, and BMI. For example, while previous studies identified relationships between difficulties in emotion regulation strategies and impaired decision-making with BMI, our study showed that the specific contribution of these variables is explained through the mediation of stress levels and severity of the ED. The second strength is the use of path analysis implemented through SEM. This analytical approach has allowed testing the invariance of the structural network/coefficients by the patients' sex and the subtypes of the ED. In etiological research, SEM has proved to be very useful for modeling complex clinical profiles (instead of focusing on bivariate associations between the variables), with the aim of visualizing the pattern of relationships and identifying both direct and indirect effects.

5. Conclusions

The results obtained in this work may contribute to the development of prevention and early detection plans, aimed at highly vulnerable populations characterized by neuropsychiatric risk and associated factors for ED (such as high impulsivity, negative mood states, and emotion dysregulation). Also, for the planning of more effective treatments for ED (concretely for BN, BED, NES, and OSFED), both prevention and intervention plans should include healthy dietary patterns and other healthy daily habits (such as adequate sleep and physical activity routines). These lifestyles can promote adequate brain health and cognitive performance, which also improve psychological well-being.

The empirical evidence of this work can also contribute to improve current psychological interventions for ED with neuronutrition research, a new scientific field that includes a subset of nutritional neurosciences to improving eating behavior, mental health and cognitive functions (in healthy and sick individuals) [86]. Reinforced psychotherapy with specific neuronutrients depending on the specific neuronutritional target may be promising multidisciplinary approach to brain health and treatment of psychiatric disorders.

Finally, we consider that the results of our study provide implications for health policy, creating a specific starting point for implementing prevention programs that jointly address mental health and eating habits, promoting early intervention on increased BMI in patients diagnosed with a subtype of ED. Health policy makers and health systems could implement more comprehensive treatments by prioritizing interdisciplinary care models, with greater investment in combined mental health and nutrition services. Meanwhile, regarding implications for clinical practice, treatments could be tailored to the individual needs of patients, considering both their psychoneurological and nutritional profile. In addition, health professionals could identify signs of psychoneurological factors that predispose and act as mediators in increased BMI in patients with ED, allowing early interventions and reducing public health costs.

Supplementary Materials: The following supporting information can be downloaded at: https://www.mdpi.com/article/10.3390/nu17020296/s1, Table S1: Structural coefficients in the multi-group model including the sex as a group; Table S2: Structural coefficients in the multi-group model including the diagnostic subtype as a group.

Author Contributions: Conceptualization, G.G.R.O.; methodology and statistics, R.G.; writing and preparation of the original draft, G.G.R.O. and R.G.; B.E. and C.T. managed the data collection. All authors have read and agreed to the published version of the manuscript.

Funding: This research did not receive external funding.

Institutional Review Board Statement: The study was carried out in accordance with the Declaration of Helsinki and was approved by the Clinical Research Ethics Committee of the Ecuadorian Ministry of Public Health, code CEISH-UCACUE-2024-064, 8 November 2022.

Informed Consent Statement: Informed consent was obtained from all subjects involved in the study.

Data Availability Statement: The raw data supporting the conclusions of this article will be made available by the authors, without undue reservation.

Acknowledgments: RG was supported by the ICREA-Academy-2021 award. G.G.R.O.: special thanks to the Ministry of Public Health of Ecuador and the Mental Health team of Zone 6 who contributed to the recruitment of the information.

Conflicts of Interest: The authors declare no conflicts of interest.

References

1. World Health Organization (WHO). A Report on Public Health. 2019. Available online: https://www.who.int/es/news-room/fact-sheets/detail/obesity-and-overweight (accessed on 5 May 2019).
2. Bernabéu, E.; Marchena, C. Emotional Eating and Perfectionism as Predictors of Symptoms of Binge Eating Disorder: The Role of Perfectionism as a Mediator between Emotional Eating and Body Mass Index. *Nutrients* **2022**, *14*, 3361. [CrossRef]
3. Bruzas, M.; Allison, K. A Review of the Relationship between Night Eating Syndrome and Body Mass Index. *Curr. Obes. Rep.* **2019**, *8*, 145–155. [CrossRef] [PubMed]
4. Agüera, Z.; Lozano-Madrid, M.; Mallorquí-Bagué, N.; Jiménez-Murcia, S.; Menchón, J.M.; Fernández-Aranda, F. A review of binge eating disorder and obesity. *Neuropsychiatries* **2021**, *35*, 57–67.
5. de Zwaan, M. Binge eating disorder and obesity. *Int. J. Obes.* **2021**, *25*, 551–555. [CrossRef] [PubMed]
6. Himmerich, H.; Kan, C.; Au, K.; Treasure, J. Pharmacological treatment of eating disorders, comorbid mental health problems, malnutrition and physical health consequences. *Pharmacol. Ther.* **2021**, *217*, 107667. [CrossRef] [PubMed]
7. American Psychiatric Association—APA. *Diagnostic and Statistical Manual of Mental Disorders: DSM-5*, 5th ed.; American Psychiatric Publishing: Washington, DC, USA, 2014.
8. Leppanen, J.; Brown, D.; McLinden, H.; Williams, S.; Tchanturia, K. The Role of Emotion Regulation in Eating Disorders: A Network Meta-Analysis Approach. *Front. Psychiatry* **2022**, *13*, 793094. [CrossRef] [PubMed]
9. Peláez-Fernández, M.A.; Romero-Mesa, J.; Extremera, N. From Deficits in Emotional Intelligence to Eating Disorder Symptoms: A Sequential Path Analysis Approach Through Self-Esteem and Anxiety. *Front. Psychol.* **2021**, *12*, 713070. [CrossRef]
10. Dakanalis, A.; Mentzelou, M.; Papadopoulou, S.K.; Papandreou, D.; Spanoudaki, M.; Vasios, G.K.; Giaginis, C. The association of emotional eating with overweight/obesity, depression, anxiety/stress, and dietary patterns: A review of the current clinical evidence. *Nutrients* **2023**, *15*, 1173. [CrossRef] [PubMed]
11. Meneguzzo, P.; Garolla, A.; Bonello, E.; Todisco, P. Alexithymia, dissociation and emotional regulation in eating disorders: Evidence of improvement through specialized inpatient treatment. *Clin. Psychol. Psychother.* **2022**, *29*, 718–724. [CrossRef] [PubMed]
12. Hayes, J.F.; Fitzsimmons-Craft, E.E.; Karam, A.M.; Jakubiak, J.; Brown, M.L.; Wilfley, D.E. Disordered eating attitudes and behaviors in youth with overweight and obesity: Implications for treatment. *Curr. Obes. Rep.* **2018**, *7*, 235–246. [CrossRef]
13. Francesconi, M.; Flouri, E.; Harrison, A. Decision-making difficulties mediate the association between poor emotion regulation and eating disorder symptoms in adolescence. *Psychol. Med.* **2023**, *53*, 3701–3710. [CrossRef]
14. van Elburg, A.; Danner, U.N.; Sternheim, L.C.; Lammers, M.; Elzakkers, I. Mental Capacity, Decision-Making and Emotion Dysregulation in Severe Enduring Anorexia Nervosa. *Front. Psychiatry* **2021**, *12*, 545317. [CrossRef]
15. de Eguilaz, M.H.R.; de Morentin Aldabe, B.M.; Almiron-Roig, E.; Pérez-Diez, S.; Blanco RS, C.; Navas-Carretero, S.; Martínez, J.A. Multisensory influence on eating behavior: Hedonic consumption. *Endocrinol. Diabetes Nutr.* **2018**, *65*, 114–125.
16. Frank, S.; Veit, R.; Sauer, H.; Enck, P.; Friederich, H.C.; Unholzer, T.; Bauer, U.M.; Linder, K.; Heni, M.; Fritsche, A.; et al. Dopamine depletion reduces food-related reward activity independent of BMI. *Neuropsychopharmacology* **2016**, *41*, 1551–1559. [CrossRef]
17. Kittel, R.; Schmidt, R.; Hilbert, A. Executive functions in adolescents with binge-eating disorder and obesity. *Int. J. Eat. Disord.* **2017**, *50*, 933–941. [CrossRef]
18. Reiter, A.M.; Heinze, H.-J.; Schlagenhauf, F.; Deserno, L. Impaired flexible reward-based decision-making in binge eating disorder: Evidence from computational modeling and functional neuroimaging. *Neuropsychopharmacology* **2017**, *42*, 628–637. [CrossRef] [PubMed]
19. Perpiñá, C.; Segura, M.; Sánchez-Reales, S. Cognitive flexibility and decision-making in eating disorders and obesity. *Eat. Weight Disord. EWD* **2017**, *22*, 435–444. [CrossRef] [PubMed]
20. Garner, D.M. Eating Disorder Inventory-3. Professional Manual. In *Psychological Assessment Resources*; Hogrefe: Amsterdam, The Netherlands, 2004.
21. Reivan-Ortiz, G.; Pineda-Garcia, G.; León, B. Psychometric Properties of The Golberg Anxiety and Depression Scale (GADS) in Ecuadorian Population. *Int. J. Psychol. Res.* **2019**, *12*, 41–48. [CrossRef] [PubMed]

22. Chan, S.F.; La Greca, A.M. Perceived Stress Scale (PSS). In *Encyclopedia of Behavioral Medicine*; Gellman, M.D., Ed.; Springer: Cham, Switzerland, 2020.
23. Gross, J.; John, O. Individual differences in two emotion regulation processes: Implications for affect, relationships, and well-being. *J. Personal. Soc. Psychol.* **2003**, *85*, 348–362. [CrossRef]
24. Plutchik, R.; Van Praag, H. The measurement of suicidality, aggressivity and impulsivity. *Prog. Neuropsychopharmacol. Biol. Psychiatry* **1989**, *13*, 523–534. [CrossRef]
25. Rubio, G.; Montero, I.; Jáuregui, J.; Martínez, M.L.; Álvarez, S.; Marín, J.J.; Santo-Domingo, J. Validación de la Escala de Impulsividad de Plutchik en población española. *Arch. Neurobiol.* **1998**, *6*, 223–232.
26. Alacreu, A.; Fuentes, M.; Abad, D.; Cano, I.; González, E.; Serrano, M. Spanish validation of General Decision-Making Style scale: Sex invariance, sex differences and relationships with personality and coping styles. *Judgm. Decis. Mak.* **2019**, *14*, 739–751. [CrossRef]
27. StataCorp. *Stata Statistical Software: Release 17*; StataCorp LLC: College Station, TX, USA, 2021.
28. Rosnow, R.L.; Rosenthal, R. Computing contrasts, effect sizes, and counternulls on other people's published data: General procedures for research consumers. *Psychol. Methods* **1996**, *4*, 331. [CrossRef]
29. Kline, R.B. *Principles and Practice of Structural Equation Modeling*, 2nd ed.; The Guilford Press: New York, NY, USA, 2005.
30. Barrett, P. Structural Equation Modelling: Adjudging Model Fit. *Personal. Individ. Differ.* **2007**, *42*, 815–824. [CrossRef]
31. Bentler, P.M. Comparative Fit Indexes in Structural Models. *Psychol. Bull.* **1990**, *107*, 238–246. [CrossRef] [PubMed]
32. Granero, R. Role of Nutrition and Diet on Healthy Mental State. *Nutrients* **2022**, *14*, 750. [CrossRef] [PubMed]
33. Zickgraf, H.F.; Hazzard, V.M.; O'Connor, S.M. Food insecurity is associated with eating disorders independent of depression and anxiety: Findings from the 2020–2021 healthy minds study. *Int. J. Eat. Disord.* **2022**, *55*, 354–361. [CrossRef] [PubMed]
34. Zhang, J.; Wang, Y.; Wu, C.; He, J. The relationship between emotional intelligence and eating disorders or disordered eating behaviors: A meta-analysis. *Personal. Individ. Differ.* **2022**, *185*, 111239. [CrossRef]
35. Mantilla, E.F.; Clinton, D.; Monell, E.; Levallius, J.; Birgegård, A. Impulsivity and compulsivity as parallel mediators of emotion dysregulation in eating-related addictive-like behaviors, alcohol use, and compulsive exercise. *Brain Behav.* **2022**, *12*, 1.
36. Benzerouk, F.; Djerada, Z.; Bertin, E.; Barrière, S.; Gierski, F.; Kaladjian, A. Contributions of emotional overload, emotion dysregulation, and impulsivity to eating patterns in obese patients with binge eating disorder and seeking bariatric surgery. *Nutrients* **2020**, *12*, 3099. [CrossRef]
37. Gluck, M.E. Stress response and binge eating disorder. *Appetite* **2006**, *46*, 26–30. [CrossRef]
38. Suliman, S.; Anthonissen, L.; Carr, J.; du Plessis, S.; Emsley, R.; Hemmings, S.M.; Seedat, S. Posttraumatic stress disorder, overweight, and obesity: A systematic review and meta-analysis. *Harv. Rev. Psychiatry* **2016**, *24*, 271–293. [CrossRef] [PubMed]
39. Vincent, H.K.; Innes, K.E.; Vincent, K.R. Oxidative stress and potential interventions to reduce oxidative stress in overweight and obesity. *Diabetes Obes. Metab.* **2007**, *9*, 813–839. [CrossRef] [PubMed]
40. Chao, A.M.; Jastreboff, A.M.; White, M.A.; Grilo, C.M.; Sinha, R. Stress, cortisol, and other appetite-related hormones: Prospective prediction of 6-month changes in food cravings and weight. *Obesity* **2017**, *25*, 713–720. [CrossRef] [PubMed]
41. Ponce, P.; Del Arco, A.; Loprinzi, P. Physical activity versus psychological stress: Effects on salivary cortisol and working memory performance. *Medicina* **2019**, *55*, 119. [CrossRef] [PubMed]
42. Holt, E.M.; Steffen, L.M.; Moran, A.; Basu, S.; Steinberger, J.; Ross, J.A.; Sinaiko, A.R. Fruit and vegetable consumption and its relation to markers of inflammation and oxidative stress in adolescents. *J. Am. Diet. Assoc.* **2009**, *109*, 414–421. [CrossRef]
43. Kim, T.J.; von dem Knesebeck, O. Income and obesity: What is the direction of the relationship? A systematic review and meta-analysis. *BMJ Open* **2018**, *8*, 819–862. [CrossRef]
44. Sutin, A.R.; Terracciano, A. Perceived weight discrimination and obesity. *PLoS ONE* **2013**, *8*, 70048. [CrossRef]
45. Imperatori, C.; Innamorati, M.; Lamis, D.A.; Farina, B.; Pompili, M.; Contardi, A.; Fabbricatore, M. Childhood trauma in obese and overweight women with food addiction and clinical-level of binge eating. *Child Abus. Negl.* **2016**, *58*, 180–190. [CrossRef]
46. Siahpush, M.; Huang, T.T.K.; Sikora, A.; Tibbits, M.; Shaikh, R.A.; Singh, G.K. Prolonged financial stress predicts subsequent obesity: Results from a prospective study of an Australian national sample. *Obesity* **2014**, *22*, 616–621. [CrossRef] [PubMed]
47. Nowicka, P.; Ek, A.; Grafström, E.; Johansson, T.; Nordin, K.; Neuman, N.; Eli, K. How do interpersonal relationships affect children's weight management? A qualitative analysis of parents' long-term perceptions after obesity treatment. *Child. Obes.* **2022**, *18*, 274–280. [CrossRef] [PubMed]
48. Danner, U.N.; Sternheim, L.; Evers, C. The importance of distinguishing between the different eating disorders (sub) types when assessing emotion regulation strategies. *Psychiatry Res.* **2014**, *215*, 727–732. [CrossRef] [PubMed]
49. Harrison, A.; Sullivan, S.; Tchanturia, K.; Treasure, J. Emotional functioning in eating disorders: Attentional bias, emotion recognition and emotion regulation. *Psychol. Med.* **2010**, *40*, 1887–1897. [CrossRef]
50. Andrei, F.; Nuccitelli, C.; Mancini, G.; Reggiani, G.M.; Trombini, E. Emotional intelligence, emotion regulation and affectivity in adults seeking treatment for obesity. *Psychiatry Res.* **2018**, *269*, 191–198. [CrossRef]

51. Ciberti, A.; Cavalletti, M.; Palagini, L.; Mariani, M.G.; Dell'Osso, L.; Mauri, M.; Miniati, M. Decision-making, impulsiveness and temperamental traits in eating disorders. *Clin. Neuropsychiatry* **2020**, *17*, 199. [PubMed]
52. Hanras, E.; Boujut, E.; Ruffault, A.; Messager, D.; Rives-Lange, C.; Barsamian, C.; Dorard, G. Binge eating disorder: What are the differences in emotion regulation, impulsivity, and eating behaviors according to weight status? *Obes. Med.* **2022**, *36*, 100462. [CrossRef]
53. Bandelow, B.; Michaelis, S. Epidemiology of anxiety disorders in the 21st century. *Dialogues Clin. Neurosci.* **2022**, *17*, 327–335. [CrossRef] [PubMed]
54. Daros, A.R.; Haefner, S.A.; Asadi, S.; Kazi, S.; Rodak, T.; Quilty, L.C. A meta-analysis of emotional regulation outcomes in psychological interventions for youth with depression and anxiety. *Nat. Hum. Behav.* **2021**, *5*, 1443–1457. [CrossRef]
55. Braden, A.; O'Brien, W. Pilot study of a treatment using dialectical behavioral therapy skills for adults with overweight/obesity and emotional eating. *J. Contemp. Psychother.* **2021**, *51*, 21–29. [CrossRef]
56. Steward, T.; Picó-Pérez, M.; Mestre-Bach, G.; Martínez-Zalacaín, I.; Suñol, M.; Jiménez-Murcia, S.; Fernandez-Aranda, F. A multimodal MRI study of the neural mechanisms of emotion regulation impairment in women with obesity. *Transl. Psychiatry* **2019**, *9*, 194. [CrossRef] [PubMed]
57. Won, Y.Q.; Christensen, K.A.; Forbush, K.T. Habitual adaptive emotion regulation moderates the association between maladaptive emotion regulation and eating disorder symptoms, but not clinical impairment. *Eat. Weight Disord.-Stud. Anorex. Bulim. Obes.* **2022**, *27*, 2629–2639. [CrossRef] [PubMed]
58. Leehr, E.J.; Krohmer, K.; Schag, K.; Dresler, T.; Zipfel, S.; Giel, K.E. Emotion regulation model in binge eating disorder and obesity-a systematic review. *Neurosci. Biobehav. Rev.* **2015**, *49*, 125–134. [CrossRef]
59. Boswell, R.G.; Potenza, M.N.; Grilo, C.M. The neurobiology of binge-eating disorder compared with obesity: Implications for differential therapeutics. *Clin. Ther.* **2021**, *43*, 50–69. [CrossRef]
60. Brogan, A.; Hevey, D.; O'Callaghan, G.; Yoder, R.; O'Shea, D. Impaired decision making among morbidly obese adults. *J. Psychosom. Res.* **2011**, *70*, 189–196. [CrossRef]
61. Farhangi, M.A. Night eating syndrome and its relationship with emotional eating, sleep quality and nutritional status among adolescents' boys. *Community Ment. Health J.* **2019**, *55*, 1411–1418. [CrossRef]
62. Lombardo, C.; Cerolini, S. Night Eating Syndrome and Nocturnal Sleep-Related Eating Disorder. In *Hidden and Lesser-Known Disordered Eating Behaviors in Medical and Psychiatric Conditions*; Springer: Cham, Switzerland, 2022; pp. 147–158.
63. Wilkinson, L.L.; Rowe, A.C.; Douglas, T.; Thirkettle, M.; Nolan, L.J. Adult attachment anxiety is associated with night eating syndrome in UK and US-based samples: Two cross-sectional studies. *Appetite* **2022**, *172*, 105968. [CrossRef]
64. Hartmann, S.; Pruessner, L.; Rubel, J.A.; Lalk, C.; Barnow, S.; Timm, C. Applying a web-based self-help intervention for bulimia nervosa in routine care: Study protocol for a randomized controlled trial. *Internet Interv.* **2022**, *28*, 100512. [CrossRef]
65. Lee, J.E.; Namkoong, K.; Jung, Y.C. Impaired prefrontal cognitive control over interference by food images in binge-eating disorder and bulimia nervosa. *Neurosci Lett.* **2017**, *651*, 95–101. [CrossRef] [PubMed]
66. Mohorić, T.; Pokrajac-Bulian, A.; Anić, P.; Kukić, M.; Mohović, P. Emotion regulation, perfectionism, and eating disorder symptoms in adolescents: The mediating role of cognitive eating patterns. *Curr. Psychol.* **2022**, *42*, 28505–28516. [CrossRef] [PubMed]
67. Bekker, M.H.; Spoor, S.T. Emotional inhibition, health, gender, and eating disorders: The role of (over) sensitivity to others. In *Emotion Regulation*; Springer: Boston, MA, USA, 2008; pp. 170–183.
68. Echeverri-Alvarado, B.; Pickett, S.; Gildner, D. A model of post-traumatic stress symptoms on binge eating through emotion regulation difficulties and emotional eating. *Appetite* **2020**, *150*, 104659. [CrossRef]
69. Balzan, R.P.; Gilder, M.; Nancarrow, T.; Mavrangelos, T.; Wade, T.D. Hasty in individuals at higher risk of developing an eating disorder. *J. Behav. Ther. Exp. Psychiatry* **2022**, *75*, 101717. [CrossRef] [PubMed]
70. Frank, G.K.W.; Shott, M.E.; DeGuzman, M.C. The Neurobiology of Eating Disorders. *Child Adolesc. Psychiatr. Clin. N. Am.* **2019**, *28*, 629–640. [CrossRef]
71. Clifton, P.G. Neural circuits of eating behavior: Opportunities for therapeutic development. *J. Psychopharmacol.* **2017**, *31*, 1388–1402. [CrossRef]
72. Lucas, I.; Miranda-Olivos, R.; Testa, G.; Granero, R.; Sánchez, I.; Sánchez-González, J.; Fernández-Aranda, F. Neuropsychological learning deficits as predictors of treatment outcome in patients with eating disorders. *Nutrients* **2021**, *13*, 2145. [CrossRef] [PubMed]
73. Lao-Kaim, N.P.; Fonville, L.; Giampietro, V.P.; Williams, S.C.; Simmons, A.; Tchanturia, K. Aberrant function of learning and cognitive control networks underlie inefficient cognitive flexibility in anorexia nervosa: A cross-sectional fMRI study. *PLoS ONE* **2015**, *10*, 0124027. [CrossRef] [PubMed]
74. Xu, J.; Harper, J.A.; Van Enkevort, E.A.; Latimer, K.; Kelley, U.; McAdams, C.J. Neural activations are related to body-shape, anxiety, and outcomes in adolescent anorexia nervosa. *J. Psychiatr. Res.* **2017**, *87*, 1–7. [CrossRef]

75. Davidovic, M.; Karjalainen, L.; Starck, G.; Wentz, E.; Bjornsdotter, M.; Olausson, H. Abnormal brain processing of gentle touch in anorexia nervosa. *Psychiatry Res. Neuroimaging* **2018**, *281*, 53–60. [CrossRef]
76. Weinstein, A.; Dannon, P. Is impulsivity a male trait rather than female trait? Exploring the sex difference in impulsivity. *Curr. Behav. Neurosci. Rep.* **2015**, *2*, 9–14. [CrossRef]
77. Ter Horst, J.P.; de Kloet, E.R.; Schächinger, H.; Oitzl, M. Relevance of stress and female sex hormones for emotion and cognition. *Cell. Mol. Neurobiol.* **2012**, *32*, 725–735. [CrossRef]
78. McMaster, C.M.; Wade, T.; Franklin, J.; Waller, G.; Hart, S. Impact of patient characteristics on clinicians' decisions to involve dietitians in eating disorder treatment. *J. Hum. Nutr. Diet.* **2022**, *3*, 1. [CrossRef] [PubMed]
79. Haber, S.N. Anatomy and Connectivity of the Reward Circuit. In *Decision Neuroscience;* Academic Press: Cambridge, MA, USA, 2017; pp. 3–19.
80. Woodside, D.B.; Colton, P.; Lam, E.; Dunlop, K.; Rzeszutek, J.; Downar, J. Dorsomedial prefrontal cortex repetitive transcranial magnetic stimulation treatment of posttraumatic stress disorder in eating disorders: An open-label case series. *Int. J. Eat. Disord.* **2017**, *50*, 1231–1234. [CrossRef] [PubMed]
81. Jobst, L.J.; Bader, M.; Moshagen, M. A tutorial on assessing statistical power and determining sample size for structural equation models. *Psychol. Methods* **2023**, *28*, 207–221. [CrossRef] [PubMed]
82. Edwards, J.R.; Lambert, L.S. Methods for integrating moderation and mediation: A general analytical framework using moderated path analysis. *Psychol. Methods* **2007**, *12*, 1–22. [CrossRef] [PubMed]
83. Wolf, E.J.; Harrington, K.M.; Clark, S.L.; Miller, M.W. Sample size requirements for structural equation models: An evaluation of power, bias, and solution propriety. *Educ. Psychol. Meas.* **2013**, *73*, 913–934. [CrossRef]
84. Pek, J.; MacCallum, R.C. Sensitivity analysis in structural equation models: Cases and their influence. *Multivar. Behav. Res.* **2011**, *46*, 202–228. [CrossRef] [PubMed]
85. Vilares, M.J.; Coelho, P.S. Likelihood and PLS estimators for structural equation modeling: An assessment of sample size, skewness and model misspecification effects. In *Advances in Regression, Survival Analysis, Extreme Values, Markov Processes and Other Statistical Applications*; Springer: Berlin/Heidelberg, Geramany, 2013; pp. 11–33.
86. Badaeva, A.V.; Danilov, A.B.; Clayton, P.; Moskalev, A.A.; Karasev, A.V.; Tarasevich, A.F.; Vorobyeva, Y.D.; Novikov, V.N. Perspectives on Neuronutrition in Prevention and Treatment of Neurological Disorders. *Nutrients* **2023**, *15*, 2505. [CrossRef]

MDPI AG
Grosspeteranlage 5
4052 Basel
Switzerland
Tel.: +41 61 683 77 34

Nutrients Editorial Office
E-mail: nutrients@mdpi.com
www.mdpi.com/journal/nutrients

www.ingramcontent.com/pod-product-compliance
Lightning Source LLC
Chambersburg PA
CBHW041417210926
51850CB00013B/3296
* 9 7 8 3 7 2 5 8 3 9 3 7 7 *